"In his enlightening new book, Bowden takes o[...]liefs
about which foods are healthy and which a[...]
some of your sacred cows mad[...]

—JOSH AXE, D.N.M., D.C., C.N.S., *New York Times* best-selling author of *Eat Dirt*

" . . . not just another rehash of conventional wisdom. Dr. Jonny isn't afraid to refute
many of our treasured beliefs about "healthy" foods and to redeem the reputation
of many foods we've wrongly demonized. Highly recommended."

—FRANK LIPMAN, M.D., *New York Times* best-selling author of
The New Health Rules and *10 Reasons You Feel Old and Get Fat*

"Jonny Bowden is my go-to nutritionist for so many reasons. If you want a vibrant,
healthy brain and body, read *The 150 Healthiest Foods on Earth*."

—DANIEL G. AMEN, M.D., *New York Times* best-selling author of
Change Your Brain, Change Your Life and coauthor of *The Brain Warrior's Way*

" . . . packed with info you can use to take control of your health,
starting with what's on your plate."

—DAVE ASPREY, *New York Times* best-selling author of *Head Strong* and *The Bulletproof Diet*

" . . . a wonderful resource and essential reading for anyone interested in their health.
Jonny Bowden provides witty and practical information that will
make eating super healthy and a pleasure."

—STEVEN MASLEY, M.D., star of PBS special
30 Days to a Younger Heart and best-selling author of *The Better Brain Book*

" . . . the indispensable guide to the best foods for your best health.
I've enjoyed this book for years and refer to it often. The new edition keeps us up to speed
with the latest research and trends as well as enticing new entries to the lineup."

—ALAN CHRISTIANSON, N.M.D., the *New York Times* best-selling author of *The Adrenal Reset Diet*

"There is no substitute for eating real, nutrient-dense foods, properly prepared and
toxin free—which is why everybody needs Jonny's excellent book!"

—JOSEPH PIZZORNO, N.D., founding president of Bastyr University and coauthor of the *Textbook of Natural
Medicine*, *Encyclopedia of Natural Medicine*, and best-selling author of *The Toxin Solution*

The 150

Healthiest

Foods

on Earth

The Surprising, Unbiased Truth
About What You Should Eat and Why

Jonny Bowden, Ph.D., C.N.S.

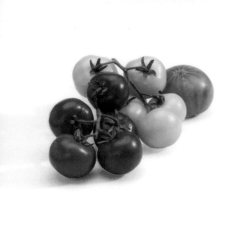 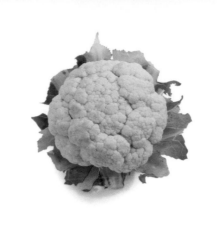 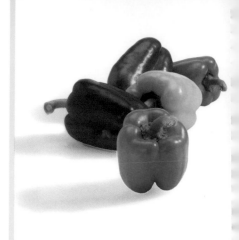

"*If you are what you eat*
and you don't know
what you're eating,
do you know who you are?"

—Claude Fischler

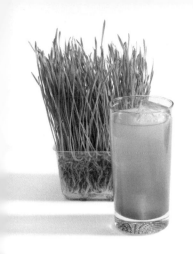
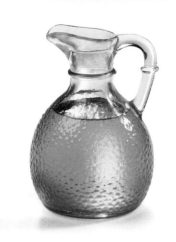
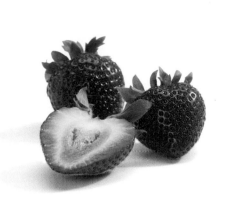

CONTENTS

Introduction

The other day someone asked me whether honey is a good sweetener.

My answer was, "It depends."

If, by honey, you mean the stuff you buy in the supermarket that comes in the cute little plastic bear, the answer is no. If, by honey, you mean raw, unfiltered, uncooked, unpasteurized organic honey, then the answer is an unqualified yes. Which reminds me of a story.

I was coming out of the multiplex at the Lincoln Center Theater in New York one Friday evening, and just as I was blending into the huge crowd, I ran into an old friend I hadn't seen in ages. We bumped smack into each other on the escalator going down to the main floor and decided to go to the local Starbucks and catch up. As soon as we sat down, we started talking about the movie. "That was so moving," I said. "Moving?" she said incredulously. "I thought it was completely maudlin and sophomoric." "What are you talking about?" I asked. "The acting was incredible, the writing was sophisticated." "Sophisticated?" she snorted. "Well, maybe if you consider Adam Sandler sophisticated!"

Silence.

We looked at each other . . .

. . . and suddenly realized . . .

. . . we saw different movies.

There's a lesson in that, and it has to do with food and language.

The person asking me about honey didn't make a distinction between the plastic bear kind and the raw unfiltered kind, yet they are two completely different foods. If I had answered the question without knowing which she was talking about, it would have been like discussing the movie, not realizing that one person had seen a drama and one had seen a comedy. You and I could be discussing what it's like to have a pet, but if you're thinking monkeys and I'm thinking daschunds, we're not talking about the same thing, even if we think we are.

I was never more aware of this issue than when I was writing and researching this book. Take salmon. Great food, right? Every nutritionist recommends it. There's only one problem: Farm-raised salmon is not the same food as wild salmon. As you'll see, one of them (the wild kind) is loaded with omega-3 fats. Its striking color is the result of it normally dining on krill, which provides it with a highly beneficial compound called *astaxanthin*, a natural carotenoid that gives salmon its rich color. Farm-raised salmon have never seen krill—they eat grain, which would be like raising lions on chocolate chip cookies. They have—by many accounts—less omega-3 fat than their wild brethren, and their color is the result of whatever selection of dye the factory farmers decide on that day. Not only that, according to the Environmental Working Group, farmed salmon are likely the most PCB-contaminated protein source in the U.S. food supply. Wild salmon and farm-raised salmon are completely different foods. Yet we unknowingly use the same word for both.

Big problem.

Without going too far afield, let me point out that this language problem has a lot to do with the difficulty in drawing conclusions from studies of meat eaters

*"Let food be thy medicine,
and medicine be thy food."*

—Hippocrates

or vegetarians. It's possible to be a vegetarian eating Twinkies and white rice, and it's possible to be a vegetarian eating nothing but vegetables, whole grains, fruits, and eggs. Similarly, meat eaters can refer to people who dine exclusively on ballpark hot dogs and have never met a vegetable they didn't hate, or it can refer to small tribes of hunter-gatherers who dine on pasture-fed wild game—when they can catch it—and tons of fresh, wild vegetables, fruits, and nuts.

See where I'm going with this?

Ten years after the first edition of this book, the problem of language and food is more critical than ever. Almost daily we hear reports about the health benefits (or dangers) of a diet—Paleo, raw food, gluten-free, vegetarian, vegan, low-carb, high-fiber—but does the average consumer even know the exact definition of those terms? The unfortunate truth is no, they don't.

Even health professionals don't have great working definitions of these diets. The most touted diet in nutrition history is the Mediterranean diet, typically described as including lots of fish, nuts, vegetables, beans, whole grains, and olive oil, but that's about as scientific a description of a diet as "it's awfully hot in here" is of temperature.

You know that low-carb diet study you heard about on CNN? Was it low-carb, high-*protein*? Or low-carb, high-*fat*? (They probably didn't tell you that.) Did the researchers control for fiber intake? And what about the precise meaning of words such as meat or soy? Is all meat the same? (It's not.) And is fermented soy the same as non-fermented soy? (Nope.) Is wild salmon the same as farmed salmon? (Nope.) Are all omega-3s created equal? (And nope.)

I think you get the picture.

We've made a huge mistake by trying to define the perfect diet in terms of protein, carb, and fat quantity—how many calories of each should I consume? We do this while neglecting the role of protein, carbohydrate, and fat quality. Endless diet and weight loss books try to come up with the perfect formula—this many carbs, that much fat, this percentage of protein—when the actual quality of the food is probably much more important for our health than the proportions of fat, carbs, and protein.

Which brings us to this book.

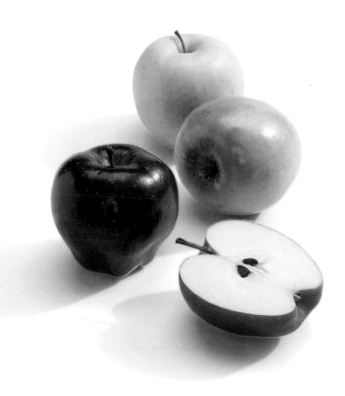

Given the mandate to choose the 150 healthiest foods on the planet, I had to make a lot of decisions. Some were easy, slam dunks, no-brainers. (Think vegetables. There are no bad ones. Unless you count french fries.) Some, because of the language issue discussed previously, required careful exposition. Milk, for example, is a great food in its raw, organic state; but, in my opinion, in its typical homogenized, pasteurized form, it's a disaster.

So when you read the entries, pay particular attention to those qualifications and caveats. You'll probably be surprised at some of the foods that made the cut, and even more surprised at some of the ones that didn't. (See, for example, the entry on soy foods. That is, if you can find it. It's pretty short.)

At one point, it was suggested that I rate the foods in each category. I didn't do it. Why? Because foods are like friends: They provide different things. You can have a friend who's great for going to basketball games with but with whom you wouldn't think of sharing your innermost feelings. Some foods provide great fats such as omega-3s, but no calcium. Others provide an abundance of vitamins and minerals, but no protein. No food provides everything. Rating them would involve deciding which essential vitamins, minerals, and macronutrients are more important, and that's impossible. You need them all. However, I did put stars on the foods I thought had exceptional nutritional value.

That said, there are four key factors to be aware of when reading this book. Having a passing acquaintance with them will enrich your understanding of the things that make foods healthy. And I'd like to go over them here, so that when I reference them in the sections on food, you'll know what I'm talking about. The first is omega-3 fats, the presence of which almost always guarantees a food makes the list. The second is fiber. The third is the glycemic load. And the fourth is antioxidants. Let's go over them one by one.

A Short Primer on Fat: The Omega-3s

Fats come in many different forms, which have varying effects on your health. Most people are aware that there are saturated fats—which they've been told to avoid—and have heard vaguely of monounsaturated fats (such as those in olive oil) and polyunsaturated fats (such as those in vegetable oils, nuts, and fish). Much as I'd love to, I don't have the space here to go into a lot of depth on fats, but I'd like to give you a few points before going into more detail about one specific class of polyunsaturated fats called the omega-3s. Here are the take-home points:

- Saturated fat is not always bad. Peer-reviewed studies in major medical and nutritional journals have shown that saturated fat does not play a causal role in heart disease as previously believed. Some sources of it—coconut oil, Malaysian palm oil, dark chocolate, the fat from grass-fed animals—are healthy. You no longer need to avoid saturated fat like it's poison. It's not.
- Trans fat, however, *is* poison. Metabolic poison, that is. It's found in cookies, crackers, baked goods and snacks, doughnuts, french fries, and most margarines. Regardless of what the label says, if there is partially hydrogenated oil in the ingredient list, it's got trans fat. Don't eat trans fats. Period. (The one single exception is the trans fat CLA, or conjugated linoleic acid, which is found naturally in grass-fed dairy and meat and is not man-made.)
- Monounsaturated fat—found in nuts and olive oil—is good stuff and heart healthy.
- Polyunsaturated fats come in two flavors: omega-6s and omega-3s. Though there are some health benefits to omega-6s, we consume too many and not nearly enough omega-3s.

There are three different omega-3 fats: One of them is found in flaxseed and called ALA (alpha-linolenic acid). It's considered an essential fatty acid because the body can't make it, so it must be obtained from the diet (more about this in the section on flaxseed and flaxseed oil; see page 341). But the other two omega-3s—DHA (docosahexaenoic acid) and EPA (eicosapentaenoic acid)—are found in fish such as wild salmon. And these two may be of even more importance to the body than the first one.

Although the body can make DHA and EPA from alpha-linolenic acid (the first, essential, one), it doesn't do a great job of it. That's why it's such a good idea to obtain these incredibly important omega-3 fats ready-made from fish or fish oil (the most potent sources). They're just so critically important to our health.

So what exactly do omega-3s do and why do we need them? Let's start with the cell membranes. Omega-3s are incorporated into cells, making their membranes more fluid so they can communicate with one another. This means, for example, that feel-good neurotransmitters such as serotonin and dopamine can get in and out of the cell more easily, translating to better mood. In fact, omega-3s are currently being studied for their positive effect on depression.

They're also being studied for their impact on behavior, feeling, and thinking. Nearly every study of behavior problems—from simple lack of concentration to actual aggressive behavior in prison inmates—has shown that people with these problems have low levels of omega-3 fats in their bloodstream. This doesn't mean that omega-3s will fix every behavior problem, but it's certainly of more than academic interest that this correlation shows up so frequently.

On a side note, the omega-3s in fish have a significant effect on the developing brain of a human fetus. Because the baby's brain, like your own, is about 60 percent fat by weight, and because most of that fat is

DHA (the very omega-3 found in fish), taking fish oil (or getting fat from healthy, wild fish) is one of the absolute best things a pregnant woman can do for her developing baby. Fish truly is brain food. The amount of omega-3's in a pregnant woman's diet helps to determine her child's intelligence, fine-motor skills (such as the ability to manipulate small objects and hand-eye coordination), and propensity to antisocial behavior.

Omega-3s are anti-inflammatory. Inflammation is a critical component of virtually every degenerative disease from heart disease to diabetes to obesity to Alzheimer's, and inflammation itself has been dubbed The Silent Killer. That makes anti-inflammatory foods and supplements of critical importance to our health. In my opinion, the anti-inflammatory power of omega-3s is one of the top reasons to consume them daily.

Omega-3s also support circulation. They transport oxygen from red blood cells to the tissues. They prevent blood cells from clumping together (remember, blood clots can be a cause of heart attack and stroke). They act as a blood thinner, much like aspirin, only without the side effects. Studies suggest that proper omega-3 intake could save 70,000 lives a year in the United States alone and reduce the number of fatal arrhythmias

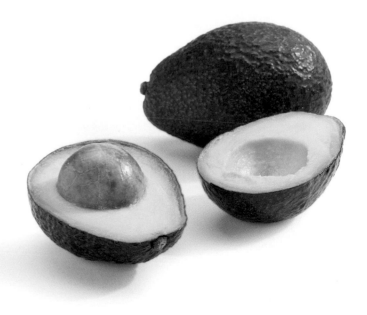

by 30 percent. Omega-3s help lower blood pressure. And they're also effective for in improving insulin and glucose metabolism in diabetics.

Fiber

Fiber—particularly soluble fiber—can also lower blood cholesterol levels and slow the absorption of sugar, which is highly important for people with diabetes, and for people with any blood sugar challenges (metabolic syndrome). A high-fiber diet reduces the risk of developing type 2 diabetes. Beans, raspberries, pure bran, oatmeal, prunes, avocado, raisins, and most green vegetables, for example, are high-fiber foods that cause less of a rise in blood sugar than foods like potatoes, or than almost any wheat-based food.

And eating a high-fiber diet may also help with weight loss. Steven Masley, M.D., and I presented a study at the 2015 annual meeting of the American College of Nutrition showing that fiber intake was one of the best predictors of long-term success on a weight loss pro-

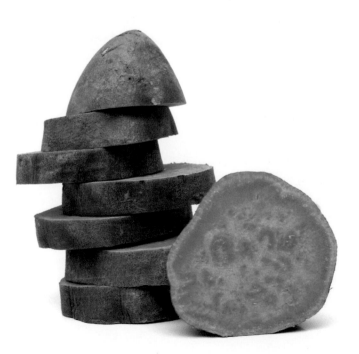

gram. High-fiber foods generally require more chewing time, giving your body extra time to register the fact that you're no longer hungry, so you're less likely to overeat. A high-fiber diet also tends to fill you up longer. And high-fiber diets tend to have more volume for fewer calories, which has been shown in research by Barbara Rolls, Ph.D., at Pennsylvania State University to be a boon to weight management. In an earlier book, I suggested that the number one supplement for weight loss is fiber. (See "The Read Deal on Fiber: It's Much More Important Than We Thought," on pages 96-97.)

The Glycemic Index: Why Do We Care?

The glycemic index is a measure of how much a given food (such as fruit) raises your blood sugar. High-sugar foods—or foods that convert quickly to sugar in the body—are considered high glycemic.

Why do we care? Because raising blood sugar raises levels of the hormone insulin, which, if raised high enough and long enough and frequently enough, contributes to diabetes, heart disease, and aging. Emerging evidence has shown that high blood sugar and correspondingly high insulin levels are implicated in Alzheimer's disease as well, which is now being referred to by researchers as "type 3 diabetes." Eating low glycemic is a strategy that is virtually guaranteed to contribute to health. When I wax eloquent about a food's low glycemic impact, that's why.

Unfortunately, the glycemic index is a misleading measure because it doesn't consider portion size. The glycemic load is a much more valuable metric, as it accounts for the actual portion size of the food being tested. For now, the take-home point is this: Eat less sugar. And eat fewer foods that convert quickly to sugar in the body (read: almost all processed carbohydrates). If you're interested in learning more about glycemic index and glycemic load—something I recommend highly that you do—you can start with a blog post I did on the subject. Just type into your search engine: "Jonny Bowden Glycemic Index vs Glycemic Load."

If you'd like to dig into the science a little deeper, try the article posted on the Oregon State University website at lpi.oregonstate.edu/infocenter/foods/grains/gigl.html.

Finally, the actual tables of the glycemic index and glycemic load for food can be found at www.mendosa.com/gilists.htm. Remember it's the glycemic load you want to pay attention to.

Antioxidants: What Are They, Anyway?

Throughout the book, I talk about compounds found in foods called antioxidants. Antioxidants do exactly what the term implies—they fight (anti) oxidation. Oxidation can be visibly seen when you leave a cut apple out in the air. When that same process happens in your body—as it does every day—it can cause significant damage to your cells and organs.

Oxidation—or oxidative stress—is a factor in nearly every degenerative disease. Antioxidants help fight oxidative damage. Deficiencies of antioxidants are implicated in the early stages of heart disease, cancer, eye disease, and age-related declines in memory. When I tell you that a food is good because it's loaded with antioxidants, now you know why.

Cholesterol: What's the Story?

I make no secret of my love for eggs. They got a star in this book for all the reasons that you'll read about. I eat them almost every day and think they are one of nature's perfect foods. And the last time I threw away the yolk and ate an egg-white omelet was around 1991.

You'll soon notice that I'm far from fanatical about recommending that you drain every drop of saturated fat from your diet. So inevitably, people ask me, "What about cholesterol?"

After the first edition of this book was published, cardiologist Stephen Sinatra M.D., and I published a

best-selling book called *The Great Cholesterol Myth.* It was featured on Dr. Oz and in a documentary on heart disease produced by the prestigious Australian Broadcasting Company. In fact, it nearly caused an international incident. In that book, we make the case for why cholesterol is wildly overrated as a marker for heart disease risk. It was—to put it mildly—a message that was not exactly embraced by the thirty-billion-dollar industry devoted to cholesterol lowering. Yet, years later, I'm happy to say, even conventional medicine is getting wise to the cholesterol myth.

Cholesterol just might be the most misunderstood molecule in the whole world. John Abramson, M.D., professor of health care policy at Harvard University, says, "It is important to keep in mind that cholesterol is not a health risk in and of itself. In fact, cholesterol is vital to many of the body's essential functions." Cholesterol is the parent molecule of some of the body's most important compounds, including the sex hormones and vitamin D. It's also an integral part of the cell membrane.

What a lot of people don't realize is that the vast majority of cholesterol is made in your body, by the liver. If you take in more from the diet, the liver makes less. If you take in less, the liver makes more. You need cholesterol. Without it, you'd die.

Doing justice to the whole cholesterol question in an introduction as short as this is a challenge, but I'd like you to have a few basic take-home points. The first is that dietary cholesterol—like the kind you find in egg yolks—has minimal impact on serum cholesterol (the kind in your blood that your doctor measures). Minimal. I'm delighted to report that since the original edition of this book was published, the U.S. government has recognized the truth of this. The most recent version of the U.S. Dietary Guidelines states that "cholesterol is not considered a nutrient of concern for overconsumption." All I can say is it's about time.

The effect of eggs on heart disease has exactly zero to do with their cholesterol content. Eggs contain many valuable nutrients, such as protein, choline (which is great for the brain), eye-nutrition superstars, such as lutein and zeaxanthin, healthy fat, and a smattering of vitamins and minerals. And the cholesterol in them is a good thing, not a negative. As Walter Willett, M.D., Dr. P.H., professor of epidemiology and nutrition at Harvard's School of Public Health and a professor of medicine at Harvard Medical School, has said, "No research has ever shown that people who eat more eggs have more heart attacks than people who eat few eggs."

The second point has to do with the demonization of saturated fat in general. Yes, saturated fat raises cholesterol but, as we point out in *The Great Cholesterol Myth*, you have to look under the hood to see that saturated fat's overall effect on cholesterol is positive. Saturated fat raises LDLa (the innocuous kind of LDL cholesterol), lowers LDLb (the "bad" kind of LDL), while raising HDL—all of which are good things. Leaving aside the relationship between saturated fat and cholesterol, the relationship between saturated fat and heart disease—which is what we really care about—has been shown in several major studies over the past few years to be basically nonexistent.

Lowering cholesterol is big business. In 2005, when the first edition of this book was being written, the cholesterol-lowering drug Lipitor was the most prescribed drug in the country. The class of cholesterol-lowering drugs to which Lipitor belongs are known as statins. In that same year, statins were the top-selling class of drugs in the country with 144.5 million prescriptions generating $16 billion, in U.S. sales alone. By 2011–2012, the most commonly used individual drug in America was simvastatin (Zocor), taken by roughly 8 percent of adults in the United States. An astonishing 50 percent of men ages 65 to 74, and 39 percent of women ages 75 and older were on statin drugs, despite evidence from the ongoing Framingham Heart Study that high cholesterol is protective in older people, and despite a complete absence of evidence that statin drugs are beneficial to people in their 70s.

It's worth noting that many researchers believe that the good that statin drugs accomplish has much less to do with their ability to lower cholesterol than their ability to lower inflammation, which is indeed a definite risk for heart disease, as well as a component of Alzheimer's, obesity, and diabetes. The foods in this book are filled with natural anti-inflammatories such as the flavonoid quercetin, for example. Spices such as turmeric are so incredibly healthy largely because they are powerful anti-inflammatories. Maybe we wouldn't need $13 billion a year's worth of drugs if we ate more of the foods that accomplish the same thing.

Finally, in my opinion, we've been way too focused on lowering cholesterol and not focused enough on lowering heart disease and mortality. They are not the same thing. In the Lyon Diet Heart Study, people who had had a heart attack were either counseled to eat a Mediterranean-type diet (fish, fruits, vegetables, whole grains, olive oil, nuts) or given routine post–heart attack advice (watch your cholesterol, eat less saturated fat). The people on the Mediterranean diet experienced

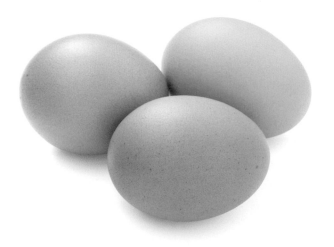

70 percent less heart disease than the group getting the standard advice, about three times the reduction in the risk of further heart disease achieved with statin drugs! Their overall risk of death was 45 percent lower than that of the group getting the conventional advice. And—get this—their cholesterol levels didn't change much. Though they had significantly less heart disease and less risk of dying, their cholesterol levels pretty much didn't budge.

Though some studies have shown a reduction in heart disease with cholesterol-lowering medications, the amount of reduction pales when compared to what's achievable with lifestyle changes. High-risk men in the WOSCOP study (a statin drug study) achieved about a 30 percent reduction in heart disease by going on drugs, but the women in the Nurses' Health Study showed 31 percent reduction in heart disease just by eating fish once a week. As Harvard's John Abramson, M.D., puts it, "Most of our health is determined by how we live our lives."

What about Organic?

I mentioned earlier in the introduction how important language is when we talk about food. It's necessary to define terms such as "grass fed," "organic," "cage-free," "free range," and the like. I'm purposely leaving out "natural," as it is the most deceptive and dishonest term in food marketing and so overused as to become utterly meaningless. "Natural" has no legal definition, and it is purely a marketing scam. Remember, poison ivy and gasoline are both natural—that doesn't mean I want to eat them!

In the section on meat and poultry, I address the issues of grass fed and free range, because the terms apply to that category. But "organic" is a label we see everywhere and it is used on everything—from fruits and vegetables to Captain Hickory's Chocolate Crunchy Cereal. What does it mean, anyway? Should we pay attention? And if so, why?

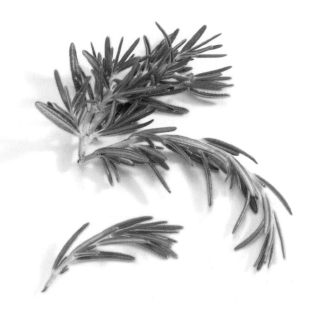

Despite the food industry's best efforts to make us think our food just magically appears in the supermarket aisle, our food comes from somewhere. And where it comes from—where and how it grows in the case of plants, and what it eats and how it was raised in the case of animals—has everything to do with its quality. So, let's start with a basic premise: The quality of the food we eat comes from the quality of the food our food eats.

This maxim even applies when we're talking about fruits and vegetables. Early studies showed that carrots grown in one section of the country did not have the same nutrient composition as carrots grown in another region. The practice of studying this sort of thing was abandoned because it outraged farmers. Grapefruit growers in one part of the country did not want data out there showing that grapefruit grown in another part of the country had more vitamin C. Agribusiness is dedicated to selling us the concept that "carrots are carrots, beef is beef." Of course, that's demonstrably not true. For example: On a gram-for-gram basis, a California avocado has 77 percent more monounsaturated fat, 44 percent more potassium, and 21 percent more fiber than its Florida counterpart.

HOW SOIL QUALITY AFFECTS FOOD QUALITY

Agribusiness interests aside, where a food comes from can make a big difference in its nutritional composition, and how it was produced can make a big difference in its chemical composition, and even its effect on blood sugar. The glycemic index/glycemic load charts show significant differences between, say, the russet potatoes from Canada and those from the United States, or between corn from New Zealand and corn from the United States.

If a fruit or vegetable is grown in soil depleted of minerals, it's going to be less nutritious than one that's grown in soil that's rich in nutrients. In fact, studies of fruits, vegetables, and wheat have revealed a 5 to 35 percent decline in some key vitamins, minerals, and protein over the last half-century. If an apple is sprayed with a ton of chemicals or pesticides—and artificially treated to make it bigger, rounder, redder, more uniform, polished, and more appealing to the eye—it stands to reason that a chemical analysis of that apple is going to look different than one of an apple growing wild on a farm somewhere.

THE ORGANIC MOVEMENT DEMANDS A RETURN TO "NATURAL" FARMING

This brings us to organic foods. The whole idea of the organic food movement—the spirit of the movement, if you will—was a desire to return to basics. It was fueled by a fervent wish to consume the healthy products of the small, sustainable farm where fruits and vegetables and cows and pigs and chickens and horses lived in an interdependent atmosphere of pastoral tranquility, where food—whether animal or vegetable—was raised or grown the old-fashioned way.

The organic movement valued—even idealized—a time and place where animals were not fed growth hormones, steroids, and antibiotics; where crops were left to fend off the elements with their own protective antioxidants and anthocyanins, rather than chemical pesticides and carcinogens; and where "Roundup Ready," genetically modified plants (GMO) were unknown. People who wanted organic food were voting for their health and against a marketplace that was increasingly providing

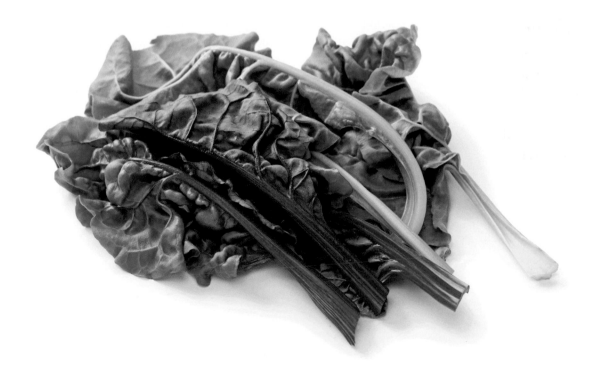

them with "food products" bearing less and less resemblance to anything that could once be considered real or whole food—stuff that grew out of the ground, fell from a tree, or was harvested from healthy animals grazing on pasture or wild fish from uncontaminated waters. Buying organic represented a return to natural—and presumably healthier—foods.

At least that was the hope.

So yes, I buy organic whenever possible. I just don't kid myself anymore that the label refers to something that came from a farm like the ones on which I collected eggs from the barnyard as a kid.

THE INCONVENIENCE OF HEALTHY ORGANIC

If you want that kind of real food, it's going to take more than just looking for the organic label on your supermarket food. You might need to join a food collective. Go to a farmer's market. Or, if you can, go to a local farm and buy your food there. See where it comes from. Say hello to the people who grow and raise it.

If you're lucky enough to be able to do that, you'll be giving yourself a real gift.

In Conclusion

So after writing this book, you'd think I'd have a definite opinion on what the best diet for human beings looks like, wouldn't you?

I do: There is no perfect diet for humans.

People have lived and thrived on high-protein high-fat diets, on low-protein high-carb diets, on diets high in raw milk and cream, and even on diets high in animal blood (the Masai). And they've done so without the ravages of degenerative diseases that are epidemic in modern life—heart disease, diabetes, obesity, neurodegenerative diseases, osteoporosis, and cancer.

Here's what they haven't done: thrived on food with bar codes. Nor, for that matter, on food you could pick up in less than a minute at a drive-through.

More than anything else, the take-home message of this book is: Eat real food. Stuff your grandmother would have recognized as food. Stuff that usually doesn't come in a package. What you eat probably doesn't ultimately matter as much as how much processing it's undergone. Real food—whole food with minimal processing—contains a virtual pharmacy of nutrients, phytochemicals, enzymes, vitamins, minerals, antioxidants, anti-inflammatories, and healthful fats, and it can keep you alive and thriving into your tenth decade.

Remember, how you eat is as important as what you eat. Mindfulness and consciousness in eating—as in everything else in life—contribute to health and well-being.

Whether you're driving a car, building a relationship, or eating a meal, paying attention to what you're doing makes a difference.

Do it. Savor each moment—and each morsel.

And enjoy the journey.

—Jonny Bowden

THE EXPERTS' TOP TEN LISTS

The Experts Speak

So much of my work centers on nutrition and health, and I'm frequently asked by friends—or even by strangers who just discovered I'm a nutritionist, probably because I was expounding too loudly on some health-related issue—the following question: "So what do you eat, anyway?"

Which got me thinking.

Not about what I eat—I already know the answer to that. But about what other experts who are conversant with the concepts in this book eat. After all, all of them know what foods are good for you and why—but it might be interesting to see what they actually do eat. One time, when I was speaking at the world-renowned Boulderfest annual conference on nutritional medicine, Robert Crayhon—the brilliant founder and organizer of Boulderfest—asked each of the speakers to write down what we had for breakfast that morning and to list a typical day's food. The seminar attendees found it interesting to read what the "experts" ate on a daily basis.

Hence my "ask the experts" sections, peppered throughout the book.

Here's what I did: I went to my database and started calling up some of the best people in the field and asking them if they'd submit a list of their top ten favorite healthy foods. The ones they actually ate, not just the ones they thought were the healthiest. All of them were kind enough to say yes, and the results are sprinkled throughout this book.

Many are authors of best-selling books on health, diet, and nutrition; others include a nationally known expert on hypertension and metabolic syndrome, an acclaimed medical educator, a well-known academic researcher in the field of diet, and an extraordinary nutritionist and media personality. Many fit into several categories—writers as well as practitioners. All are, in my humble opinion, brilliant.

I gave them all one mandate: Tell me your top ten healthy foods. Then I allowed them to interpret that instruction in any way they chose, including extending the list to eleven or twelve. I think you'll find the results amusing and instructive.

For those of you who are inclined toward statistics and graphs and like betting on the office pool for the Academy Awards, it's amusing to notice which foods got the most votes and which were bypassed completely. The clear winners were blueberries (and other berries), spinach (and kale), nuts (especially almonds), broccoli, and wild salmon, with grass-fed beef a very close runner-up. There were some surprises (coffee got mentioned twice), some new stars (pomegranate and sea vegetables), and some notable absences (not one person mentioned soy—not as surprising as you might think—see my essay on soy, page 186). Anyway, I thought it was interesting, and I hope you do, too.

If you're aching to know what I personally eat, I'll tell you: oatmeal, pastured bacon, raw certified organic milk, eggs, blueberries, spinach, cherries, sardines, kale, whey protein powder, free-range beef, apples, wild salmon, turmeric, full-fat yogurt, figs, cheese, nuts, watermelon, fresh cold-pressed juices, Malaysian palm oil, coconut oil, avocado, green tea, fresh vegetable juice, and green drinks. There, now you know. And, of course, if I'm being honest, ice cream.

Read the entries and you'll know why I—and so many of the experts—love those foods. I hope you will, too.

CHAPTER 1

VEGETABLES

Let's get one thing straight right away: There are no bad vegetables. Maybe I need to clarify just a bit, because the most consumed "vegetables" in the United States include ketchup, iceberg lettuce, and french fries. I'm talking about anything that has a leaf. I'm talking about anything that makes a crunch when you bite it. I'm talking about anything that's green, red, orange, or, in rare cases, white (cauliflower and mushrooms). Get the point? I'm not talking about french fries.

So, if the title of this book were *The 500 Healthiest Foods on Earth* instead of the 150 healthiest foods, probably every member of the vegetable family you can possibly think of would be listed—which is not the case with dairy, grains, or some other categories in this book. Even corn and potatoes make the cut. (And they wound up on no one's top ten list, I'm happy to say.) The thirty-six vegetables that made the A-list here are those that I felt represented the absolute best nutritional bang for the buck in a crowded field in which most entries are already winners.

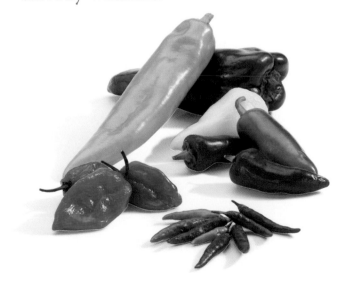

Aren't Some Vegetables Fattening?

We're currently experiencing an obesity and diabetes epidemic in most of the Western world (and even in some parts of the non-Western world), and a reasonable question to ask would be this: Are some vegetables more fattening than others, and should they be avoided?

Generally speaking, the answer is no.

There's a lot of confusion about certain starchy vegetables that have a high glycemic index, vegetables that people following lower-carb eating plans have been told to avoid. The short answer is this: If you're a person for whom blood sugar management is a real issue, yes, some vegetables on this list—sweet potatoes, for example—might be worth limiting. But, in my opinion, the argument about vegetables and sugar is a tempest in a teapot.

There are two real culprits in the obesity crisis: one, the fast-acting carbs and sugars in breads, cereals, pastas, desserts, cakes, rolls, crackers, and fast food; and two, the obscenely large portions of everything else. As my wisecracking pal, the brilliant nutritionist and U.S. Department of Agriculture (USDA) researcher C. Leigh Broadhurst, Ph.D., says, "No one ever got fat on peas and carrots."

So of course, watch your sugar content. But most vegetables don't have that much, particularly compared to the real culprits in the American diet. (Potatoes and corn are exceptions.) You can't go wrong with a single vegetable on this list, and you would do well to consume a variety of all of them.

So here's my list of top winners in the vegetable sweepstakes. Argue with them, if you like. Add some favorites of your own, and throw out a couple you really hate. Just eat as many as you can.

You'll be giving yourself a real gift of health.

 ## The Stars

It was difficult deciding which foods to give a star to, and I'm sure you could argue that some good foods didn't get stars. You'd be right. Remember, everything on this list is already a star in its respective category. For example, in this chapter I gave stars to the superstars— the vegetables that are so uniquely loaded with nutrients, fiber, cancer-fighting phytochemicals, or some combination thereof, that they deserved some special mention, even among the company of great foods.

Artichokes

Artichokes are kind of like the lobster of the vegetable community—you must really work to get at the good parts. The part that contains the meat is called the heart, even though it's technically the bottom of the plant. And it takes some digging to get there. Is it worth it? Definitely.

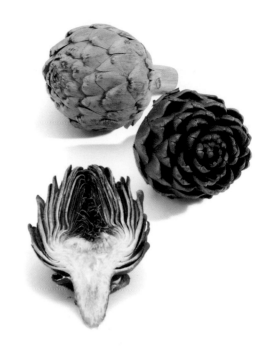

Artichokes are a liver-cleansing food. If you've ever looked at the ingredients on a supplement specifically designed for liver health or for detoxification, you're likely to have seen artichoke extract listed on the label. Why? Because this plant is a wonderful source of silymarin, the active ingredient in milk thistle. Silymarin has a long and distinguished pedigree as a plant compound that helps protect and nourish the liver. And artichokes have plenty of it.

Artichokes Bring Stomach Relief

That's not all they have. The artichoke leaves contain several active chemical compounds that have been found to be beneficial across a range of health issues. For example, the bile-stimulating action of the plant has been well documented in at least one controlled trial in which, after administration of artichoke extract directly into the duodenum, liver bile increased significantly. This may be why artichokes are often used for indigestion. According to herbal experts Joe and Teresa Graedon, Ph.D. (authors of *The People's Pharmacy*), patients with chronic gastrointestinal (GI)

upset who were given artichoke extract showed amazing improvement. In one study, researchers reported that 85 percent of patients experienced substantial relief from stomach pain, nausea, and vomiting.

The standardized extract has also been used to treat high cholesterol and triglycerides, and in test-tube studies, the flavonoids from the artichoke (especially luteolin) have prevented the oxidation of LDL ("bad") cholesterol, a definite risk factor for cardiovascular disease.

Although artichoke extract has a distinguished history as an herbal supplement, the vegetable itself is a healthy food. It contains 72 mg of magnesium, 425 mg of potassium, a little folate, the eye-friendly carotenoids lutein and zeaxanthin, and best of all, a substantial 6½ g of fiber per one medium artichoke. (If you go for a large one, you get almost 9 g of fiber!) And that's all for a miserly 60 calories. (Okay, 76 if you're going for the big guy.) A good nutritional deal no matter how you slice it. Or, in the case of the artichoke, how you dig for it.

Arugula

Arugula sure doesn't look like an aphrodisiac, but that's exactly what the ancient Egyptians and Romans considered it to be. I don't know about that, but I do know that it's the überfood of nutritional bargains: One cup (20 g) of arugula contains … get ready … 5 calories. For that you get some folate (folic acid), vitamin A, and a surprisingly decent amount of the extremely eye-healthy carotenoids, lutein, and zeaxanthin.

There's also about the same amount of calcium as there is in spinach, but arugula is actually lower in oxalates, a substance that inhibits calcium absorption.

Arugula has a nice amount of vitamin K: One cup (20 g) contains almost half the recommended daily allowance (which in my opinion is too low). Vitamin K is essential for clotting and is a key player in developing strong bones. The Framingham Heart Study, for example, found that people who consumed approximately 250 mcg of vitamin K a day had a 35 percent lower risk of hip fractures compared to those who consumed just 50 mcg a day. True, you'd have to consume 10 cups (200 g) of arugula to get that much, but still, a few cups (33 mg) in a salad is a good start.

The arugula plant, like many others in the cruciferous family, contains glucosinolates. When you chew the plant, the glucosinolates mix with an enzyme (myrosinase) that turns them into other compounds called isothiocyanates, which have documented anticancer properties. Isothiocyanates combat carcinogens by neutralizing them, reducing their poisonous effect, and stimulating the release of other substances that help combat them. Isothiocyanates also inhibit cell proliferation. Studies have shown that they help prevent lung and esophageal cancer and can lower the risk of other types of cancers, including gastrointestinal cancer.

That's an awful lot of good stuff to pack into a cup of food that contains only 5 calories.

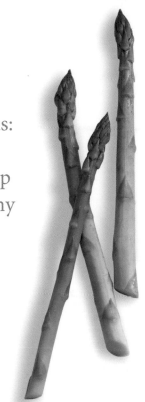

Asparagus

Here's an interesting piece of trivia about asparagus: They're one of the only plants that have distinct male and female versions. And if you'd like a dollop of irony with that factoid, the male plants are skinny and the females are … well, Rubenesque. To compound the political incorrectness, it's the fresh young plants that are the most desirable—they taste the best. On the other hand, when allowed to mature, a gorgeous fern develops. You can't eat it, but it makes one of the most beautiful hanging plants around.

The asparagus has two parts—a thick root and the tender stalks. The root is used in traditional Indian medicine as a diuretic and to strengthen the female reproductive system. The asparagus root is also believed to help develop peace of mind, a loving nature, a good memory, and a calm spirit. Chinese traditionalists save the best roots of the plant for their families and friends, believing that it will increase feelings of compassion and love. Meanwhile, in India, it's used to promote fertility, reduce menstrual cramping, and increase milk production in nursing mothers. These customs have some basis in science—the root contains steroidal glycosides that affect hormone production and possibly influence emotions. In India, the racemosa species is used to increase sperm count and nourish the ovum.

In the Western world, asparagus has long been touted as an aphrodisiac. I was unable to find any scientific evidence for its ability to make people amorous, but the legend remains, probably due to the vegetable's phallic shape. It's worth noting that asparagus is also known in India by the name Shatavari, which means "she who possesses 100 husbands." Draw your own conclusions.

Low in Calories, High in Nutrients

Asparagus, like most fruits and vegetables, has a favorable ratio of potassium to sodium. A cup (180 g) of cooked asparagus contains a whopping 404 mg of potassium, as well as 268 mcg of folate, an important B vitamin that helps prevent neural tube defects and helps reduce a harmful blood chemical called homocysteine. It's also high in vitamin K, essential for healthy clotting and for strong bones. There's also rutin, which helps protect blood vessels, and the anti-inflammatory, cancer-fighting flavonoid quercetin. And finally, a cup (180 g) of cooked asparagus gives you a decent 4 g of fiber, all for a ridiculously low number of calories (40).

Best of all, there's serious published research showing that compounds in asparagus have antitumor activity. A study from Rutgers University, published in *Cancer Letters*, showed that crude saponins from asparagus inhibited the growth of human leukemia cells. Asparagus is also high in glutathione, one of the body's most important antioxidants. And asparagus contain inulin, a special kind of fiber that feeds the good bacteria in your gut and helps support gastrointestinal health.

The only downside to asparagus is that it makes your pee smell funny. This is because it contains the amino acid asparagine. It's weird and annoying, but completely harmless.

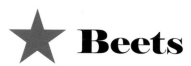 # Beets

Since the original edition of this book, beets have attained something of a superstar status in the nutrition world, particularly among athletes. Beets are rich with nitrates, which metabolize into an important (and desirable!) molecule called nitric oxide. Beets have become extremely popular with cutting-edge nutrition buffs largely because of growing appreciation for the importance of nitric oxide, which relaxes the arteries, lowers blood pressure, and may increase circulation to exercising muscles. Athletes now take beetroot juice supplements in the hope that the nitric oxide they produce will help their energy and performance.

In many holistic, integrative, and Eastern traditions, beets are believed to be an excellent liver tonic and blood purifier. They're a staple of the juicing crowd, for good reason (more in a moment). Beets get their red color from a compound in them called *betacyanin*, which is the messy stuff that stains your clothes and hands. Betacyanin also turns your urine red, so if you juice with beets, don't be alarmed—you're not bleeding internally!

The Heart-Healthy Benefits of Beets

Beets are an important dietary source of betaine and a good source of folate. These two nutrients work synergistically to reduce potentially toxic levels of homocysteine, a naturally occurring amino acid that can be harmful to blood vessels, thereby contributing to the development of heart disease, stroke, dementia, and peripheral vascular disease (reduced blood flow to the legs and feet).

Beets are also loaded with potassium, a vitally important mineral for heart health. Our caveman ancestors consumed a diet high in potassium and low in sodium. A high potassium-to-sodium ratio is ideal for human health, but these days the ratio is reversed. The potassium in beets can help correct this imbalance. Potassium is found in fruits (such as bananas) and vegetables; beets, weighing in at a whopping 528 mg of potassium for two beets, are an excellent source. They also have magnesium and a tiny amount of vitamin C.

Beets got a bad rap from the low-carb folks (with whom I'm sometimes allied) because they are high in sugar. That's true, but not significant unless you're really, really sugar sensitive. That said, they're on the "no-no" list of a lot of docs who specialize in diabetes, such as Richard Bernstein, M.D. (author of *The Diabetes Diet*). For the rest of us, they make a terrific addition to the menu. They can be baked, boiled, steamed, or shredded raw and added to salads and slaws. The leaves are even higher in nutritional value than the roots, especially in calcium, iron, vitamin A, and vitamin C.

Beets make a delicious juice, but have a strong flavor and are usually best mixed with some combination of carrots, apples, spinach, and ginger.

Bok Choy
(Chinese cabbage, pak-choi, Chinese chard)

Bok choy is an Asian member of the cabbage family that has long, thick stalks topped by blue-green leaves. You probably know it as an ingredient in wonton soup, but despite that decidedly mundane use, it's a real health food.

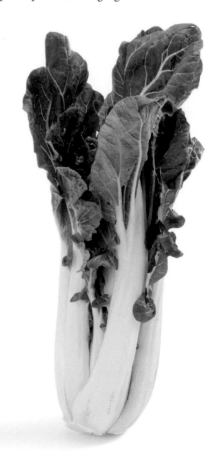

Is It Really a Cabbage?

There's some minor controversy about whether bok choy, also known as Chinese cabbage, should even be called a cabbage in the first place. Technically, it's not a cabbage, because it doesn't form a head. In many circles, it's more properly referred to as Chinese chard. But who cares? Whatever you choose to call it, this vegetable is a card-carrying member of the *Brassica* family, which means it contains indoles, compounds that have been shown to significantly lower the risk of cancer. Not only that, it's loaded with calcium, potassium, beta-carotene, and vitamin A. All for fewer than 20 calories a cup (170 g), and even fewer if it's raw.

Bok choy has a high-water content, so it becomes limp quickly if you overcook it. Instead, cook it quickly over a high temperature so that the leaves become tender and the stalks stay crisp. Stir-frying is ideal, but bok choy stalks are also terrific raw, used with a dip.

Raw bok choy might just be the lowest-calorie vegetable on the planet—one cup (70 g) of the shredded vegetable has exactly 9 calories. Because a cooked cup of the stuff is more concentrated, it gives several times the potassium and twice the calcium, beta-carotene, and vitamin A, plus almost 2 g of fiber. Either way—cooked or raw—it's a bargain.

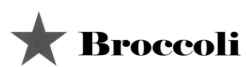

★ Broccoli

Broccoli is vegetable royalty. When I sent out a request to the best nutritionists, medical doctors, naturopaths, and researchers asking for their personal list of "top ten" healthy foods, it was almost a given that broccoli would be among the most frequently mentioned (and it was). No wonder. This superstar vegetable has been lauded for its cancer-fighting power so many times that it's a celebrity in the nutrition world.

Broccoli is a member of the *Brassica* family of cruciferous vegetables—the same vegetable royalty that includes bok choy, cabbage, kale, kohlrabi, and Swiss chard. These vegetables are excellent sources of a family of anticancer phytochemicals called isothiocyanates. Isothiocyanates fight cancer by neutralizing carcinogens—the bad guys of the cancer battle. They do this

by reducing their poisonous effects and stimulating the release of "carcinogen killers," speeding up their removal from the body. Studies have shown that isothiocyanates help prevent lung and esophageal cancer and can lower the risk of other cancers, including gastrointestinal cancer. Several isothiocyanates have been shown to inhibit tumors induced by chemical carcinogens. Broccoli in particular contains a potent isothio-cyanate that is an inhibitor of mammary tumors.

Why Women Should Eat More Broccoli

The anticancer properties of broccoli are well established. Even the American Cancer Society recommends eating it and other cruciferous vegetables. Though there are many compounds responsible for its impact on our health, one that deserves special mention is the indoles. Broccoli contains indole-3-carbinol, which, in addition to being a strong antioxidant and stimulator of detoxifying enzymes, seems to protect the structure of DNA. It also reduces the risk of breast and cervical cancer.

Indole-3-carbinol is of particular importance to women. Estrogen has three basic metabolites, and they behave somewhat differently in the body. Two of the metabolites—16-alpha-hydroxyestrone and 4-hydroxyestrone—have carcinogenic action, but the third, 2-hydroxyestrone, is benign and has protective effects. Indole-3-carbinol increases the ratio of the "good" (benign) estrogen metabolite to the potentially harmful ones. Men have estrogen also, and it stands to reason that broccoli and other cruciferous vegetables containing indoles should be helpful and protective to them as well. In addition, indole-3-carbinol has been shown to protect against the carcinogenic effect of pesticides and other toxins.

Note: Indole-3-carbinol is available as a supplement, but I don't recommend it. Instead, I always recommend DIM, a metabolite of indole-3-carbinole that is safer and more reliable as a supplement and accomplishes the same thing.

Cruciferous vegetables such as broccoli also contain high levels of a phytochemical called sulforaphane. Sulforaphane increases the activation of enzymes known as phase-2 enzymes, which help fight carcinogens. It's believed that phase-2 enzymes may reduce the risk of prostate cancer. Per research from the Department of Urology at Stanford University published in *Cancer Epidemiology Biomarkers and Prevention*, sulforaphane is the most potent inducer of phase-2 enzymes of any phytochemical known to date.

A Nutritional Powerhouse

Even apart from its demonstrated cancer-fighting ability, broccoli is a nutritional powerhouse. One cup (71 g) contains more than 2 g of protein, 2 g of fiber, 288 mg of potassium, 43 mg of calcium, 81 mg of vitamin C, plus folate, magnesium, phosphorus, beta-carotene, vitamin A, and 1,277 mcg of the superstars of eye nutrition, lutein and zeaxanthin. Lutein and zeaxanthin, both members of the carotenoid family, are being extensively researched for their demonstrated ability to reduce or prevent macular degeneration, the number one cause of blindness in older adults.

And, by the way, the broccoli head is actually the flower of the plant. But according to natural foods expert Rebecca Wood, cofounder of the East West Center in Boulder, Colorado, there are plenty of nutrients in the stalks as well. She suggests peeling the fibrous skin off the stalks and using them. She also suggests using the leafy greens, which offer tons of nutrients as well.

WORTH KNOWING

The Environmental Working Group, a consumer advocate and protection nonprofit research organization, in 2017 ranked broccoli as thirty-six out of fifty-one of the most contaminated foods with pesticides.

Broccoli Rabe

Broccoli rabe is a distant relative of broccoli, and is in fact a lot more closely related to the turnip (it's often called a turnip green). But from the point of view of taste, you might think of it as broccoli on steroids. To put it mildly—no pun intended—it's aggressive and bitter. The Chinese variety, also known as flowering cabbage, is milder.

But make no mistake—this peppery little plant is a card-carrying member of one of the largest edible-plant families —the *Brassica* family—which includes such nutritional and health heavyweights as cabbage, broccoli, Brussels sprouts, bok choy, and kohlrabi. And it shares many of their amazing health benefits. Like all cruciferous vegetables, broccoli rabe contains flavonoids, sulforaphane, and indoles, which help prevent cellular degeneration and may help protect against cancer. Sulforaphane, for example, has been shown to induce powerful enzymes that protect rodents from tumors. And flavonoids in general have extensive biological properties that promote human health and help reduce the risk of disease.

Great for Healthy Bones and Superb Vision

This immune-boosting vegetable packs an incredible nutritional wallop for a tiny number of calories. One serving, a mere 28 calories, contains 100 mg of calcium, 292 mg of potassium, 31 mg of vitamin C, 60 mcg of folate, 217 mg of bone-building vitamin K, and more than 3,800 IUs of vitamin A, including 2,300 mcg of beta-carotene. Also, there are 1,431 mcg of the superstars of eye nutrition, lutein and zeaxanthin, which are being investigated for their ability to fight macular degeneration, the number-one cause of blindness in elderly adults. For its paltry 28 calories, broccoli rabe also contains a healthy helping of fiber—2.4 mg per single serving. This is one great vegetable!

How to Prepare Broccoli Rabe

About the taste: Blanching the leaves and shoots before cooking will tame their flavor, though many people like it and use it to spice up dishes. Sophie Markoulakis of the *San Francisco Chronicle* recommends sautéing blanched broccoli rabe in olive oil and garlic for about 10 minutes and adding it to cooked pasta with a little cooking liquid, finely chopped dried figs, and toasted pine nuts. "Sprinkle with ricotta salata or other dried salted sheep's milk cheese and pass the pepper grinder," she says. Does that not sound amazing?

Brussels Sprouts

Brussels sprouts are not really sprouts at all, but members of the cabbage family, which makes sense because that's exactly what they look like: tiny little miniature cabbages, growing tightly packed together on a tall, thick stalk. They were first widely cultivated in sixteenth-century Belgium, which accounts for their name.

Members of the cruciferous vegetable family, they have many of the same nutritional benefits of other cabbages. Cabbages in general probably contain more cancer-fighting nutrients than any other vegetable family. One of the key dietary recommendations of the American Cancer Society is to include these cruciferous vegetables in your diet on a regular basis.

Brussels Sprouts May Ward Off Colon Cancer

Brussels sprouts contain a chemical called sinigrin, which suppresses the development of precancerous cells. The breakdown product of sinigrin (allyl isothiocyanate) is the active ingredient in Brussels sprouts and is responsible for the characteristic smell of sprouts. It works by persuading the precancerous cells to commit suicide—a natural process called *apoptosis*—and so powerful is the effect that it's entirely possible that the occasional meal of Brussels sprouts could help reduce the incidence of colon cancer.

Brussels sprouts are high in isothiocyanates and sulforaphane, which are compounds known to help fight cancer by inhibiting cell proliferation, neutralizing carcinogens, and helping to detoxify nasty environmental toxins. Sulforaphane, a particularly potent member of the isothiocyanate family, increases the production of certain enzymes known as "phase-2 enzymes," which can disarm damaging free radicals and help fight carcinogens. It's believed that phase-2 enzymes may reduce the risk of prostate cancer. Department of Urology at Stanford University research published in *Cancer Epidemiology Biomarkers and Prevention*, says that sulforaphane is the most potent inducer of phase-2 enzymes of any phytochemical known to date. And in a review article from the 11th Annual Research Conference on Diet, Nutrition, and Cancer from the American Institute of Cancer Research, the authors stated that "isothiocyanates are well-known protectors against carcinogenesis."

HARD ON THE NOSE, EASY ON THE BODY

Unfortunately, the sulfur content of allyl isothiocyanate gives these veggies their less-than-pleasant odor, often known affectionately as "eau d'New Jersey." (Luckily, the smell has nothing to do with their taste.)

Brussels sprouts also supply good amounts of folate, potassium, and bone-building vitamin K, and a small amount of beta-carotene.

★ Cabbage

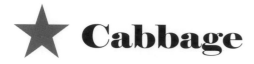

In the world of vegetables, the *Brassica* family is true royalty. And the reigning king of the brood—which includes broccoli, kohlrabi, cauliflower, bok choy, Brussels sprouts, and chard—is the cabbage. When we speak of cabbage, we're really talking about the large, lettuce-like head that has been a staple for at least two millennia. Eaten raw, it's the stuff of slaws. Cooked, it is hard to ignore, as even slight overcooking produces the smell of rotten eggs. But cabbage can be a delicious vegetable. And even more to the point, the cabbage family is probably the most important vegetable in the world from the point of view of nutritional benefits and cancer-fighting ability.

Cabbage Keeps Breast Cancer at Bay

Cabbage first came to the attention of researchers after they observed that women in Eastern European countries surrounding Poland and Russia were much less likely to develop breast cancer than American women, according to author and researcher Laurie Deutsch Mozian, M.S., R.D. An analysis of their diet revealed a much higher intake of cabbage, and when the cabbage was analyzed, likely candidates for the effect were the phytochemicals called indoles. Years of research have now demonstrated that these indoles, in fact, alter estrogen metabolism in a favorable way, one that is likely to reduce the risk of cancer.

Here's how it works. Estrogen has three basic metabolites, and they behave somewhat differently in the body. Two of the metabolites—16-alpha-hydroxyestrone and 4-hydroxyestrone—have

carcinogenic action, but the third, 2-hydroxyestrone, is benign and has protective effects. Indole-3-carbinol, one of the main indoles in cabbage, increases the ratio of the "good" (benign) estrogen metabolite to the potentially harmful ones. Men have estrogen also, and it stands to reason that the indoles in cabbage should be helpful and protective to them as well. In addition, indole-3-carbinol has been shown to protect against the carcinogenic effect of pesticides and other toxins.

Note: Indole-3-carbinol is available as a supplement, but I don't recommend it. Instead, I always recommend DIM, a metabolite of indole-3-carbinole that is safer and more reliable as a supplement and accomplishes the same thing.

The anticancer benefits of cabbage don't stop with the indoles, though. Other phytochemicals that pack an anticancer wallop and are plentiful in cabbage include dithiolethiones, isothiocynates, and sulforaphane. Sulforaphane, a particularly potent member of the isothiocyanate family, increases the production of certain enzymes known as phase-2 enzymes, which can disarm damaging free radicals and help fight carcinogens. It's believed that phase-2 enzymes may reduce the risk of prostate cancer. Sulforaphane is the most potent inducer of phase-2 enzymes of any phytochemical known to date, according to research from the Department of Urology at Stanford University published in *Cancer Epidemiology Biomarkers and Prevention*. And in a review article from the 11th Annual Research Conference on Diet, Nutrition, and Cancer from the American Institute for Cancer Research, the authors stated that "isothiocyanates are well-known protectors against carcinogenesis."

More Than Just a Pretty Plant

Red or purple cabbage is also a source of anthocyanins, pigment molecules that make blueberries blue and red cabbage red. They're found in many colorful fruits such as grapes and berries. Turns out they do a lot more than make our produce pretty. Anthocyanins belong to a group of plant compounds called flavonoids, and they have considerable bioactive properties, including acting as powerful antioxidants. In one study anthocyanins were found to have the strongest antioxidizing power of 150 flavonoids studied (more than 4,000 different flavonoids have been identified). And the anthocyanins in red cabbage were found in another study to protect animals against the damages produced by a known toxin. There's every reason to think that they're equally protective for us.

Anthocyanins' ability to act as antioxidants and to fight free radicals make them powerful weapons against cardiovascular disease. And anthocyanins are also known for their anti-inflammatory effects. Anti-inflammatory anthocyanins can help dampen allergic reactions as well as help protect against the damage to connective tissue and blood vessel walls that inflammation can cause.

On top of all its phytochemical power, cabbage is a darn good source of everyday vitamins and minerals. It contains calcium, magnesium, potassium, vitamin C, vitamin K, beta-carotene, and even a little of the eye-healthy carotenoids, lutein and zeaxanthin. And let's not forget the fiber. One cup (150 g) of the cooked stuff gives you almost 4 g of fiber. One cup (89 g) of raw cabbage gives you 2 g. All this in one of the lowest-calorie foods on the planet.

WORTH KNOWING

Many members of the cabbage family contain goitrogens, naturally occurring substances that may interfere with the function of the thyroid gland. People with hypothyroidism would be wise to consume moderately. In the absence of thyroid problems, there is no research whatsoever to indicate that goitrogenic foods will have any negative impact on your health.

★ Carrots

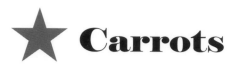

What's the very first thing you think of if someone uses the term "healthfood?" For many people, it's carrots. Well-known naturopathic physician Michael Murray, N.D., calls carrots "the king of the vegetables," and for good reason. Human studies have indicated that as little as one carrot a day could possibly cut the rate of lung cancer in half.

The cancer-fighting properties of this great vegetable should be taken seriously. Carrots are high in carotenoids, antioxidant compounds found in plants that are associated with a wide range of health benefits. You've probably heard good things about beta-carotene, but that's only one of about 500 members of the carotenoid family. Some research suggests that other carotenoids may be even more important. High carotenoid intake has been associated with a decrease of up to 50 percent in bladder, cervical, prostate, colon, larynx, and esophageal cancer, as well as up to a 20 percent decrease in postmenopausal breast cancer.

Carrots are also high in alpha-carotene, another carotenoid that appears to have health benefits of its own. In fact, one report published in *NCI Cancer Weekly* by Michiaki Murakoshi, who led a team of biochemists at Japan's Kyoto Prefectural University of Medicine, contends that alpha-carotene may be more powerful than beta-carotene in inhibiting processes that may lead to tumor growth.

Although one badly designed study a few years ago seemed to indicate that beta-carotene by itself had no value in preventing cancer, what wasn't well publicized is that the study subjects were heavy smokers and that the beta-carotene given to them was a synthetic kind that behaves differently in the body than the real deal. The real lesson from that study is that the carotenoids perform best working as a unit, and should be obtained in their natural—not synthetic—form. Dozens of studies show beneficial associations between eating fruits and vegetables high in carotenoids and less cardiovascular disease, not to mention less prostate, lung, stomach, colon, breast, cervical, and pancreatic cancer, according to Walter Willett, M.D., Dr. P.H., professor of epidemiology and nutrition at Harvard's School of Public Health.

Why Your Mom Was Right about Carrots

Put carrots in the column labeled "things mother was right about after all." Carrots really are good for your eyes. They're a great source of lutein and zeaxanthin, two other carotenoids that, when working together, have shown enormous promise in protecting the eyes and helping to prevent macular degeneration and cataracts. Both alpha-carotene and beta-carotene convert in the body to vitamin A, which, in addition to being a great antioxidant and immune system stimulator, turbocharges the formation of a purple pigment in the eye called rhodopsin. Rhodopsin is needed by the eye to see in dim light—it raises the effectiveness of the light-sensitive area of the retina—so not getting enough vitamin A can lead to night blindness.

Three medium carrots contain 60 mg of calcium, 586 mg of potassium, a little bit of magnesium, phosphorus, and vitamin C, and of course, a whopping 30,000 IUs of vitamin A, including 15,000 units of beta-carotene and 6,000 of alpha-carotene. They also have 5 g of fiber.

Cooked Carrots Prevail

Cooking slightly changes the nutritional content and makes some of the nutrients more bioavailable. But both raw and cooked carrots are healthy.

To get the most out of the carotenoids found in carrots, eat them with a little fat. The carotenoids and vitamin A are fat-soluble nutrients and are better absorbed that way.

Finally, carrots are a favorite ingredient for juicing, and carrot juice is often used as part of a detoxification program. Just be aware that when you juice carrots you're using a lot of them, plus you're removing the fiber, both of which increase the concentration of sugar. That doesn't mean it's not a fantastically healthy juice ingredient, just something you should be aware of if you're sensitive to blood sugar fluctuations. Juicing carrots with some low-sugar vegetables such as spinach and broccoli lessens the impact.

WORTH KNOWING

Carrots got a bad and totally undeserved rap by the low-carb folks because of their high glycemic index. Actually, the glycemic index isn't very important—the glycemic *load* is. The glycemic index tests are done on a 50-g portion of carbohydrate, whereas the load tests are done on real-life portions. A carrot has only about 4 g of carbohydrate, so its glycemic load—the only number that matters—is ridiculously low (about 3 on a scale of 0–40+). You'd have to eat a ton of carrots to get a significant rise in blood sugar. Even so, some very careful diabetes doctors whose opinion I respect still tell patients to beware. For everyone else, I think carrots are absolutely fine.

Cauliflower

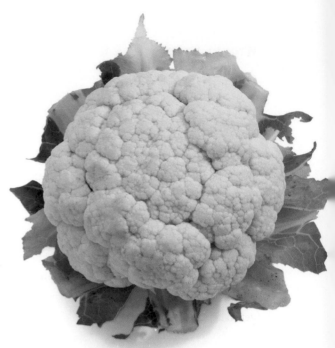

For a long time now, common nutritional wisdom has held that the best diets are rich in colors (green as in spinach, blue as in blueberries, red as in peppers) and low in "the white stuff" (sugar, potatoes, white bread, rice, Twinkies, spaghetti, and the like). I agree with that wholeheartedly. But there are three exceptions to "anti–white stuff" dictum: whitefish, mushrooms, and cauliflower.

Cauliflower is a member of the *Brassica* or cabbage family and, as such, contains many of the compounds, like indoles, that have given this vegetable family its rightly deserved reputation as a potent cancer fighter.

In addition to indoles, cauliflower contains sulforaphane, a breakdown product of compounds in the cauliflower called glucosinolates. While glucosinolates themselves typically have low anticancer activity, sulforaphane has plenty! Sulforaphane was first identified in broccoli sprouts by scientists at the Johns Hopkins University School of Medicine. It's one of a class of chemicals in plants called isothiocyanates and is a potent antioxidant and stimulator of natural detoxifying enzymes in the body.

How Does Cauliflower Fight Cancer?

Here's how it works: Within minutes of being eaten, sulforaphane enters the bloodstream and turbocharges the body's antioxidant defense systems. When it reaches the cells, it activates phase-2 detoxification enzymes in the liver, which then "disarm" carcinogenic molecules and help remove them from the cells. Sulforaphanes, along with other isothiocyanates and indoles is believed to be responsible for the lowered risk of cancer that's associated with the consumption of cruciferous vegetables such as cauliflower, kale, cabbage, and, of course, broccoli and broccoli sprouts.

How to Make Fake Mashed Potatoes

A cup (124 g) of cauliflower is ridiculously low in calories, and contains 3 g of fiber as well as over 50 mg of vitamin C, 176 mg of potassium, and 55 mcg of folate.

The vegetable got a much-deserved boost when the author of *The South Beach Diet*, Arthur Agatston, M.D., popularized a fabulous fake mashed potatoes made using cauliflower in place of the potatoes. With a little butter, lemon, and sea salt, it is beyond delicious. (Of course, my friend and fellow author Dana Carpender was making "fauxtatoes" way before *The South Beach Diet* was ever published, but don't get me started.)

Celery

I'm a big fan of celery for a lot of reasons. It's terrific for appetite control and can be used at the end of a meal (or any time) to stem carb cravings. Smear a spoonful of almond butter or natural peanut butter on it and you have a perfect low-sugar snack that's pretty filling. Celery—with or without the almond butter—travels well in plastic or glass containers. Chewing it stimulates saliva and can aid in digestion. It's a terrific addition to fresh juice (more about that in a moment). And that's just for openers.

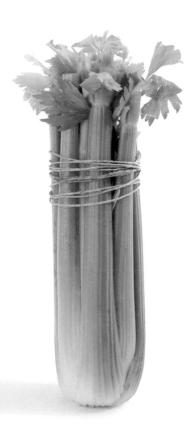

Celery Number One for Treating High Blood Pressure

Celery just might be the number one medicinal food for blood pressure. It's been recommended in traditional Chinese medicine for high blood pressure for centuries, and experimental evidence has confirmed its usefulness.

In one study, injecting lab animals with celery lowered their blood pressure by 12 to 14 percent. If you're a human, you'd get that effect with about four ribs. Mark Houston, M.D., director of the Hypertension Institute in Nashville and my go-to guy for all things related to hypertension, has celery at the top of his list of foods for his patients with high blood pressure. The substances in celery that seem to produce the benefit are phytochemicals called *phthalides*. Clinical studies show that they work by relaxing the muscle tissue in artery walls and therefore increasing blood flow. Phthalide also helps lower levels of stress hormones.

The Celery Hangover Cure

Here's a little folk legend for you: In ancient Rome, they used to wear celery around the neck to ward off a hangover after a particularly demanding night of Roman-style partying. It might be that this is where the practice of putting a stick of celery in a Bloody Mary came from, but that could just be urban legend.

Celery is also a great source of silicon, which is getting a lot of attention recently as a very important nutrient for bone health. Because of its silicon content, celery can help renew joints, bones, arteries, and all connective tissue.

There's also an ingredient found in celery called acetylenics, which has been shown to stop the growth of cancer cells. Celery also contains phenolic acids. These have been shown to block the actions of prostaglandins, which are known to encourage the growth of cancerous tumors.

Give Celery Juice a Try

In Asian traditions, celery is one of the few vegetables that combines well with fruit. Personally, I love it as a base for fresh juice. One of my absolute favorites: Combine a few ribs with one pear and a couple of inches of gingerroot.

Collard Greens

If you've ever wondered what people mean when they use the expression "soul food," this is the food they're talking about. This cabbage-family vegetable was brought to these shores by African slaves and is a staple of Southern cooking. Its flavor lies somewhere between cabbage and kale. It's your quintessential green leafy vegetable, and, in fact, is usually sold as a loose bunch of leaves, though you can get it frozen as well. The fresh version needs to be cleaned thoroughly before cooking.

Typically, collards are simmered for several hours, which makes them tender. But you can also boil them in water for 15 to 30 minutes if you don't mind them being a bit firmer. In Southern cooking, they're often cooked with bacon or salt pork, but they don't have to be; they're often served with beans, especially black-eyed peas (also optional). Personally, I think they're outstanding with just sweet butter and sea salt.

Collards are members of the family of cruciferous vegetables and provide valuable cancer-fighting phytochemicals. One cup (190 g) of collards provides almost the same amount of calcium as 8 ounces (235 ml) of milk, and 5 whopping grams of fiber in the bargain. In addition, they've got magnesium, phosphorus, more than 200 mg of heart-friendly potassium, vitamin C, and a ton of vitamins A and K. There's also a meaningful amount of beta-carotene. And if all that weren't enough, they are a significant source of lutein and zeaxanthin, two carotenoids that are fast becoming the go-to nutrients for eye health.

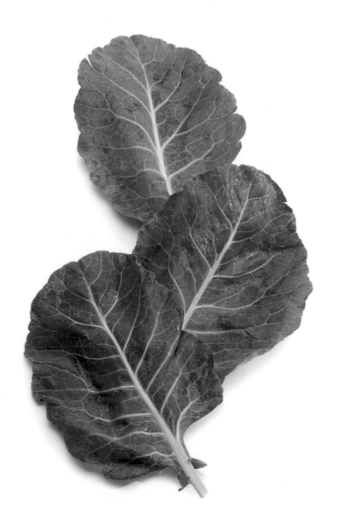

★ Dandelion

The Latin name for dandelion—*Taraxacum officinale*—is your first clue as to what this plant is about. Loosely translated, it means "official remedy for the disorders." (In Greek, taraxons means "disorder," and akos means "remedy." The Arab physicians of the eleventh and twelfth centuries who were the first to write about this miracle plant called it taraxacon.) Dandelion is used in herbal traditions all over the world, including by Native Americans, Arabs, Chinese, and Europeans.

Louis Vanrenen, in his excellent little book *Power Herbs*, lists it as one of the top fifty power herbs. Yup, we're talking about the same dandelion that many people consider a weed. But as Ralph Waldo Emerson said, a weed is just a plant whose virtues have not yet been discovered. This weed has a distinguished history of medicinal use in China, Japan, Russia, and Europe, and it has been used for detoxification for more than a century.

Dandelion Improves Your Liver and Your Moods

Probably at the top of the list of dandelion's health benefits is its profound effect on the liver. Dandelion ranks right alongside milk thistle as the most frequently recommended herbs to help patients who need liver detoxification, says Mark Stengler, N.M.D.

The liver's job is to detoxify every chemical, pollutant, and medicine that we're exposed to—according to some experts it performs more than 5,000 enzymatic reactions. That means keeping it strong and functioning smoothly is of prime importance to our health. "Just by treating the liver we can sometimes resolve numerous conditions ranging from physical problems such as indigestion and hepatitis to the emotional imbalances that contribute to irritability and depression," says Stengler. Dandelion root figures prominently in many natural nutritional support programs for hepatitis C.

One of the chemical components of dandelion, taraxacin, is thought to stimulate the digestive organs and help prompt the liver and gallbladder to release bile. This can be useful in constipation and indigestion—bowels move more easily with increased bile flow, and unlike pharmaceutical laxatives, dandelion can be taken for a few months. Christopher Hobbs, a licensed acupuncturist and fourth-generation herbalist and botanist with more than 35 years of experience with herbs, writes that clinical and laboratory research on dandelion shows "a doubling of bile output with leaf extracts and a quadrupling of bile output with the root extract." Bile helps with the digestion and absorption of fats; this might explain how effective dandelion is in helping with heartburn and indigestion.

Dandelion Root for Diabetes

Dandelion root is also helpful in the treatment of diabetes. It contains inulin, which is a naturally occurring type of soluble fiber known to have a positive effect on blood sugar levels. Inulin also increases calcium absorption and possibly magnesium absorption while promoting probiotic bacteria. In addition, dandelion also contains some pectin, another type of fiber that helps relieve constipation and reduce cholesterol. (Pectin is also found in apples.)

Dandelion is a natural diuretic. Want something for bloat and water retention? This is your natural medicine. One of the nice benefits of using it as a diuretic is that it does not cause loss of potassium. Dandelion leaf extract works great for the water retention of PMS, and Stengler routinely uses it for edema of the lower legs and ankles that he sees in elderly patients (edema is swelling or bloating caused by fluids in the extremities).

Dandelion also contains two hormone-balancing constituents, taraxerol and taraxasterol. "It's one of the premier herbs recommended for hormone-related conditions like PMS," says Stengler. Because it's a natural diuretic, dandelion leaf is a wonderful aid in reducing high blood pressure. (Note: *Never* discontinue a blood pressure medication without the approval of your health professional.)

Why It Ranks in the Top Four of All Green Vegetables

If all this weren't enough, dandelion is one of the most nutrient-rich vegetables on the planet. They rank in the top four green vegetables in overall nutritional value, according to the USDA. One cup (105 g) of cooked dandelion greens contains 147 mg of calcium, 244 mg of potassium, 203 mg of bone-building vitamin K, and a respectable 3 g of fiber. Dandelions are nature's richest green-vegetable source of beta-carotene and the third richest source of vitamin A of all foods after cod liver oil and beef liver. One cup of the stuff contains more than 10,000 IUs of vitamin A! And just for good measure, the same cup contains 4,944 mcg of the new superstars of eye nutrition, lutein and zeaxanthin, which are being investigated for their ability to protect against the number-one cause of adult blindness, macular degeneration. Fresh dandelion greens make an excellent salad, alone or with other garden greens. You can use the bittersweet root the same way you would a carrot—in stir-fries, in soups, or sautéed with onion and garlic, says natural-foods expert Rebecca Wood. The root also makes a terrific, liver-friendly, detoxifying tea.

WORTH KNOWING

Those with gallstones should consult a health professional to determine which herbs to use and in what doses.

Eggplant

Whenever you see a richly colored vegetable or fruit, you can be sure of one thing: Nature put those colors in there to protect against something in the environment, usually the intense rays of the sun, which can cause free-radical damage if unchecked. The blue pigment in blueberries, the red pigment in raspberries and watermelon, the yellow pigments in peppers . . . all contain a potent array of phytochemicals that not only protect the plant from damage in its environment but also do the exact same thing for the cells and DNA in your body. And, of course, the deep, rich purple pigment in eggplant skins is no exception.

The Nutritional Power of Purple

A substance called nasunin has been isolated from that deep purple pigment. Nasunin, a member of the anthocyanin category, is a powerful antioxidant. Studies show that it literally eats up free radicals, rogue molecules in your body that can cause serious damage to your cells and your DNA and are partly responsible for aging.

In addition, nasunin protects against lipid per-oxidation—that means it helps keep fats from turning rancid, including the fats in your body (such as LDL cholesterol). The brain is particularly vulnerable to oxidative damage, and studies have shown that antho-cyanins in general are highly protective of animal brain tissue. Other studies show that nasunin binds to iron, which is a very good thing, as too much iron in the system can cause all kinds of problems.

Eggplant isn't a nutritional superstar, but it's a nice vegetable with 2.5 g of fiber in a cup (99 g) that only costs you 35 calories. Plus it's filling. I go to an amazing little Japanese restaurant in Studio City, California, that looks exactly like the restaurants on the side streets of Tokyo, and they serve cooked eggplant in a miso-ginger sauce that will knock your socks off. You can easily make a meal out of an entire eggplant eaten that way. The eggplant itself is only 132 calories, and all you have to do is use the sauce judiciously and you've got a great dish. Add a couple of eggs for protein—I know it's unconventional, but it's great— and you've got a terrific and complete meal with very moderate calories.

Eggplant is also great sprinkled with olive oil. And if you're making a big salad for the family and you can manage to include one whole eggplant sliced up, you'll be adding a whopping 18½ g of fiber and 1,260 mg of potassium to the mix, not to mention niacin, folate, calcium, magnesium, phosphorus, and phytosterols.

Here's an interesting fact: Eggplant is consid-ered a fruit, but botanically it's a berry. Go figure. It's related to the potato and tomato and is a member of the nightshade family.

WORTH KNOWING

Like all nightshades, eggplant contains a substance called *solanine*. In theory, if solanine is not destroyed in the intestine, it could be toxic. This is generally not an issue, but Norman Childers, Ph.D., chairman of the Arthritis Nightshades Research Foundation and professor emeritus at the University of Florida, hypothesizes that some people with osteoarthritis may not be able to destroy solanine in the gut, leading to solanine absorption and aggravating osteoarthritis. Though this has never been put to a strict clinical test, I believe that individual variations in metabolism and detoxification abilities account for many problems with foods and chemicals—some people can get rid of the problem compound just fine, others simply can't. Proponents of the "solanine aggravates arthritis" theory claim you need to eliminate it for six months before potential benefit can be seen. I think this information is only applicable to a tiny number of people, but it's worth knowing.

Endive

(Belgian endive, escarole, French endive)

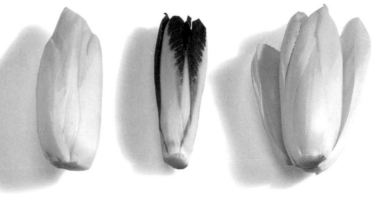

Endive is a member of the botanical family Chicorium and is a close relative of chicory, with the same characteristic of being fresh yet slightly bitter in flavor. Belgian endive—also called French endive or witloof—is a small, cylindrical head of pale, tightly packed leaves. Curly endive—sometimes wrongly called chicory—has lacy, green-rimmed, curly leaves with a prickly texture (and slightly bitter taste). Then, of course, there's escarole, which has a milder flavor than either Belgian or curly endive.

Two cups (100 g) of endive have an awful lot of nutrients for a paltry 8 calories. There's 26 mg of calcium, about ½ mg of iron, 157 mg of potassium, 71 mcg of folate, more than 1,000 IUs of vitamin A (650 of beta-carotene), and 115 mg of bone-strengthening vitamin K. Now that's a healthy salad green!

My favorite: Toss them with some walnuts and sliced pears and maybe a little blue cheese and olives. Olive oil is a nice addition to the mix.

Fennel

Fennel is a perfect example of how sometimes a plant will show its medicinal properties in the most unexpected conditions. Consider colic. Although common enough and thought to be benign, it's a significant problem in infants and imparts a psychological, emotional, and physical burden on parents. The only medicine that has been shown to be effective is dicyclomine hydrochloride. But there's one little problem. Five percent of infants treated with it develop serious side effects, including death. So if there were a benign plant-based medicine that got the job done, that would be a pretty terrific thing.

Babies Benefit from Fennel

A study published in volume 9 of the 2003 *Journal of Alternative Therapy Health and Medicine* tested the effect of fennel seed oil on infantile colic. Fennel eliminated colic in 65 percent of the infants, produced a significant improvement in the treatment group, and lowered the NNT (number needed to treat), all without a single side effect reported. If it can do that for infant colic, one might be forgiven for thinking that it could have other benefits as well.

And if you had that thought, you'd be right. Supplements containing different combinations of various natural herbs including fennel seed extract were tested in a study in anticancer research and found to suppress the growth of certain tumors. The dried fruit of the fennel contains an essential oil that has a rich mix of health-promoting compounds, including anethole (responsible for the licorice flavor), limonene, and quercetin (an anti-inflammatory flavonoid). In laboratory studies, fennel oil counteracts spasms of smooth muscle in the gut. It seems to relieve gas and help with cramps, and in Indian restaurants, it's often offered on a plate after dinner for its soothing effect on the digestion and its sweetening effect on the breath. It also makes a nice tea—pour boiling water over a couple of spoonfuls of the dried fruit, crushing it immediately before using. Steep for 10 minutes and strain.

WORTH KNOWING

Pregnant women should not use fennel oil or fennel extracts, say herbal experts Joe and Teresa Graedon, Ph.D., authors of *The People's Pharmacy*. Also, anyone allergic to celery, carrots, dill, or anise should avoid fennel as well.

FENNEL TRIVIA

Fennel is the Greek name for marathon. Seems that back around 490 B.C.E., the Greeks defeated the Persians in a fennel field exactly 26 miles (42 km) and 385 yards (352 m) from Athens. They sent a runner bearing the good news back home, and ever since then the length of a marathon race has remained the same as the distance from the fennel field into town.

Green Beans

**(and their cousins:
French beans, runner beans,
and Italian beans)**

Let's face it: Green beans are not a superstar of the vegetable community. Rather, they're a good, solid utility player. If they were in an investment portfolio, they'd be Ginny Maes or savings bonds. You're not likely to get rich on them, but they're good, reliable performers, and they belong in your portfolio.

Yesterday's String Beans Are Today's Green Beans

For the purposes of this book I'm lumping all the beans in the *Phaseolus vulgaris* category together: that's French beans, runner beans, snap beans, green beans, wax beans, Italian beans . . . you get the picture. When I was a kid we called them string beans, because in the old days (before I was born, of course) there used to be a fibrous string running the length of the pod seam, which you had to remove before cook-

ing. Nowadays the folks who breed these things have genetically engineered them so the string is a thing of the past.

Green beans contain folate (about 10 percent of the RDI, which is too low anyway). An RDI, or Reference Daily Intake, is the replacement standard for the old RDA. But as traditional naturopath Regina Wilshire points out, the folate in green beans is bound in the proper ratio to two amino acids in the green beans, which makes it much more highly absorbed than the folate from enriched cereals. Folate is a critically important B vitamin that not only helps prevent neural tube defect, but also helps bring down homocysteine, a naturally occurring amino acid that can be harmful to blood vessels and contributes to the development of heart disease, stroke, dementia, and peripheral vascular disease (reduced blood flow to the legs and feet).

Green (string) beans have a bunch of other vitamins and minerals—a little bit of calcium, a little bit of vitamin A, and a nice dose of potassium. They also contain about 20 percent of the daily value for manganese, an important trace mineral that's essential for growth, reproduction, wound healing, peak brain function, and the proper metabolism of sugars, insulin, and cholesterol. Throw in some beta-carotene and the eye-friendly carotenoids lutein and zeaxanthin for good measure, and about ½ of the daily requirement for bone-building vitamin K. And a cup (125 g) of them will give you about 4 g of fiber (better than the average slice of bread and a whole lot better for you). You can eat them raw or cooked—the vitamin content changes marginally for the better when they're cooked. They age fast once harvested, so use them quickly.

Horseradish

The first time I tasted horseradish was also the first time I attended a Passover Seder, where it occupies a place of honor on the dinner plate as one of the five bitter herbs representing the bitterness of slavery. Little did I imagine that decades later I would be writing about its health benefits.

Horseradish is a relative of the mustard family that acts as a digestive stimulant. It's also great for clearing up the sinuses! It inhibits bacterial infection and increases circulation. (You might notice that you start sweating when you eat a lot of it!)

And for its tiny number of calories (14 for 2 tablespoons [30 g]) it contains a nice assortment of minerals, particularly potassium. But that's the least of the benefits this cabbage-family member has to offer.

Why Horseradish Beats Broccoli

Horseradish is a member of the distinguished Cruciferae family, which I call "the Medici of vegetables," whose relatives include broccoli, Brussels sprouts, cabbage, cauliflower, kale, rutabaga, and turnip. If you've read about any of the above vegetables in this book, you know that a significant body of research exists showing the health benefits and cancer-fighting properties of many of the compounds that have been isolated from this food family. And horseradish is one of the richest sources of allyl isothiocyanate, which is believed to play a role in the prevention of tumors and in the suppression of tumor growth.

A study from the University of Illinois shows that horseradish has substantial quantities of glucosinolates, compounds that are the parent molecules of substances that increase human resistance to cancer. Glucosinolates in food increase the liver's ability to detoxify carcinogens and, according Mosbah Kushad, Ph.D., associate professor in the department of crop sciences at the University of Illinois, they may suppress the growth of existing cancerous tumors. Kushad, who has been involved in studies of many cruciferous vegetables, says that horseradish contains ten times more glucosinolates than broccoli, so you don't need as much to benefit. "A little dab on your steak will go a long way to providing the same health benefits as broccoli," he says.

Horseradish may be one of the few foods in this book that improves with processing. It contains an enzyme that breaks down these valuable glucosinolates into other compounds—isothiocyanates—that are responsible for the anticancer benefits: When you process the stuff, that enzyme is released. The enzyme, in turn, encounters the glucosinolates, and presto, you've got the nutritionally beneficial isothiocyanates.

WORTH KNOWING

If you've ever eaten sushi or sashimi, you've encountered wasabi, also known as Japanese horseradish—it's that very strong-tasting green stuff they put on the plate to mix with the soy sauce. Bioactive chemicals in wasabi are said to act as an antidote to food poisoning, one factor that might have led to the use of wasabi with raw fish dishes in Japan. Wasabi contains isothiocyanates, which, like the other compounds from the Cruciferae family, have significant health benefits. One research report specifically done on the isothiocyanates in wasabi found that they had a significant anti-inflammatory effect and killed many human stomach cancer cells in a test tube.

Jerusalem Artichokes

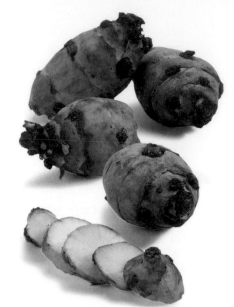

Jerusalem artichokes aren't really artichokes; plus, they're not even from Jerusalem. They're a member of the sunflower family and are also referred to as sunchokes, kind of a cross between artichoke and sunflower. They probably got the name Jerusalem because it sounded like *girasol*, which is the Italian name for sunflower. This large yellow flower—which is very pretty, by the way—was cultivated by the Native Americans, who prepared the tubers for Lewis and Clark in 1805 (in what is now North Dakota). The tuber—or underground stem—resembles a gnarly potato or a piece of ginger, and it has a nice taste. The baked tubers are delicious.

Feeding the Good Bacteria for a Healthy Gut

Whatever the genesis of its odd name, this vegetable lands on the list because of its high content of fructooligosaccharides and inulin. What are those, you ask? They're what we now call prebiotics—extremely healthy food for the "good" bacteria in your gut.

You know how antibiotics wipe out all the bacteria in your gut garden, including the healthy kind like acidophilus? Well, the good bacteria in your gut love to dine on fructooligosaccharides—they're health food for those good bacteria, and thereby help you to maintain a healthy gut ecology. That's why they're referred to as prebiotics. And inulin is a form of soluble fiber that, in one study published in the *Journal of Nutrition*, was found to lower blood glucose, triglycerides, and LDL cholesterol as well as inhibit the growth of various kinds of cancer.

Jerusalem artichokes are one of a handful of foods that are good sources of resistant starch, a form of prebiotic fiber that the good bacteria in your gut go absolutely nuts over. When the gut bacteria feast on resistant fiber, they produce something called butyric acid, which the gut cells use as a source of energy. This whole ecological system is very important, not just for gut health, but for health in general.

Be aware that inulin may cause flatulence in some people. If you're sensitive to that, you might want to avoid eating Jerusalem artichokes raw.

Jicama

Okay, I admit it—I had never even heard of jicama until it showed up on the top ten list from my friend Ann Louise Gittleman, Ph.D., C.N.S. (see page 78).

Coincidentally, the next day I was in Whole Foods, where they had sliced fresh jicama in a package in the produce center, ready to eat. Of course I had to buy it. And here's my verdict: Jicama is so fresh, clean, refreshing, and crispy tasting that you feel healthier after eating it.

What on Earth Is Jicama?

Jicama is a root vegetable that is a staple in Mexican food. It's sold as a street food in South America, with a squeeze of lime and a bit of fiery chili powder. It's a white-fleshed tuber that can weigh anywhere from half a pound to more than five pounds. Some people have characterized it as a cross between an apple and a potato. It looks like a turnip, has a thin brown skin that you can peel, and its taste is something like an apple but not quite. By itself, it's a bit bland, but that allows it to be used in a zillion ways, because it takes on the flavor of whatever you dip it in or cook it with. And you're still getting all the nutrition that jicama has to offer.

Jicama is a low-calorie, low-fat, high-fiber food. It's mostly water (about 90 percent), yet a cup (120 g) of it contains more than 6 g of fiber! That alone would probably garner it a place among the world's healthiest foods, but jicama also has calcium, magnesium, potassium, vitamin C, vitamin A, and beta carotene. And all for its measly 49 calories per cup (120 g). An entire medium-size jicama has only 250 calories, and it contains an astonishing 32 g of fiber, almost three times the amount most Americans get in a day.

How Is Jicama Prepared?

You can bake or broil a jicama just like a potato, and it has a lot less starch. It fits nicely into stir-fries. It's also fantastic raw, the way I discovered it. Gittleman recommends trying it with a dash of lime juice and cayenne pepper, Mexican style, for a snack that really satisfies.

Kale

Kale is definitely a superstar vegetable. It's a green, weird-looking leafy vegetable that is a form of cabbage. This vegetable is a nutritional powerhouse. And since the original publication of this book in 2007, the world seems to have caught on to kale's amazing nutritional résumé. Kale has become the new superstar of the health-conscious crowd. A quick unscientific check on Google Shopping yielded at least a half a dozen brands of kale crisp snack foods, and kale is showing up on menus everywhere.

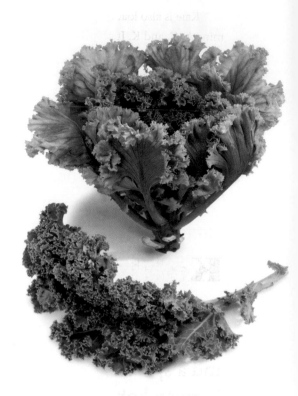

Why Kale Is Number One

When this book was first published, the USDA used a now-retired testing procedure to determine the antioxidant capacity of fruits and vegetables. The procedure looked at all the antioxidants and phytochemicals found in a plant food to determine how well everything worked together as a team—how much ability the "team" has to fight cell-damaging free radicals. The foods received an oxygen radical absorbance capacity, or ORAC, rating. Though there were different versions of the test, the best known had kale as number one among the vegetables, with an ORAC value of 1770. The next highest rated vegetable was spinach, with an ORAC value of 1260. Though the test isn't used anymore, kale continues to score high rankings on nearly all the tests that have replaced it.

Prevent Cancer as You Chew

Because it's a cabbage, kale has even more benefits than its antioxidant power alone would indicate. Like others in the *Brassica* family, it contains powerful phytochemicals like cancer-fighting indoles, plant compounds that have been found to have a protective effect against breast, cervical, and colon cancer. In addition, kale is high in sulfur and contains something called sulforaphane, which helps give a boost to the body's detoxification enzymes and may help fight cancer as well. Sulforaphane is formed when the vegetables containing it are chopped or chewed, and it triggers the liver to remove free radicals and other chemicals that may cause DNA damage. In fact, a study in the *Journal of Nutrition* demonstrated that sulforaphane helps stop breast cancer proliferation.

Kale is also loaded with calcium, iron, and vitamins A, C, and K. It contains seven times the beta-carotene of broccoli and ten times as much lutein and zeaxanthin, carotenoids known to help protect against macular degeneration. And 2 cups (134 g) of the stuff contain about 4 g of protein and 3 g of fiber.

Secrets to a Great Kale Salad

Tender kale greens can provide a terrific addition to salads, especially when mixed with strong flavored ingredients such as tamari-roasted almonds or red pepper flakes.

Kale is one of my favorite foods. The Sherman Oaks (California) Whole Foods deli manager mixes kale leaves with pine nuts and cranberries, then softens the whole mixture by tossing it well in olive oil. It's become so popular the deli can't keep it in stock, and because of that recipe, I eat kale about five times a week. It's amazing.

Kohlrabi

Kohlrabi is a member of the cabbage family, and it looks like a cross between an octopus and a space capsule. The name comes from the German kohl (cabbage) plus rabi (turnip) because of the resemblance of the cabbagelike stem to the turnip. The stem can be crisp and juicy, almost as sweet as an apple, and similar to a turnip in taste. You can eat it raw or cooked. It makes a great crudité. It comes in two "flavors," green and purple, with the purple kind tending to be somewhat spicier. Both the leaves and the stem are edible.

Kohlrabi's membership in the cabbage family of cruciferous vegetables gains it an automatic place among the world's healthiest foods. Like its relatives (broccoli, Brussels sprouts, cabbage), kohlrabi contains important phytochemicals such as cancer-fighting indoles, sulforaphane, and isothiocynates. It's also a good source of vitamin C (83 mg per cup [135 g]) and an excellent source of potassium (472 mg). And for a measly 36 calories per cup, you get a whopping 5 g of fiber.

In case someone ever asks you, Hamburg Township in Michigan has christened itself the "Kohlrabi Capital of the World." No, I'm not making this up. At one time, back in the 1980s, they had a kohlrabi festival that drew six hundred people.

Leeks

One way to think of a leek is as a sweeter version of an onion. They really are delicious, and most people add them to recipes like stir-fries for their marvelous flavor. But leeks have a serious side as well—they're members of the allium family, which includes onions, garlic, and shallots. These vegetables contain a whole pharmacy of compounds with health benefits, including thiosulfinates, sulfides, sulfoxides, and other sulfur compounds.

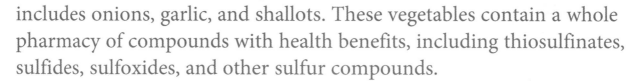

The active substances in leeks, including allyl sulfides, help provide protection against cancers. Allyl sulfides block the action of hormones or chemical pathways within the body that promote cancer. Regular consumption of allium vegetables is associated with a reduced risk of both prostate and colon cancer. The sulfides of the allium family also decrease the tendency for blood clots to form—a significant risk for strokes and cardiovascular events. Plus, they lower levels of LDL ("bad") cholesterol. Allium vegetables have also been shown to lower high blood pressure.

Good Down to the Roots

There is more to the leek than just the flavorful white bulb, which is the part most people use in cooking. Natural-foods expert Rebecca Wood uses the many tiny rootlets that hang from the base of the plant like little mop strings. She claims these mineral-dense filaments add valuable flavor and more nutrients and suggests cutting the cluster of stringy roots from the base, soaking them to loosen any embedded sand, rinsing, mincing, and sautéing in any vegetable dish or soup.

Leeks are also a good source of two of the most important carotenoids for eye health, lutein and zeaxanthin. One 54-calorie leek contains 1,691 mcg of these two superstar nutrients, which are currently the subject of extensive research for their ability to prevent macular degeneration, the number-one cause of blindness in adults. Leeks also have fiber, calcium, iron, magnesium, phosphorus, potassium, vitamin K, and more than 1,400 IUs of vitamin A.

★ Maca

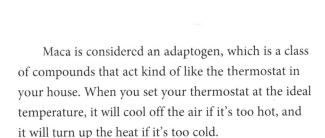

The first thing you need to know about maca is its nickname: Peruvian Viagra.

Okay, let that one sink in for a minute.

The reason they call it Peruvian Viagra is that it's best known for its use in treating fatigue and sexual dysfunction. Research has shown that maca can be effective in improving both sexual desire and function. That alone makes it worth the price of admission.

But there's a lot more.

Maca is one of those herbs that have been used in indigenous cultures (such as the ancient Incas) for thousands of years, mostly for its legendary ability to stimulate mental clarity and energy while enhancing sex drive. And although there's a ton of anecdotal evidence of its benefits, there's not a lot of Western science to prove its effectiveness.

Nonetheless, there's great wisdom in the ancient cultures and, let's face it, an herb doesn't hang around for a couple thousand years and gain a solid reputation for being effective if it doesn't work.

The late integrative and functional medicine psychiatrist Hyla Cass, M.D., said, "In my practice I have seen maca restore hormonal imbalance and related sexual desire and fertility in both men and women."

My pal Chris Killiam, the Medicine Hunter, says, "The question is not whether it works—because we know it works with certainty—but *how* it works."

Maca is considered an adaptogen, which is a class of compounds that act kind of like the thermostat in your house. When you set your thermostat at the ideal temperature, it will cool off the air if it's too hot, and it will turn up the heat if it's too cold.

That's exactly how adaptogens work. They help you adapt to fluctuating levels, of, say stress hormones.

"Consuming maca often makes people feel more alive, energetic, and leaves them with a sense of well-being, all of which are thought to be due to its ability to restore proper hormone balance and elevate 'feel good' endorphins," says noted health expert Josh Axe, D.N.M., D.C., C.N.S. Axe—a big fan of maca—points out that it provides over twenty amino acids, including eight essential ones, twenty free-form fatty acids (such as the antimicrobial lauric acid), vitamins B1, B2, C, and E, calcium, magnesium, and about nine other minerals. Maca is also a rich source of phytonutrients.

What's more, maca stimulates the immune system. It's antiviral, and may help to protect against the influenza virus. It's believed to help women with Polycystic Ovary Syndrome (PCOS) by helping to control and balance estrogen levels. And a 2008 study showed that maca had positive effects on boosting mood and decreasing anxiety and depression in menopausal women. Maca root is a natural antioxidant, boosting your body's levels of two of the most important antioxidants in the human body, glutathione and SOD (superoxide dismutase). It even lowers blood sugar.

And then, of course, there's energy.

Energy is one of maca's big selling points. Maca helps to regulate the hypothalamus, which in turn helps balance focus and energy. Many people feel better and brighter on a daily dose of maca—me included!

Personally, I start every single day with a maca drink. (This is separate from my protein drink, which I'll often have after two hours on the tennis court.) I use Mighty Maca Plus, by Vida Pura, which was formulated by my good friend and colleague, Anna Cabeca, D.O., after years of research. I like it, number one, because it tastes good, and number two, because I trust Anna Cabeca, who is scrupulously conscientious in creating her products.

Mighty Maca Plus is a lot more than just maca, though. It's also got spirulina, chlorella, mangosteen, a bunch of enzymes (such as bromelain and papain), oat bran, milk thistle, resveratrol, quercetin, flaxseed, turmeric, grape seed extract, and green tea extract, making it one of the most complete green drinks I've ever come across.

I use one or two heaping scoops a day, and I mix it in the NutriBullet with pomegranate juice, some powdered brain formula, five or six drops of liquid vitamin D, my Oligo30 prebiotics, a packet of ResVitále Collagen Renew, and a squirt of Omega Swirl by Barlean's, in either key lime or mango peach.

Consuming it is a great way to start the day. You can order Mighty Maca Plus on my website, www.jonnybowden.com.

I'm sure you're going to love it as much as I do.

★ **Mushrooms**

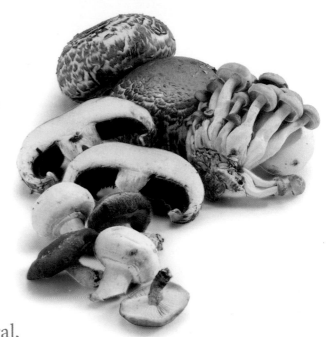

Although mushrooms have been used medicinally in Eastern medicine for eons, Western medicine is now beginning to catch up as the healing properties of mushrooms are beginning to be demonstrated scientifically. Medicinal mushrooms contain potent antiviral, anti-inflammatory, antimicrobial, and antibacterial compounds. Some of the polysaccharides found in medicinal mushrooms activate cytokines and natural killer cells, which in turn latch onto cancer cells, causing them to die. They also possess anticancer and immune system enhancing capabilities.

The three specific types with the greatest health benefits are maitake, shiitake, and reishi. All three have powerful effects on the immune system, and all three act as medicine. Ganoderma, turkey tail, and chaga mushrooms have also been used medicinally.

When you think about it for a minute, it makes an awful lot of sense that mushrooms have medicinal properties. Mushrooms are fungus. They scavenge on organic matter. Where do you find them? Growing on decaying matter, such as wood. That means they can absorb—and then safely eliminate—toxins. I don't know about you, but I'd like to put them to work doing that in my own body, and eating them appears to be a great way to do it.

Maitake

Maitake comes from the Japanese word meaning "dancing mushrooms"—an urban legend says foragers danced with joy when they found it. According to some legends, the little mushroom could be traded for its weight in precious metals.

In addition to being loaded with vitamins, maitake has a special polysaccharide component called beta-1,6 glucan, a very close relative of the beta-1,3 glucan in the shiitake (see below). Beta-glucans stimulate the immune system. Many of the compounds in the cell structures of mushrooms are classified as HDPs—host defenses potentiators. They're used as adjunctive cancer treatments throughout Asia. In fact, Maitake is approved by the Japanese government for just this purpose.

Maitake is especially good for counteracting the toxic effects of radiation and chemotherapy, such as extreme fatigue and nausea. Maitake extract can shrink tumors in mice, my friend Robert Roundtree, M.D., author of *Immunotics*, says. He also points out that several studies in Japan showed that maitake and chemotherapy together can boost the effectiveness of standard chemotherapy for several types of cancer. He personally feels that maitake is the most potent of the three medicinal mushrooms discussed here, though he uses all of them for different things.

Shiitake

The shiitake mushroom is one of the most widely cultivated specialty species of mushroom in the world and is deeply valued for its medicinal effects as well as for the fact that it tastes delicious. It contains enzymes and vitamins that do not normally appear in plants, such as all eight essential amino acids and one of the essential fatty acids, linoleic acid. The caps contain more nutrients than the stems.

This superstar mushroom contains a chemical component especially worth noting: lentinan, which is approved as an injectable drug in Japan and usually used to prolong survival of patients in cancer therapy. It doesn't work directly against cancer, but it is believed to help prevent some of the damage that results from anticancer drugs.

Lentinan is also referred to as beta-1,3 glucan, a polysaccharide that has potent immune-stimulating effects, and a close relative of the beta-1,6 glucan found in maitake (see above). When beta-glucans bind to immune system cells like natural killer (NK) cells,

T-cells, and macrophages, the activity of these cells is increased. No one is quite sure why, but Roundtree speculates that the beta-glucans trick immune system cells into thinking they're under attack. (Mushrooms are, after all, fungus, and maybe the cells think the harmless little critters are dangerous. Who knows? The point is, the immune system is stimulated by them.) Many studies have confirmed beta-glucans' wide range of protective effects, including improved resistance to infections, liver protection, and cardiovascular benefits. It also appears to help inhibit tumor growth in mice.

Japanese researchers have reported that consumption of shiitake mushrooms lowers blood cholesterol by as much as 45 percent, due to an active compound in them called eritadenine.

Reishi

Sometime in the third century BCE, the Chinese emperor Shih Huang was reputed to have sent a fleet of ships to search for a mushroom called the "Elixir of Immortality." That mushroom? The reishi. Its special chemical makeup was thought to be a tonic for a long and healthy life. In traditional Chinese medicine, reishi is still considered to be among the highest class of tonics.

Now we're finding out that they may have been on to something. One study at Cornell Medical College found that reishi reduced side effects during chemotherapy while improving the quality of life. Its beneficial components—specifically ganodermic acids classified as triterpenoids, plus a number of polysaccharides—seem to benefit everything from blood pressure to liver detoxification to adrenal function.

REISHI HAS EARNED ITS CANCER-FIGHTING REPUTATION

Even the conservative and highly regarded Memorial Sloan Kettering Cancer Center has reishi mushroom listed on the "about herbs" section of its website, where it states that reishi mushrooms stimulate the immune system through their positive effect on macrophages and other immune compounds. Sloan Kettering also references clinical studies showing that reishi increases antioxidant capacity and enhances the immune responses in advanced-stage cancer patients.

And then there's stress.

Reishi mushrooms appear to be a natural stressbuster. Reishi is the mushroom of choice for people under extreme physical or emotional stress, Roundtree says. He recommends it for endurance athletes as well. Reishi mushrooms have a high level of antioxidants, largely due to their ganodermic acid.

Cremini (white button mushrooms)

I almost omitted cremini mushrooms from the list completely—I mean, after all, how could these little prosaic mushrooms possibly hold a candle to the downright medicinal value of their famous siblings? But, my friend, traditional naturopath Regina Wilshire, sent me this missive, just in time for press. It's so complete, I'm going to reprint it right here in its entirety:

"Cremini mushrooms are superdense with nutrients. One 5-ounce serving (dry weight before cooking) gives you more than 50 percent of the Daily Value for the cancer-fighting trace mineral selenium, 40 percent of the Daily Value for riboflavin, 35 per-

cent of copper, 30 percent of niacin, 20 to 25 percent of pantothenic acid, phosphorus, and zinc, plus 10 to 15 percent Daily Value of manganese and thiamin. They also have trace amounts of magnesium, calcium, folate, B_{12}, and iron."

Now I don't feel so bad counting mushrooms as a vegetable!

The Mushroom Weight Loss Plan?

Mushrooms in general also contain a powerful antioxidant called L-ergothioneine. L-ergothioneine neutralizes dangerous free radicals called hydroxyl radicals and increases enzymes with antioxidant activity. In at least two studies, it seems to act as a metabolic energy enhancer, stimulating the breakdown of sugar in red blood cells and mimicking carnitine in its ability to transport fat into the mitochondria of the cells where the fat can be burned for energy. That's exactly what most over-the-counter weight loss supplements promise but rarely deliver.

Three studies also showed L-ergothioneine to be a protector of environmental UV-radiation damage. Though shiitake and maitake have much more of it, even our friend the lowly white button mushroom has many times more L-ergothioneine than wheat germ and chicken liver, the other two sources of this incredible antioxidant.

Okra

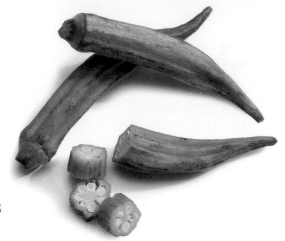

For generations, okra has been a staple of traditional Southern cooking. This nutritious green vegetable arrived in the United States in the mid-1600s and became an important part of the colonial diet. Its seeds were even used to brew a coffee substitute that was consumed by Southern Americans during the Civil War, when they couldn't obtain coffee beans. Today it's still very much a part of what is lovingly called "soul food."

Okra contains a unique combination of valuable nutrients. It's one of a select group of foods that include naturally occurring glutathione, arguably the most important antioxidant in the body. Optimal amounts of glutathione are necessary for supporting the immune system; glutathione is required for replication of the lymphocyte immune cells. It also helps the liver detoxify chemicals.

Okra Beats Cereal for Fiber Content

Okra's also a high-fiber food. People often ask me where they should get their fiber from, given that our standard diet is so deficient in this important compound. My standard answer is fruits, vegetables, and legumes, and okra is a perfect example of what I'm talking about. One cup (160 g) of cooked okra—which is a tiny 35 calories' worth—provides 4 g of fiber, way more than the average slice of bread or the average cup of commercial cold cereal. And for a vegetable, it's also high in protein. That same 35-calorie cup also provides almost 3 g of protein.

Calorie for calorie, okra is high in calcium, magnesium, potassium, vitamin A, vitamin K, and folic acid, which helps prevent neural tube defects in developing fetuses. In Ayurvedic medicine, okra is considered tridoshic, meaning it is good for balancing all metabolic types. It can be steamed, pickled, broiled, baked, or even fried and goes well with tomatoes and highly seasoned vegetable dishes. When you boil it, it gives off a kind of viscous substance that adds a lot of smooth thickness to soups and stews, making okra a favorite for gumbo.

Note: The larger pods are tough and fibrous. Look for smooth, firm, unblemished, brightly colored pods smaller than 3 inches long.

★ Onions

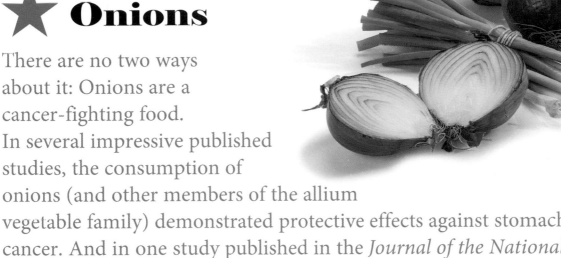

There are no two ways about it: Onions are a cancer-fighting food. In several impressive published studies, the consumption of onions (and other members of the allium vegetable family) demonstrated protective effects against stomach cancer. And in one study published in the *Journal of the National Cancer Institute*, eating onions (as well as other members of its family such as garlic, scallions, chives, and leeks) significantly lowered the risk for prostate cancer. Onions (and their close relatives) have also been shown to have the same effect against esophageal cancer.

In Vidalia, Georgia, where the Vidalia onion comes from and where onions are consumed in large quantities, the death rate from stomach cancer is 50 percent lower than the national mortality rate from stomach cancer. One theory is that onions contain diallyl sulfide, which increases the body's production of an important cancer-fighting enzyme, glutathione-S-transferase.

Onions Help Build Strong Bones

At least two important studies show that onions help build strong bones. In one, published in the prestigious journal *Nature*, male rats fed a small amount of dried onion daily had a 17 percent increase in calcium; female rats that had had their ovaries removed (which would rapidly induce bone loss and osteoporosis) had stronger bones when fed onions. And in another study, published in the *Journal of Agriculture and Food Chemistry*, a compound in onions inhibited the activity of the cells (osteoclasts) that break down bones. The popular drug Fosamax works in a similar way, but onions have no side effects, unless you count the need to have a breath mint before kissing someone!

Onions belong to the allium family, which also includes leeks, garlic, and shallots. They contain a whole pharmacy of compounds with health benefits, including thiosulfinates, sulfides, sulfoxides, and other smelly sulfur compounds. But those same smelly compounds offer a lot of nutrition bang for the relatively small price of a little eye-watering. In a study in the *European Journal of Clinical Nutrition*, onions are one of a very select group of foods that in combination reduced mortality from coronary heart disease by an impressive 20 percent. The others included broccoli, tea, and apples.

Why Allergy and Asthma Sufferers Benefit from Onions

Onions contain powerful antioxidants, and they are anti-inflammatory, antibiotic, and antiviral. They are a great source of quercetin, one of my favorite anti-inflammatory compounds and one that is associated with beneficial effects on chronic diseases like cancer and heart disease. The class of chemicals that quercetin belongs to—flavonoids—have antiallergic properties as well. Quercetin is frequently used by nutritionists as part of their arsenal for treating allergies with natural substances. It can help relieve asthma and hay fever by blocking some of the inflammatory responses in the airways. Our bodies absorb quercetin from onions very easily, though you'll probably need quercetin supplements if your main interest is using it therapeutically as an anti-inflammatory. Onions also contain several sulfides similar to those in garlic, which may lower blood lipids and blood pressure.

The type of onion affects the content of the health-promoting chemicals, and the stronger-tasting ones have superior properties.

Peppers

Hot peppers: cayenne, chile, jalapeño

You would think that hot peppers—such as chile peppers or cayenne peppers—would be exactly what you'd want to avoid if you had heartburn. Maybe, maybe not. At least one study demonstrated that the active ingredient in hot peppers may protect the stomach lining from damage. Granted, that study was done in rats, but still. The active ingredient—capsaicin—has a host of benefits and uses.

Capsaicin peppers are rich in a host of nutrients, including beta-carotene, eye-friendly carotenoids lutein and zeaxanthin, and vitamin C. Their vitamin C content is probably the reason they have been used as a popular natural remedy for colds and coughs.

Hot peppers also may make you feel good.

Capsaicin interacts in the body with a protein called TRPV1, which normally gets "turned on" by physical heat. That causes a chain reaction in which messages get sent to the brain ("we're on fire!"). One of the substances released during this chain reaction is called Substance P, which basically transmits pain signals to the brain.

When those pain signals are received, the brain responds by releasing endorphins, a class of neurotransmitters that makes you feel good. Endorphins are thought to be responsible for the euphoric sensation known as "runner's high." And that's why eating capsaicin peppers can make you feel good.

One of the neurotransmitters released in response to substance P is dopamine, the neurotransmitter of excitement and anticipation. This is why peppers can sometimes give you a pick-up, and is probably what Hillary Clinton was talking about when she told the *New York Times* (back in 2008) that she got a lot of energy from eating them.

Peppers for Pain Relief?

That same active ingredient, capsaicin, produces a feeling of warmth when applied to the skin, and it is used a lot in pain-relieving creams. Capsaicin is a vasodilator, which enhances circulation and increases body temperature. Hot peppers, and their respective powders, may act as a metabolism booster. In one study on mice, the active ingredient promoted energy metabolism and suppressed body fat accumulation. Makes sense when you think of how eating hot peppers makes you sweat.

Traditionally, some hot peppers such as cayenne were used to aid digestion and stimulate the appetite. Counterintuitive though it seems, they probably do not irritate the stomach. In fact, they may help prevent ulcers by killing bacteria, and they also simulate the lining of the stomach to secrete powerful protective juices. In Ayurvedic medicine, they are used for healing, but with care. They're definitely not recommended for anyone with an inflamed colon.

Red chiles have a nice amount of vitamin A, and both red and green chiles contain fiber, potassium, folic acid, and iron. Some people with sensitive skin are warned to wear rubber gloves when handling them. In general, the smaller and more pointed the pepper, the hotter the taste.

WORTH KNOWING

Both animal and human studies have indicated that consumption of chile-containing meals increases both fat burning and calorie burning. And a study in the July 2006 *American Journal of Clinical Nutrition* showed that chile pepper has a beneficial effect on insulin levels. Subjects fed a meal containing a cayenne chile blend had less insulin in their bloodstreams after eating, meaning something in the chile helped clear the insulin from their bloodstreams after it did its job. High insulin is emerging as a risk factor for everything from heart disease to obesity to Alzheimer's, so that's an awfully important side effect. The researchers think that capsaicin is responsible. And by the way, the insulin-lowering results were even more dramatic in the subjects with the highest body weights.

Sweet Peppers

On Saturdays in the summertime you can walk around the city—at least in Los Angeles and New York, which are the only two cities I've lived in—and see gorgeous mountainous displays of fresh vegetables at the local farmers' market. If you look closer, you'll usually find that the vibrant colors that catch your attention are brought to you courtesy of the peppers.

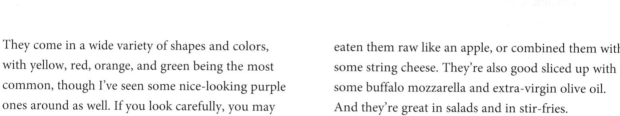

They come in a wide variety of shapes and colors, with yellow, red, orange, and green being the most common, though I've seen some nice-looking purple ones around as well. If you look carefully, you may even be able to spot a rarer black variety.

The Sweet and Spicy Difference

Both chile peppers and sweet peppers belong to the capsicum family, which is Latin for "box." The major difference between the two is that chiles contain fiery capsaicin (see hot peppers, 58-59) and are used mainly as a spice. The sweet ones lack capsaicin and are mainly used as vegetables. The riper the pepper, the greater its nutrition and the better its flavor. In general, the thinner the skin the more peppery the taste; the thick-skinned ones are sweeter. Many peppers start life as a green vegetable and, when they fully mature, they change colors. Red is the sweetest of the bell peppers; it is a fully ripened green pepper with a milder flavor.

Peppers are low in calories and a well-kept secret as a snack food. They blend with everything. I've eaten them raw like an apple, or combined them with some string cheese. They're also good sliced up with some buffalo mozzarella and extra-virgin olive oil. And they're great in salads and in stir-fries.

Nutritionally, peppers are an excellent source of vitamins C and A (beta-carotene) and the mineral potassium. They also contain vitamin K, which is increasingly being recognized as a vitally important component of bone health. Peppers are also one of the few foods around that contain lycopene, a member of the carotenoid family that has been shown in quite a bit of research to be associated with lower risk of prostate cancer. The amount of lycopene in the average pepper isn't substantial, but it's more than in most foods, and every little bit helps.

Though early studies using supplemental beta-carotene with smokers did not turn out the way we had hoped, the natural vitamin A and other compounds in peppers are, in fact, turning out to be protective. Red peppers contain beta-cryptoxanthin, a carotenoid that may lower the risk of developing lung cancer. One study, in *Cancer Epidemiology Biomarkers and Prevention*, followed more than 63,000 people in China and found that those eating the most cryptoxanthin-rich foods had a 27 percent lower risk for lung cancer. And some research indicates that exposure to a carcinogen in cigarettes—either directly or secondhand—induces a vitamin A deficiency, so foods rich in vitamin A may help counter that and provide some level of protection. Vitamin A is also a great immune system stimulator.

The Dark Side of Peppers

Now here's the dark side, which really isn't all that dark. Peppers are a member of the nightshade family along with eggplants and tomatoes. Nightshades are high in alkaloids, chemical substances that can have a strong physiological effect. In fact, many (but

not all) alkaloids are frequently found in drugs: coffee, opium, morphine, heroin, belladonna. That said, mature fruits such as eggplants, tomatoes, and peppers contain only faint traces: you won't get stoned from eating peppers! And cooking lowers alkaloid content by almost half. Nonetheless, one substance in nightshades—solanine—may have an impact on those with arthritis, and many arthritics are told to follow a "no-nightshade" diet. There isn't really any strong research evidence to back this up, but there are many folks walking around whose symptoms have improved when they eliminated nightshades. Norman Childers, Ph.D., the chairman of the Arthritis Nightshades Research Foundation, has theorized that some people with osteoarthritis may not be able to destroy solanine in the gut.

Pumpkin

We tend to think of pumpkins only at Thanksgiving and Halloween, but it's time to ditch that limited view of this great vegetable and expand its portfolio. Pumpkin is an unheralded superfood—it's ridiculously low in calories while high in nutrients.

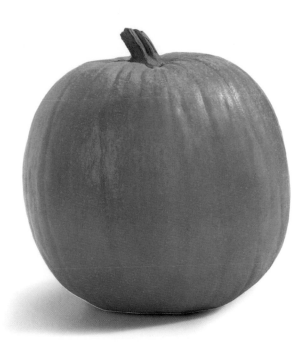

For example, pumpkin is a potassium heavyweight—for a measly 49 calories per cup (245 g) of mashed pumpkin, you get a whopping 564 mg of potassium, that's about 33 percent more than a medium banana.

Why should you care? Because the balance between potassium and sodium is of critical importance to our health. Potassium works with sodium to maintain the body's water balance, and that in turn affects all sorts of important things—such as blood pressure, for example.

One possible explanation for potassium's protective effect against hypertension is that increased potassium may increase the amount of sodium excreted from the body. Several studies indicate that people who consume high amounts of potassium have lower blood pressure than people who don't. In primitive cultures, salt intake is about seven times lower than potassium intake, but in Western industrialized cultures, salt intake is about three times higher than potassium intake.

Can Pumpkins Decrease Your Risk of Stroke?

Consider this: Several large epidemiological studies have suggested that increased potassium intake is associated with decreased risk of stroke. A study of more than 43,000 men followed for 87 years found that men in the top 20 percent of potassium intake (averaging 4,300 mg per day) were only 62 percent as likely to have a stroke than those in the lowest 20 percent of potassium intake (averaging 2,400 mg per day). This inverse association was especially high in men with high blood pressure.

Four large studies have reported significant positive associations between dietary potassium intake and bone mineral density. This isn't surprising if you think about it. When we eat a highly acid diet,

the body has to buffer that acid, and it does this by mobilizing alkaline calcium salts from the bones to neutralize the acids consumed in the diet. Increased consumption of high-potassium fruits and vegetables, such as pumpkin, reduces the net acid content of the diet and may help preserve calcium in the bones, where it belongs.

The Choice of Champions

Finally, athletes may need more potassium to replace what is lost from muscle during exercise and the smaller amount lost in sweat. Low potassium can cause muscle cramping and cardiovascular irregularities. When clients tell me they have muscle cramps, the first thing I think is that they're low on minerals, especially potassium, magnesium, and calcium.

Pumpkin would be a great food just on the basis of its high amount of potassium. But there's much more to pumpkin than potassium. One cup (245 g) of mashed pumpkin contains more than 5,000 mcg of beta-carotene, another 853 of alpha-carotene, and more than 3,500 mcg of beta-cryptoxanthin, a member of the carotenoid family that seems to reduce the risk of lung and colon cancer. Studies have shown that beta-cryptoxanthin can reduce the risk of lung cancer by more than 30 percent. Other studies have shown that it reduces the risk for rheumatoid arthritis as well (by 41 percent in one study). It appears to have strong antioxidant properties.

Your Eyes Will Thank You

Pumpkin has more than 2,400 mcg of the carotenoids lutein and zeaxanthin, which are fast becoming the star nutrients in eye health and vision protection programs. Pumpkin also has more than 12,000 IUs of vitamin A, plus a little bit of calcium, iron, magnesium, and phosphorus just for good measure. And a cup (245 g) of the stuff also provides more than 2½ g of fiber.

Remember that the carotenoids need fat for absorption, which makes it all the easier to consume some pumpkin on a regular basis. Just cook it with a dab of butter or olive oil. If you like it sweet, try adding some xylitol. It's an extraordinary substitute for mashed white potatoes; way healthier, and in my opinion, way more delicious.

The Fiber Connection

For decades, I've railed against the conventional wisdom that grains are an important source of fiber. They're not—just read the label on any cereal box. Pumpkin, however, is a whole different story. Consider that the average slice of bread or the average portion of commercial cold cereal has between 1 to 3 g of fiber, and it comes with a whole host of blood-sugar-raising starch, not to mention gluten and (frequently) high-fructose corn syrup. Pumpkin, on the other hand, has 49 calories per cup (245 g), and a whopping 7 g of fiber. Bread is about 100 calories a slice, and, with few exceptions, has virtually nothing of nutritional value to recommend it. And no bread on Earth provides the amount of fiber that a cup of mashed pumpkin provides.

In case you think this doesn't matter, consider that just about every epidemiological study ever done shows much better health outcomes for people who consume large amounts of fiber in their diet. Since the publication of this book, Steven Masley, M.D., and I presented a study at the annual conference of the American College of Nutrition showing that fiber intake was one of the best predictors of success on a weight loss program. Fiber matters—it slows the entrance of sugar into the bloodstream (blunting its glycemic impact), helps with digestion, and provides "food" for bacteria in the gut. When bacteria in the gut dine on fiber, they produce critically important nutrients such as butyric acid, which helps support the integrity of the gut wall and may have positive metabolic effects as well. Adding a cup (245 g) of pumpkin to your daily intake is a great way to get about 20 to 25 percent of the fiber you should be getting daily.

WORTH KNOWING

Pumpkin seeds have medicinal properties of their own—see page 177.

Purslane

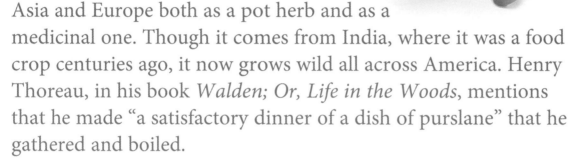

If you Google purslane, you'll find all kinds of agricultural sites that tell farmers how to get rid of it because many people confuse it with a weed. It's an incredibly nutritious vegetable that is valued in Asia and Europe both as a pot herb and as a medicinal one. Though it comes from India, where it was a food crop centuries ago, it now grows wild all across America. Henry Thoreau, in his book *Walden; Or, Life in the Woods*, mentions that he made "a satisfactory dinner of a dish of purslane" that he gathered and boiled.

Purslane Highest in Omega-3s

The real claim to fame of purslane as a health food is that its omega-3 concentration is the highest of any green leafy vegetable. About one cup (100 g) of fresh purslane leaves can contain up to 300 to 400 mg of alpha-linolenic acid, the same omega-3 found in flaxseed. Purslane also contains small amounts of the longer-chain omega-3s (DHA and EPA), which are rarely found in anything but fish and fish oil. Omega-3 fatty acids are anti-inflammatory, heart-healthy fats that have been found beneficial in hypertension, type 2 diabetes, coronary heart disease, and depression. The more omega-3s we eat, the better! (Note: For more on the benefits of omega-3 fats, see page 330.)

Purslane has plenty of other nutrients besides its omega-3 content. In fact, Artemis Simopoulos, M.D., author of *The Omega Plan*, devoted an entire article in the *Journal of the American College of Nutrition* to the health benefits of this vegetable ("Common purslane: A source of omega-3 fatty acids and antioxidants"). One cup (115 g) of the cooked leaves contains 90 mg of calcium, 561 mg of potassium, and more than 2,000 IUs of vitamin A.

Purslane leaves and stems are great raw in salads, but they can also be steamed or added to soups, stews, and vegetable dishes. You'll frequently see it in health food stores as part of mesclun salad. It's got a mild, sweet-and-sour flavor and a chewy texture.

Spinach

Calorie for calorie, green leafy vegetables such as spinach provide more nutrients than almost any other food on the planet. Spinach is loaded with vitamins, and it is one of the best sources of vitamin K. Vitamin K is critically important for building strong bones; it activates a compound called osteocalcin that anchors calcium molecules inside the bone. In the ten years since the original publication of this book, vitamin K (particularly K_2) has taken its rightful place as one of the most important nutrients we can consume.

So see, you can take all the calcium you want, but if it's not getting into the bones, it's not going to do you very much good, and it can do you some harm by being deposited in other places in the body, like the arteries. I believe this is a big part of the reason why studies have shown increases in heart disease with people taking large doses of calcium, the way we've been advised to for years. That calcium doesn't do you any good if it winds up in the arteries instead of the bones, and in the absence of vitamin K, that's exactly what happens. Vitamin K (especially K_2) makes sure that you get the minerals into the bone where they belong. And 1 cup (30 g) of fresh spinach leaves provides 200 percent of the Daily Value of vitamin K.

Worth noting: Most of the vitamin K found in green leafy vegetables such as spinach is in fact vitamin K_1. Vitamin K_2, on the other hand, is found mainly in fermented foods. While vitamin K_2 is important for heart health (probably by keeping calcium out of the arteries), vitamin K_1 is still critically important for bone health, so don't make the mistake of dismissing its importance just because of all the buzz about K_2.

Great Alternative to Milk for Vitamin C

Speaking of calcium, spinach is a fine source, and it is a great alternative to dairy for people who don't want to drink milk. It's also got vitamin A, manganese, folic acid, magnesium, iron, vitamin C, and the powerful anti-inflammatory compound quercetin.

Researchers have identified at least thirteen different compounds in spinach—they're called flavonoids—that function both as antioxidants and as anticancer agents. The anticancer properties of these compounds in spinach have been so impressive that researchers have created specialized spinach extracts that could be used in controlled studies. These extracts have been shown to slow down cell division in stomach cancer cells and, in studies on mice, have been shown to reduce skin cancers. And one study on adult women living in New England in the late 1980s showed that the more spinach women ate, the less the incidence of breast cancer. Powerful stuff, right?

Popeye Had It Right

For men, a carotenoid in spinach fights prostate cancer in two different ways. Research published in the September 2004 issue of the prestigious *Journal of Nutrition* showed that this spinach compound—it's called neoxanthin—causes prostate cancer cells to self-destruct. It also helps prevent their replication. That alone is a pretty good reason to make like Popeye.

Spinach is a great source of vitamin C and vitamin A, which are vitally important antioxidants that help prevent cholesterol from becoming oxidized. Oxidized cholesterol is the only kind of cholesterol you need to worry about (see *The Great Cholesterol Myth* by Stephen Sinatra and myself). Oxidized cholesterol is damaged cholesterol, the kind that goes hand in hand with inflammation and ultimately contributes to heart disease. Getting plenty of vitamin C and beta-carotene can help prevent this.

One cup (180 g) of boiled spinach gives you an awesome 294 percent of the Daily Value for vitamin A. It's also a great source of folic acid, which helps bring down a dangerous chemical in the body called homocysteine, which is harmful to blood vessels and puts you at risk for heart disease, stroke, and dementia. And spinach is also loaded with magnesium, a mineral that helps lower high blood pressure and protect against heart disease at the same time. When given to rats, spinach produced a blood pressure–lowering effect within just two to four hours. And to get that effect, the rats only had to eat the human equivalent of one main course–sized spinach salad for lunch or one side serving of steamed spinach.

Sharp Minds for Spinach Eaters

Spinach can also help prevent colon cancer because its vitamin C and beta-carotene help protect the colon cells from the damaging effects of free radicals. Those vitamins also help reduce inflammation, and they may help protect the brain from the kinds of age-related declines we often see in brain function. In fact, one study in the May 2005 issue of the *Journal of Experimental Neurology* showed that rats fed diets enriched with spinach and blueberries lost a lot fewer brain cells after a stroke and recovered significantly more than rats that weren't eating the spinach and blueberry-enriched diets. To get these protective benefits, the rats in the experiment only had to eat a measly 2 percent of their diet as spinach and blueberries!

Spinach is a great source of iron. That's especially important for menstruating women, who are a lot more at risk for iron deficiency. Sure, the iron in vegetables isn't as potent and absorbable as the heme iron (found in animal foods), but it still counts!

Finally, spinach contains lutein, a carotenoid that protects against eye disease and vision loss, like the kind caused by cataracts and macular degeneration. Now here's something interesting: Lutein can't be absorbed unless fat is also present. (That's why the lutein in egg yolks is so powerful.) So, to really get the vision protection that the lutein in spinach has to offer, I suggest enjoying your spinach steamed, sautéed, or fresh in a salad with a little olive oil and a topping of chopped hard-boiled eggs. One of my favorite ways to eat it is to stir-fry it in coconut oil. Even if you think you hate spinach, you'll find that way of preparing it to be delicious! And spinach is one of the lowest-calorie foods on the planet. You'd have to eat barrels of the stuff to equal the calories in even one small serving of french fries.

Squash (winter and summer)

Squash comes in two basic categories: winter and summer. While they share characteristics, there are significant differences. Summer squash comes in several different varieties, including zucchini, crookneck, and pattypan. It was first cultivated for its seeds; the squash of 10,000 years ago didn't have much flesh, was bitter and inedible, and didn't bear any resemblance to the squash we see in supermarkets today. The more modern version started as a wild squash in South America, spread throughout the Americas, and was brought back to Europe by old Christopher Columbus himself. Now it's produced around the world.

Summer and Winter Squash Go Head to Head

Like most vegetables, summer squash is high in the heart-healthy mineral potassium. One cup (180 g) of cooked summer squash gives you more than three times the amount of potassium in the typical potassium supplement. There's also a decent amount of vitamin A, and beta-carotene, and best of all, more than 4,000 mcg of lutein and zeaxanthin, two members of the carotenoid family that are getting serious research attention for their ability to protect the eyes against macular degeneration and other vision problems.

Winter squash comes in many varieties also, the most well known being acorn squash, butternut squash, and spaghetti squash. Pumpkin is technically in this category also, but gets its own listing because of its many specific benefits. Winter squash is higher in carbohydrate content than summer squash, and there are some specific differences among the winter varieties. Acorn squash is a fiber heavyweight—1 cup (245 g) of cooked acorn squash gives you 9 g of fiber, which makes it one of the highest-fiber foods in this book, especially calorie for calorie (1 cup of acorn has 115 calories). It also has a whopping 896 mg of potassium and almost 2 mg of iron. Spaghetti squash, on the other hand, has almost no calories (42 calories per cup [155 g]!) but also less fiber (2.2. mg) and a lot less potassium and vitamin A.

Butternut squash is a vitamin A giant, weighing in at a whopping 22,868 IUs per cup (240 g).

Butternut is also high in both beta-carotene and its less well-known brother, alpha-carotene, which has many health benefits of its own. And butternut is unique among the squashes in that it has a substantial amount of beta-cryptoxanthin, a carotenoid that may lower the risk of developing lung cancer. One study in *Cancer Epidemiology Biomarkers and Prevention* followed more than 63,000 people in China and found that those eating the most cryptoxanthin-rich foods had a 27 percent lower risk for lung cancer. And research indicates that exposure to a carcinogen in cigarettes—either directly or secondhand—induces a vitamin A deficiency. So foods rich in vitamin A, such as squash, may help counter that and provide some level of protection. Vitamin A is also a great immune system stimulator.

Squash Can Help with Weight Loss

One of the good things about squash in general is that it has a high-water content. Research by Barbara Rolls, Ph.D., at Pennsylvania State University, shows that foods with high water content are classified as high-volume foods; there's a lot there for a very little bit of calories. Because they're both filling and low-calorie, high-volume foods are an integral part of successful weight loss programs. And though some varieties are higher in fiber than others, squash gives you a nice amount of fiber overall for a low number of calories. Higher-fiber diets are associated with a king's ransom of benefits, including lower risk of heart disease and

cancer. And higher-fiber foods, including squash, are frequently recommended for digestive disorders such as diverticulosis.

Since the original publication of this book, the case for fiber has only grown stronger. In 2015, Steven Masley, M.D., and I presented a paper at the annual conference of the American College of Nutrition showing that, over the course of ten years of follow-up, fiber consumption was one of the best predictors of success on a weight loss program. And the exploding research on the microbiome—certainly to be one of the hottest topics in the next decade—has shown us that fiber plays a crucial part in microbiome health. Which should matter to you because the research has demonstrated a connection between an unhealthy microbiome and, anxiety, depression, obesity, and even schizophrenia.

Here's something amazing you can try with squash, especially butternut. Peel it and seed it and then cut it into the shape of french fries. Spray a cookie sheet with nonstick cooking spray, or better yet, lightly coat the tray with olive oil or butter, then place the "fries" on the sheet and bake for about 40 minutes (turn them over halfway). You can season with sea salt or any spice you like—call me crazy, but I put turmeric on everything (see page 325). Then feed them to your kids the next time they're jonesing for fast food! They are way healthier, and they taste amazing.

For reasons that I can't figure out, a lot of people think squash should be avoided if they're trying to control their blood sugar because they are sure the vegetable has a high glycemic index or glycemic load. But here's the thing: No reputable source that has published glycemic ratings for squash—not the authoritative Mendosa listing, not the University of Sydney (where the glycemic research was first done), and not the famous 2002 issue of the *American Journal of Clinical Nutrition*—has found squash to have a high glycemic rating. So, everyone else is basically guessing. That said, it's probably a good bet that winter squash has a higher glycemic load than most green vegetables (probably a "medium" ranking), and summer squash, which has about one-third the carb content, has a lower rating. But remember: I'm guessing like everyone else.

In any case, I think that for all but the most severe cases of carb intolerance, the argument over squash is a tempest in a teapot. Squash is a good high-fiber, low-calorie, nutrient-rich vegetable that you can enjoy on a low-carb diet as well as any other kind of eating plan. As my pal the nutritionist and USDA researcher C. Leigh Broadhurst, Ph.D., once said, "No one ever got fat on peas and carrots." The same could be said of squash.

Sweet Potatoes

Sweet potatoes are not actually related to the potato—they're a member of the morning glory family. (Which is a great thing to know if you're ever on *Jeopardy*.) They're sweet, dark, and one of the oldest vegetables known to man, having been around since prehistoric times. And there are many reasons to eat them.

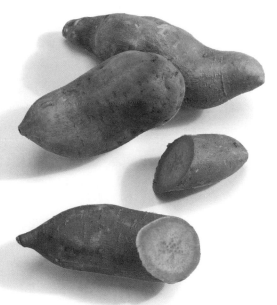

As starchy vegetables go, this is probably my absolute favorite. Back in the days when I spent more hours in the gym than I want to think about, I used to bake a week's worth of them in advance, wrap them individually, put them in the fridge, and take them with me along with some grilled chicken for an after-workout snack. Something about letting them sit on ice like that for a day makes them sweeter, and they make just about the most delicious snack you can imagine. Note: This is not for people with blood sugar problems (more on that in a moment). For everyone else, it's light years better than anything in the snack machine, and very portable in the bargain.

This starchy carbohydrate is high in fiber (half of which is soluble) and a rich source of powerful antioxidants in the carotenoid family, especially beta-carotene.

Sweet potatoes are loaded with vitamin A and heart-healthy potassium, and they even have a dollop of calcium. An article in the *Journal of Agriculture and Food Chemistry* found that an extract from a baked sweet potato has chemopreventive (cancer-fighting) properties. Finally, sweet potatoes contain other phytochemicals like quercetin, a powerful anti-inflammatory, and chlorogenic acid, an antioxidant. And a medium-size baked sweet potato has only 103 calories (the operative word there is "medium").

Potatoes Take a Hit in the Low-Carb Craze

Back in the low-fat 1980s, potatoes were the darling of the fitness set because they are pretty much a fat-free item. Potatoes have since suffered a reversal of fortune, swept out of the diet—along with bread, cereal, and pasta—by a lot of carb-conscious eaters. When consumers began to be (rightly) concerned with controlling their blood sugar, potatoes became vegetable non-grata at the dinner table, because they raise your blood sugar quickly, producing a lot of the fat-storing hormone insulin. That's why white potatoes didn't make my list of the healthiest foods. I don't think they have enough nutritional wallop to counterbalance their effect on blood sugar. By the time a bite of white potato gets to your stomach, the body sees it as just a big lump of sugar. Though they may not be the worst food on the planet, they're not among the best foods on the planet. (From a health perspective, french-fried potatoes are probably one of the three worst.)

A short course in blood sugar management: The impact of food on blood sugar is of great concern to those trying to lose weight, and of even greater concern for those with either diabetes or metabolic syndrome. The impact of food on blood sugar is most accurately measured by its glycemic load. (The higher the glycemic load, the more it raises blood sugar and the fat-burning hormone, insulin.) Although some people claim that sweet potatoes have a lower glycemic load than regular potatoes, the truth is that only a certain variety from Australia (*ipomoea batatas*) has anything like what could be called a low glycemic load. (Low glycemic load is technically 10 or under; the Australian variety has 11.) All the rest run between 16 and 20. That is not a bad thing if you aren't diabetic or prediabetic. But if blood sugar control is an issue for you, either because of stubborn weight problems or medical ones such as diabetes, the glycemic impact of this delicious potato needs to be considered.

So let me be clear: If you don't have blood sugar issues, sweet potatoes are a great food. And even if you do, eating them in reasonable amounts, as part of a mixed meal with some vegetables and some protein and fat, is hardly the worst thing you could do. And if you're a bodybuilder at the gym and you're looking for a great after-workout meal, you can't do much better than tuna, broccoli, and sweet potatoes.

What's the Difference between Sweet Potatoes and Yams?

There are two basic types of sweet potato: moist (orange fleshed) and dry (yellow fleshed). Both are delicious. The sweeter orange-fleshed varieties dominate the U.S. market. The moist-fleshed potatoes are often called yams, but this is a misnomer. True yams (botanical family *Dioscoreaceae*) are large root vegetables grown in Africa and Asia and rarely seen in the Western world.

Whatever you do, don't forget to eat the skin. It's the best part and has the most fiber.

★ Swiss Chard

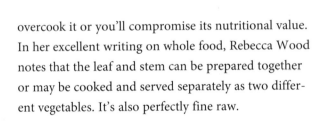

When I first looked up the lab analysis of the nutritional content of Swiss chard, I had to go back and check twice to be sure there wasn't a mistake. The amount of nutrition in this baby is so spectacular I thought it was a misprint; but no, it's true. Swiss chard is an excellent example of a nutritional powerhouse that delivers the goods for almost no calories.

Easy on the Eyes

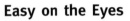

A cup (175 g) of cooked chard gives you almost 4 g of fiber, more than 100 mg of calcium, an incredible 961 mg of potassium, and more than 30 mg of vitamin C. And that's just the beginning. You also get more than 10,000—that's right, 10,000—IUs of vitamin A, more than 6,000 of beta-carotene (plus some alpha-carotene as well), and a staggering 19,000 mcg of lutein and zeaxanthin, two members of the carotenoid family that are getting significant research attention for their ability to protect the eyes and guard against vision problems like macular degeneration. And did I mention that one cup—the amount that provides all those nutrients—has 35 calories?

Chard is a member of the goosefoot family of plants, is a relative of beets, and comes in red and white. The red kind is a standout in supermarkets. It's very quick cooking—like spinach, in fact—so don't overcook it or you'll compromise its nutritional value. In her excellent writing on whole food, Rebecca Wood notes that the leaf and stem can be prepared together or may be cooked and served separately as two different vegetables. It's also perfectly fine raw.

WORTH KNOWING

Swiss chard—like spinach, beets, rhubarb, and some other foods—contains oxalates, which are not a concern for most people, but may be for those who have a particular type of kidney stone. Calcium oxalate kidney stones can result from excessive oxalates being absorbed through the gut and then binding with calcium in the urine and precipitating out to form the stones. Unfortunately, cooking doesn't do very much to reduce them. Oxalates should be watched by people with hyperoxaluria, a rare, inherited metabolic disorder that often causes the stones. Let me repeat that this is not a problem for 99 percent of people.

Tomatoes

Botanically speaking, tomatoes are a fruit; technically, they're a berry, and legally, they're a vegetable. No, I'm not making this up. In an 1893 ruling of the U.S. Supreme Court, the tomato became legally classified as a vegetable because it's used as one.

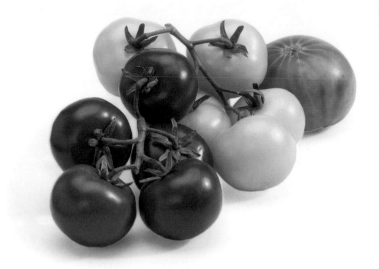

Tomato-Eating Men Have Fewer Prostate Cancers

Cooked tomatoes, especially those cooked with oil, are a rich source of the carotenoid lycopene. There is promising research showing that lycopene is associated with significant reduction in prostate cancer. As far back as 1995, the *Journal of the National Cancer Institute* published the results of a study conducted by Harvard University researchers that looked at the eating habits of more than 47,000 men between the ages of forty and seventy-five. They found that the men eating ten servings or more a week of tomatoes, tomato sauce, tomato juice, and even pizza had 45 percent fewer prostate cancers than men who ate fewer than two servings a week.

In another study done a few years later at the Karmanos Cancer Institute in Detroit, researchers gave lycopene supplements to thirty men who already had prostate cancer. Those given the lycopene supplements had smaller tumors and less spreading of the cancer. Best of all, the tumors in the participants who consumed lycopene supplements showed signs of regression and decreased malignancy.

And it's not just prostate cancer that the lycopene in tomatoes protects against. Strong evidence indicates that lycopene protects against lung and stomach cancers as well, and preliminary research shows protection against pancreatic, colorectal, esophageal, oral, breast, and cervical cancers. Lycopene also protects the heart against oxidative damage, thereby reducing the risk of heart attacks. And one study published in *American Heart Journal* showed that treatment with antioxidant-rich tomato extract can reduce blood pressure in patients with grade 1 hypertension.

Get the Most Out of Your Tomatoes

The anticancer properties of lycopene are especially beneficial when consumed with fat-rich foods, such as avocado, olive oil, or nuts. Why? Because carotenoids are fat-soluble nutrients. To get maximum absorption of them, you need to eat them with a little fat!

Besides lycopene, tomatoes contain a variety of other powerful phytochemicals that fight disease. A trio of antioxidants—zera-carotene, phytoene, and phytofluene—are found together in many fruits and vegetables, including tomatoes, and scientists believe that this triple-threat antioxidant team has strong disease-fighting potential. And if that isn't enough, phenolic acids found in tomatoes have the potential to fight lung cancer with their ability to inhibit the formation of nitrosamines (carcinogenic compounds) in the body.

Tomatoes also have a compound in them called *lutein*, which is great for your eyes. Lutein is important for eye health—we have lutein in the retina of our eyes and we need it for healthy vision. The lutein in tomatoes may help prevent macular degeneration, a leading cause of blindness in older adults, and may help improve vision. Lutein may also help prevent or slow down the thickening of arteries that we know as atherosclerosis.

Not bad for a fruit—I mean a berry—I mean a vegetable—that up until about 100 years ago was thought to be poisonous!

The Benefits of Vine-Ripened Tomatoes

Tomatoes are an excellent source of vitamin C, though the vitamin C is most concentrated in the jellylike substance that surrounds the seeds. Tomatoes also contain vitamin A, B-complex vitamins, potassium, and phosphorus. Note: A tomato grown in a hothouse has half the vitamin C content as its vine-ripened cousin.

And speaking of vine-ripened: Tomatoes are one of those foods that people rarely appreciate because the commercial kind are picked when green and then artificially ripened with ethylene gas, leaving a food product that may look great, but has negligible taste. You're best off buying tomatoes from local farmers and getting vine-ripened tomatoes whenever possible. They taste a lot better.

WORTH KNOWING

Tomatoes are a member of the nightshade family. Green tomatoes contain a substance called *solanine*, which may be aggravating to those with arthritis. Many health professionals counsel people with arthritis to avoid nightshades altogether, though some say there isn't any solid research to support this. If you have pain from arthritis, cutting out nightshades is probably worth a try. Be aware, however, that some very respected health professionals believe that you need to do this for at least six weeks (maybe more) to really see results from the elimination of nightshades. Tomatoes are usually avoided by people with GERD (gastroesophageal reflux disease) as well.

Turnips

Whenever I think of turnips, I can't help recalling that line in Tennessee Williams's famous play, *Cat on a Hot Tin Roof*, where Big Daddy calls the little kids "no-neck monsters"! Sure enough, turnips have no necks, and the fact that they grow just about anywhere, in the poorest soil, has made them kind of like the catfish of vegetables, endearing them to the poor and giving them pretty low status among snobbier folk who haven't tasted them. But they're anything but a poor country cousin when it comes to nutrition.

Turnips and rutabagas (see page 77) are among the most commonly grown and widely adapted root crops. They are members of the Cruciferae family and they both belong to the genus *Brassica* (cabbage), members of which are widely acclaimed for their cancer-fighting indoles and isothiocyanates and other health-giving phytochemicals. And, along with rutabagas, turnips are particularly high in anticarcinogenic glucosinolates.

Turnip Greens Promote Bone Health

Turnips are another of those high-volume foods that fill you up without costing you a lot of calories. A cup (156 g) of cooked turnips (without the greens) has all of about 35 calories, with 3 g of fiber, more than 250 mg of potassium, 18 mg of vitamin C, and 51 mg of calcium. Add the nutritious bone-building greens to the mix and your calcium nearly triples to

148 mg, plus you get a whopping 14,000 IUs of vitamin A, more than 8,000 IUs of beta-carotene, and an incredible 676 mcg of bone-friendly vitamin K. In the bargain, you also get more than 15,000 mcg of lutein and zeaxanthin, two members of the carotenoid family that have been shown (in a study known as the AREDS-2 Study) to help protect the eyes from vision problems like macular degeneration.

Turnip greens are sometimes available by themselves, usually next to other greens like kale and collards, but sometimes at a farmers' market you'll be able to find the turnips with the tops attached. Buy them!

Raw, grated turnips serve as a digestive aid similar to radish and daikon and are good for general detoxification, says natural-foods expert Rebecca Wood.

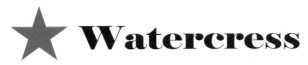 # Watercress

Irish monks used to refer to the watercress plant as "pure food for sages." And with good reason. This pungent, stimulating herb, frequently found in salads that bear its name, truly deserves the name superfood.

Watercress Contains Four Times the Calcium of Milk

If you were to compare an equal number of calories of watercress with an equal number of calories of 2 percent milk, the watercress would give you four times the calcium and six times the magnesium. Gram for gram, this little plant contains as much vitamin C as oranges and more iron than spinach. It's also as close to a calorie-free food as you're likely to find. A full cup (34 g) of the stuff contains only 4 calories, and for those 4 calories you get an amazing 1,500 IUs of immune system–building vitamin A (including 950 mcg as beta-carotene), 85 mcg of bone-building vitamin K, 14 mg of vitamin C, and, as a bonus, more than 1,900 mcg of the new superstars of eye nutrition, lutein and zeaxanthin. Both lutein and zeaxanthin are members of the carotenoid family, and they are being extensively researched for their demonstrated ability to prevent or reduce macular degeneration, the number-one cause of adult blindness.

Watercress Neutralizes Carcinogens

The health benefits of watercress have been known since ancient times. Watercress is a member of the family of vegetable superstars, the *Brassica* family of cruciferous vegetables, which counts among its members such vegetable royalty as broccoli, cabbage, kale, kohlrabi, and Swiss chard. These vegetables are now known to be excellent sources of a family of anticancer phytochemicals called isothiocyanates. Isothiocyanates literally fight cancer by neutralizing carcinogens—the bad guys of the cancer battle. They do this by reducing their poisonous effects and stimulating the release of "carcinogen killers," speeding up their removal from the body. Studies have shown that isothiocyanates help prevent lung and esophageal cancer and can lower the risk of other cancers, including gastrointestinal cancer.

Watercress is unique among the cruciferous vegetables in that it contains high concentrations of one particularly potent isothiocyanate, PEITC (phenethyl isothiocyanate). It also contains another group of compounds with anticancer potential belonging to the sulforaphane family (also found in broccoli). Research

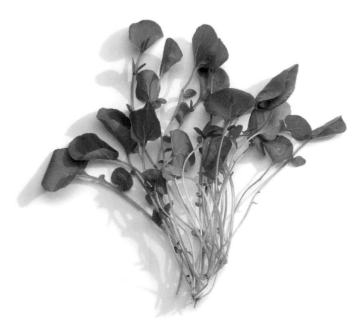

published in two separate cancer journals—*Cancer Research* and *Carcinogenesis*—concluded that the potent combination of PEITC and sulforaphanes had a "triple whammy" effect: zapping cancer cells by inducing their death (apoptosis), stopping potential carcinogens from becoming active, and stimulating cell defenses against assaults from carcinogens.

Watercress can be eaten raw and most frequently is, but it can also be cooked. Natural-foods expert Rebecca Wood says cooking eliminates its bite and leaves a vegetable that is pretty sweet. Remember that when you cook it, its volume is reduced by three-fourths. The raw version probably contains more enzymes and live energy.

Vegetable Runners-Up

Parsnips

The unassuming-looking but amazingly flavorful parsnip has been revered since ancient times, when the first-century Roman emperor Tiberius had them specially imported and served them gently cooked in honeyed wine. A parsnip looks a lot like a carrot that doesn't get out much—pale and almost white. But there's a world of difference in the taste.

USE PARSNIPS IN PLACE OF MASHED POTATOES

Parsnips are sweet. Personally, I think they're a great replacement for white potatoes—they're nutty and flavorful, and unlike white potatoes, have a lot of nutrition. Plus they lend themselves to mashing really well, making them the ideal substitute for mashed potatoes. Put on a little organic creamy butter, some lemon pepper, and maybe some sea salt, and you're good to go!

Parsnips are a member of the umbelliferous vegetable group, which the National Cancer Institute has identified as possessing cancer-protective properties. Parsnips have polyacetylenes, plant compounds that help protect against carcinogens. They also contain phthalides, a group of phytochemicals that provide health benefits by stimulating beneficial enzymes and inhibiting inflammatory ones.

(Note: Don't confuse the beneficial phthalides with the similar sounding phthalates. The two compounds differ in spelling by only two letters, but there's a world of difference. Phthalates are bad guys. Of all the bad things about fast food, one of the worst is the creation of phthalates from the way the food is prepared. Research from 2015 shows that the phthalates formed in the cooking of fast food increases the risk of cancer.)

Parsnips are high in folate, calcium, potassium, and especially fiber. One little cup (156 g) of cooked parsnips has 5½ g of fiber, 58 mg of calcium, 45 mg of magnesium, 90 mcg of folate, and a whopping 573 mg of potassium. And it weighs in at slightly more than 100 calories. That's not insignificant. A cup (156 g) of parsnips has more potassium than a banana.

And let's not forget the fiber, either. The research on the benefits of fiber continues to explode, and Americans don't get nearly enough of the stuff because most of our foods have had the fiber processed out of them. Putting parsnips in heavy rotation on your menu helps to correct that deficit.

Here's a secret lesson about parsnips I learned in my own kitchen—they're amazing when you juice them. Their nutty flavor adds a lot of richness to a standard apple-carrot-spinach-ginger mix. And, as most cooks know, parsnips are amazing in soups. They have a strong dominating flavor, though, so use with discretion.

Rutabagas

A rutabaga is a strange-looking root vegetable that looks like a cross between a turnip and a wild cabbage. They're an important part of Scandinavian cuisine and are sometimes referred to as "Swedes." They can be steamed, boiled, or mashed; baked, roasted, or sautéed; and they're good in soups. They also make a great puree.

Rutabagas are an amazing source of potassium: One cup (240 g) of the cooked vegetable has 782 mg (about 1½ times the amount in an extra-large [9-inch or 23 cm] banana!). It also has 115 mg of calcium, 55 mg of magnesium, 45 mg of vitamin C, and a little more than 4 g of fiber. Not too shabby for a mere 94 calories per cup. In Asian medicine, root vegetables are considered "warming" foods that strengthen the digestion and help detoxify the liver.

Here's a bachelor-friendly dish that'll make you fall in love with rutabagas: Cut them into cubes, boil them till tender, and toss them with chopped walnuts, raisins, and a little cold-pressed organic honey. You'll never miss chocolate cake again. Well, okay, I lied, but seriously, that dish will knock your socks off.

Snow Peas

The French name for this tender legume is *mange-tout*, meaning "eat it all." Unlike the pod in sugar snap peas, the pod in snow peas tastes as good as the seeds it contains. Almost anyone who has eaten Chinese food has eaten snow peas—they're flat green pods containing five to seven seeds, and although most Americans know them from Chinese takeout, they've been around for centuries—the tender-crisp, jade snow pea was first mentioned in 1597, though pea seeds were found in archaeological digs in Turkey as far back as 5700 B.C.E.

One cup (160 g) of cooked (frozen) snow peas has 5 g of fiber, almost half of the amount most Americans are getting on a daily basis. Remember, that's way too little—I recommend an absolute minimum of 25 grams a day of fiber, with more being better! They contain lutein and zeaxanthin, two carotenoids that have been shown to be extremely protective of the eyes. They also have 94 mg of calcium and 347 mg of heart-healthy potassium, plus a little vitamin C (35 mg), folate (56 mcg), and a respectable 2,098 IUs of vitamin A, including 1,216 of beta-carotene. Snow peas are also a good source of bone-building vitamin K: One cup (160 g) of the cooked peas contains 48 mg. All this for about 80 calories. That's a nutritional bargain if there ever was one.

Snow peas can be found in the produce section of most health food stores and specialty markets. They're even beginning to make their way into your general-purpose supermarket, especially in the frozen vegetable section. Look for brightly colored, crisp pods that have fresh-looking leaflets and small seeds. Use as soon as possible or store in the fridge for up to three days.

Note: When you stir-fry them, be sure not to overcook. They taste best—and are most nutritious—when they are bright green. And by the way, they're very tasty raw, in salads.

THE EXPERTS' TOP TEN LISTS

Ann Louise Gittleman, Ph.D., C.N.S.

Ann Louise Gittleman is the *New York Times'* award-winning author of more than twenty-five books, including *The Fat Flush Plan* and *Before the Change*. She was one of the first authors I read when I got interested in nutrition, and she and I now have a mutual admiration society. She has a unique gift for clear explanation and for motivating people, and her fans are legion. She's appeared on dozens of national television shows, including *Dr. Phil* and *The View*.

1. **Ground flaxseed:** Flaxseeds provide 800 times more cancer-fighting lignans than any other food, which protect against breast and prostate cancer. Delicious in salads, smoothies, and as a topping on veggies.

2. **Unsweetened cranberry juice:** Rich source of phytonutrients such as phenol-based antioxidants that are so helpful in supporting cardiovascular health and preventing urinary tract infections. Mix in a 1:2 ratio with water!

3. **Lemons:** High in limonene, lemons are an old-time remedy for thinning the bile and enhancing digestion.

4. **Whey:** Undenatured, unheated whey protein provides the aminos from which the body makes glutathione, its premier antioxidant.

5. **Grass-fed beef:** High in the healthy, fat-burning fat CLA (conjugated linoleic acid) plus omega-3s; grass-fed beef is also antibiotic and hormone-free and a great source of zinc and vitamin B_{12}.

6. **Spaghetti squash:** My personal favorite substitute for pasta, especially for the gluten or carb intolerant. Delicious as spaghetti squash and meatballs!

7. **Jicama:** Crunchy, juicy, and low calorie, jicama is delightful in salads and as a veggie for dips. Naturally sweet to satisfy the most sophisticated sweet tooth!

8. **Peanut butter:** Preferably organic, peanut butter is a quick snack that satiates the appetite. High in stress-busting pantothenic acid (vitamin B_5).

9. **Blueberries:** One of the least pesticide-ridden fruits, blueberries are exceptionally high in proanthocyanidins, so helpful in preventing degenerative disease.

10. **Organic cream:** Organic cream from grass-fed cows is not only a treat but a terrific source of fat-burning CLA! It nourishes the nerves and is a wonderful accompaniment for all sorts of berries.

CHAPTER 2

GRAINS

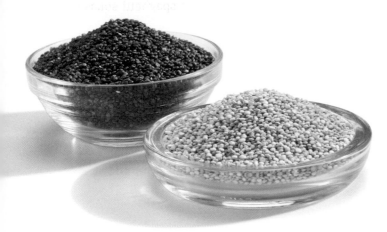

You may be puzzled by the almost complete absence of grains on my list of 150 healthiest foods on the planet. In fact, it may seem like nutritional heresy. After all, aren't whole grains supposed to be nutritious and healthy? We all know that refined grains aren't any good for you, but aren't whole grains among the world's most perfect foods? Doesn't research show that people eating them get tremendous health benefits?

Let's see . . .

In the decade since the original publication of this book, there has been a virtual explosion of public awareness about gluten and about grains in general. As a result, questioning the value of grains is no longer confined to fringe nutritionists (as it was when the first edition of this book came out). Cardiologist William Davis' blockbuster best seller, *Wheat Belly* was published in 2011, hit number one on the New York Times bestseller list in 2012, and continues to sell briskly. *Wheat Belly* was perhaps the first successful mass market book that took a stand against wheat (and grains), but it was hardly the last. *Grain Brain* by the integrative neurologist David Perlmutter—another book that presented powerful evidence against grains—also reached bestseller status, as did *Eat Dirt* by Josh Axe, D.N.M., D.C., C.N.S., and *The Autoimmune Fix* by Tom O'Bryan, D.C., C.C.N., D.A.C.B.N. And the rise of the Paleo movement—which shuns grains of any kind—has only served to reinforce a growing suspicion—when it comes to the value of grains, we have not been told the whole truth.

That said, it's worth repeating some of the arguments in favor of grains. Keep in mind while reading the following section that grains may have been necessary or beneficial for the development of civilization, but that does not mean they are beneficial—or even necessary— for your personal health.

Grains Allow Modern Civilization to Flourish

Loren Cordain, Ph.D., is one of the world's most renowned scientists doing groundbreaking research into the original human diet. He's a professor in the health and exercise science department at Colorado State University and a member of the American Society for Clinical Nutrition. In 1999, he wrote a groundbreaking 100-plus-page paper that was published in the *World Review of Nutrition and Dietetics.* It was called "Cereal Grains: Humanity's Double-Edged Sword." In essence, here's what he said.

The human genetic constitution has not changed much in the past 40,000 years.

The vast majority of humankind rarely, if ever, consumed cereal grains.

The natural diet of humans is food that could be hunted, fished for, gathered, or plucked.

The natural diet served us well as long as populations were limited and wildlife was plentiful.

As the population of the world increased and the supply of wild game became more limited, it became necessary to provide an alternative or supplementary means of nourishment—and about 10,000 years ago, agriculture was born.

Agriculture has made it possible for humans to live in cities, and literally, for civilization to flourish.

Eight cereal grains (wheat, corn, rice, barley, sorghum, oats, rye, and millet) now provide 56 percent of the calories and 50 percent of the protein consumed on Earth. Without these crops, the planet could not support nearly 8 billion people.

So here's the double-edged sword: Without cereal grains, we would not have cities, civilization, industry, or the planet as we know it. Take away rice, wheat, and corn, and half the people on Earth will not eat. As one researcher said, "Cereal grains literally stand between mankind and starvation." The dwindling supplies of our natural diet of wild animals and wild plants, together with the huge expansion of the planet's population, made agriculture a necessity for survival.

Why Cereal Grains Are a Nutritional Compromise

On the other hand, cereal grains are a nutritional compromise. They are not nearly as healthy, nor as nutritionally complete, nor as perfectly suited to our ancient digestive wiring, as the foods they have replaced. And the health implications of eating a diet so high in cereal grains—and so different from the diet we were designed to eat—are just now beginning to be fully understood.

So, cereal grains are a recent addition to the diet of humanity. Agriculture didn't really take hold until ten to twelve thousand years ago, which is less than a nanosecond in the twenty-four-hour time clock that represents the 2.4 million years the human genus has been on the planet. As Cordain points out, we have had little time since the inception of the agricultural revolution to adapt to a food type that now represents humanity's major source of calories and protein.

Are Whole Grains Any Better?

Truth be told, grains have a host of nutritional shortcomings. It's now accepted wisdom that the refined grains—which constitute most of our cereals, pastas, and breads—are useless nutritionally. The problem is that whole grains are only marginally better (if at all).

One reason is that no grain can be eaten in a completely unrefined state. No one plucks wheat from the ground and starts chowing down. All edible grains have to be milled and ground because in their natural state they contain antinutrients, substances that interfere with the absorption and assimilation of nutrients in the grain, especially minerals. It's not a matter of whether to refine them, it's a matter of how much.

Ostensibly, whole grains have been less processed and less milled than the really refined junk and therefore contain more of the bran—the outer coating—of the grains, providing fiber for the diet. (Oats are different from barley, wheat, and other grains in that they retain the bran and germ layers where most of the nutrients are found.)

But read the label of most whole grain cold cereals—they are fiber lightweights. It's rare to find a cereal with 5 g of fiber per serving—most have 1 or 2, making it a pretty bad nutritional bargain. Compare that to an avocado (11 to 17 g) or a serving of beans (11 to 17 g) or a guava (8 g).

Then there's the gluten issue. Gluten is a primary component of grains such as barley, rye, oats, and especially wheat. A full-blown allergy to gluten is called celiac disease, and at one time it was thought to affect 1 in 200 people. Now it's 1 in 133, 1 in 56 for people with related symptoms, with 60 percent of diagnosed children and 41 percent of diagnosed adults not showing any symptoms. But what has become increasingly clear is that full-blown celiac disease is just the extreme case of gluten sensitivity. There is now a condition called Non-Celiac Gluten Sensitivity (NCGS), and many experts—such as Tom O'Bryan—speak of gluten intolerance. The point is that people with celiac disease are not the only ones who have serious problems with gluten.

Many people have undiagnosed or delayed food sensitivities, and wheat and gluten are prime triggers. (Wheat is one of the seven top allergens in the diet.) I can tell you that among nutritionists, naturopathic physicians, and doctors practicing integrative and functional medicine, one of the first dietary orders of business with patients who have multiple complaints is to take them off wheat, dairy, and sugar. Although I can't prove it scientifically beyond a shadow of a doubt, in the experience of thousands of people the removal of wheat (and dairy and sugar) produces remarkable relief

from a very wide variety of symptoms, not the least of which is unwanted weight and bloat.

The Myth of Whole Grains

This brings us to the whole connection between grains and obesity, diabetes, and blood sugar. It's worth noting that the old (thankfully discredited) food pyramid, which had six to eleven servings of grains at the bottom of the structure, was suspiciously similar to the pyramid used by farmers to fatten up cattle. Ask any farmer on the planet—if you want to fatten up farm animals, you feed them grain, not grass.

Think it's all that different with people? Think again. While the urban legend is that whole grains raise blood sugar much more slowly than their refined cousins, an examination of the glycemic index and glycemic load tables shows this is not always the case. Brown rice and white rice have virtually the same glycemic impact. So do whole wheat and white bread. Grains, by and large, are starch juggernauts and almost all of them raise blood sugar (and insulin) quickly.

Personally, I've seen very few grain-foods that could hold a candle—nutritionally speaking—to most of the vegetables or legumes in this book. Grains can be prepared deliciously, and many people are very attached to them. But the notion that grains should be an essential part of any diet is far from the truth.

Choose Your Grains Wisely

So do I want to wipe grains off the face of the earth? Of course not. Nor do I think we should never eat them. But between their very modest nutritional content, their propensity to trigger gluten and grain intolerances, their connection (for many) to carbohydrate addiction, and—despite good PR campaigns—their limited delivery of fiber, it's hard to see how grains are among the best foods on the planet.

Sure, there are plenty of studies of healthy diets

that show that people eating fruits, vegetables, fish, omega-3 fats, and whole grains do much better health-wise than those eating the Standard American Diet. But it's a real stretch to attribute those health benefits to the grains. In my opinion, if people were eating plenty of fish, vegetables, fruits, omega-3 fats, and M&Ms they'd still be much healthier than most of America.

Let's put it this way: If you ate a great balance of foods from the 150 that make up the list of the healthiest foods on the planet, and you never touched a grain for the rest of your life, you wouldn't be missing a thing, nutritionally speaking. The same cannot be said of the fruits, vegetables, eggs, oils, spices, meat, fish, and poultry.

And in any case, there's always oatmeal. That's a minimally processed grain that's truly worth eating.

Oatmeal

Oatmeal has a place on virtually everyone's "best foods" list. It's like the Muhammad Ali of foods—universally loved, no matter where you stand in your dietary philosophy. Even those who are stringent about keeping carbs low soften a bit when it comes to oatmeal. The guru of diabetic diets, Richard Bernstein, M.D., who, one might say jokingly, "never met a carb he didn't dislike," allows oatmeal once a day for his diabetic patients. And of course, it's been a staple of the high-carb folks for decades. I can still remember seeing the bodybuilders at Gold's Gym with their Tupperware full of the stuff, usually mixed with scrambled eggs.

What is it about oatmeal that makes it go to the head of the list for everyone's favorite health foods? Let's start with fiber. Oats are simply a great source of fiber and contain a nice mix of both essential kinds (55 percent soluble and 45 percent insoluble). But the soluble fiber in oats, known as beta-glucan, makes oatmeal special.

Oatmeal Turbocharges Your Immune System

Beta-glucan is a type of polysaccharide (a long string of glucose molecules). Beta-glucan significantly reduces the risk of cardiovascular disease and stroke. The USDA ruled that companies making oats for cereal can make the claim that their product helps reduce the risk of heart disease, though certain stipulations exist, one of which is that a serving must have at least a ½ gram of beta-glucan.

Beta-glucans enhance the body's immune system by turbocharging its response to bacterial infection. They do this by activating certain white blood cells called macrophages, which act like hungry little Pac-Men, gobbling up foreign invaders like fungi and bacteria. Research is currently going on to determine whether beta-glucans might boost the ability of the body to kill cancer cells, in addition to their ability to lower bad cholesterol and triglycerides, some of this research is quite promising.

Oatmeal also has a very low glycemic load, meaning it has a very, very modest effect on blood sugar. Type 2 diabetics also seem to benefit from the beta-glucan, as it appears to be helpful in stabilizing blood sugar, which is probably why diabetes expert Richard Bernstein, M.D., allows it on his programs.

Oats contain avenanthramide, a polyphenol antioxidant unique to oats and believed to have anti-inflammatory and heart-healthy properties. Many people believe that it's the avenanthramides in oats that are responsible for the healing properties of a traditional oatmeal bath.

Oatmeal Has More Protein Than Any Popular Cereal

In addition to its 5 g of fiber content, oatmeal has the highest protein content of any popular cereal: 8½ g of protein in ⅔ cup (54 g) of oats. It also contains phosphorus, potassium, selenium, manganese, and a couple of milligrams of iron.

There are two groups of people who should be very cautious in their consumption of oats. First, those who are gluten sensitive. Celiac disease is the most dramatic example of gluten intolerance, but many people are gluten sensitive without having full-blown celiac disease. Oats themselves do not contain gluten; however, they are frequently processed in facilities that also process wheat products, and gluten contamination can occur through farming, storage, and transportation. That's why people with gluten-issues are frequently warned to be careful with oats.

The second group needing to be careful are those suffering from uric acid–related problems (i.e., gout and kidney stones). Oats contain purines, which are substances that break down to uric acid in the body.

Choosing the Best Oats

Besides the packs and the instant oatmeal, both of which are, in my opinion, worthless, there are several great ways to get oatmeal. Groats are dehulled oats, probably the least processed, but you don't see them around much. Steel-cut oats, also known as Irish or Scottish oats, require less cooking time than the whole oats, but have all the great oatmeal health benefits. So do rolled oats, but make sure they're old-fashioned and thick, which means they're less processed.

One more thing: It seems to be a well-kept secret that oats do not need to be cooked. Spoiler alert: You do not have to cook them. Ever see the Swedish cereal muesli in the supermarkets? It's basically raw oats, dried fruit, and nuts!

Raw oats are amazing—I have them all the time, lightly moistened in either raw milk or juice, or even hot water. I let them sit a few minutes, then throw on the berries and nuts. And don't let the package instructions put you off—while that 20-minute cooking time does give you a rich, hearty flavor, it's completely unnecessary to get the health benefits or even the rich taste. I make them on the stove in less than 5 minutes. They taste just fine.

WORTH KNOWING

The type of oatmeal you buy makes all the difference in the world. Forget about the instant packs. They're usually sweetened, making their potential benefits for diabetics disappear. They're also the most processed. Remember, the less processing, the higher the fiber, the lower the glycemic load (sugar impact), and the better the oatmeal is for you.

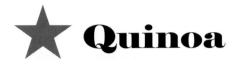

Quinoa

Quinoa is another of those foods that keeps getting miscategorized—everyone thinks it's a grain, everyone uses it like a grain, but it's actually a seed. Anyway, who really cares? You know how the old saying goes . . . if it looks like a grain and it acts like a grain . . . same principle.

The Stuff War Balls Are Made Of

Quinoa was known by the Incas as the "mother of grains." They used the seeds of this plant as one of their chief sources of nutrition. In fact, legend has it that the Incan armies frequently marched for days at a time eating a mixture of quinoa and fat known as "war balls," and at planting time tradition demanded that the Incan leader would plant the first quinoa seed using a gold shovel.

Quinoa is a highly nutritious food, and it is considered a high-protein "grain." The protein quality and quantity in quinoa seed is often superior to those of more common cereal grains, and the nutritional quality of this crop has been compared to that of dried whole milk by the Food and Agriculture Organization (FAO) of the United Nations. Quinoa is higher in lysine than wheat (lysine is an amino acid that's scarce in the vegetable kingdom), and the amino acid content of quinoa seed in general is considered well balanced for human and animal nutrition, and like that of casein.

In the decade since the original publication of this book, quinoa has gone mainstream. It's become a staple of the whole foods set, it's popping up on the menus of more and more restaurants, while an increasing number of people are becoming aware of it. And it's about time. It makes a great base for a salad, it's terrific as a hot side dish, and it's ideal for breakfast. It's high protein, low glycemic, and generally delicious. What's not to like?

Preparing and Eating Quinoa

You can use quinoa to make flour, soup, or breakfast cereal. Most quinoa sold in the United States has been sold as whole grain that is cooked separately as rice or in combination dishes such as pilaf. Noted natural-foods expert and author Rebecca Wood suggests cooking about 2 cups (473 ml) of stock or water per cup (340 g) of quinoa, which should yield about 3 cups (555 g) of cooked grain and take only about 15 minutes to prepare. She reminds us that it is as versatile as rice and much more nutritious. Try substituting quinoa for rice in any recipe, or use it alone as a side dish.

Quinoa has a lower sodium content and is higher in calcium, phosphorus, magnesium, potassium, copper, manganese, and zinc than wheat, barley, or corn. It's particularly high in iron—½ cup (93 g) contains almost 8 mg, way more than any other cereal grain. And last but hardly least, it contains a hefty 5 g of fiber.

Teff

Teff is a grain, but it's a grain with an old soul. It was one of the earliest plants to be domesticated, probably between 4,000 and 1,000 B.C.E. in the Ethiopian highlands, and it continues to be a staple of traditional Ethiopian cooking. Along with spelt, amaranth, barley, kamut, and millet (and a few others), teff is considered an ancient grain.

It also has the distinction of being the smallest grain in the world. A single kernel of wheat is as big as one hundred grains of teff! In fact, the word "teff" comes from the Ehio-Semitic root *tff* which basically means "lost"—because of the size of the grain! Get it?

Teff is a nutritional heavyweight, certainly as far as grains go. One cup of cooked teff (252 g) has 10 grams of protein and 7 grams of dietary fiber, not to mention a whole bunch of nutrients like potassium, phosphorus, calcium, and magnesium. And it's one of the best food sources for manganese.

One reason we're hearing a lot about teff these days is that it's naturally gluten-free. The National Research Council of the United States suggested that teff seeds are more nutritious than wheat (National Research Council, 1996), and that they contain higher amounts of the essential amino acids. The overall amino acid profile of teff is regarded as well balanced.

Teff is known to have a subtle yet nutty flavor. It can be used as a cereal—it makes a great porridge—or it can be used to thicken soups and stews. It's also used as a flour, and it makes a great wheat alternative.

WORTH KNOWING

You only need a few seeds of teff to sow an entire field. Plus it's able to grow in tricky climates (e.g., the arid lands of Ethiopia). It requires only a small amount of land, and it produces a high yield, making it a great grain for the planet.

Grain Runner-Up

Rice (brown)

Depending on which of the different varieties we're talking about—and how it's prepared—rice can be a great food or it can be a useless waste of time. There are thousands of strains of rice today, including those grown in the wild and those that are cultivated as a crop; more than 550 million tons of the stuff are produced annually around the world, 92 percent of it in Asia. So, two folks may both be talking about eating rice, but, from a nutritional point of view, they may in fact be eating entirely different foods.

While white rice accounts for most of the rice eaten worldwide, brown rice is by far the more nutritious of the two, mainly because brown rice is the entire grain of rice, while white rice has had the bran layer removed. Stripping the grain of its bran layer strips it of many its fiber content along with many of its vitamins and minerals. Brown rice only has the outer hull removed, and it retains such nutrients as niacin, vitamin B6, magnesium, manganese, phosphorus, selenium, and even some vitamin E.

A cup (195 g) of cooked brown rice contains about 4 g of fiber (four times the amount in white rice). Even better, most of it is insoluble fiber that helps protect against various types of cancers, including colon, breast, and prostate.

Rice in general is pretty much a no-no on low-carb diets because of its high glycemic impact. In general, rice raises blood sugar quickly, causing all sorts of problems for those concerned with diabetes or weight. The fiber in brown rice does help lower the glycemic index of some varieties, but still does not make rice a low-glycemic food.

So what's the best advice? If you eat rice, stick with whole grain. Forget about white, and avoid instant rice. Consider using rice the way the Europeans and Asians do, as a small side dish, about the size of an ice cream scoop.

Rice can be a decent food, but not if it's been processed to death like most of the rice we see in industrial nations. In my opinion, the best use of conventional, processed, instant white rice is as a packing material.

WORTH KNOWING

There's a substance in brown rice called oryzanol that's mainly found in the rice bran oil. Back in the day, oryzanol was touted for its ability to interfere with cholesterol absorption. It was also rumored to increase testosterone and to be good for menopause, neither of which has ever been confirmed in any reputable study. Because of the oryzanol content, a lot of people promote rice bran oil as a health food. It's not. Rice bran oil is highly refined and has a terrible ratio of omega-6s to omega-3s (27:1). And the health benefits of oryzanol range from nonexistent to highly exaggerated. Take a pass.

THE EXPERTS' TOP TEN LISTS

Mark Houston, M.D., M.S., F.A.C.P.

Mark Houston is my go-to guy for anything at all to do with hypertension or metabolic syndrome. He's a clinical professor of medicine at Vanderbilt University Medical School and director at Hypertension Institute in Nashville. His book, *What Your Doctor May Not Tell You about Hypertension: The Revolutionary Nutrition and Lifestyle Program to Help Fight High Blood Pressure,* should be required reading—I recommend it to everyone. I love his practice philosophy, "A wise healer uses that which works," and I love him!

1. **Spinach:** This vegetable contains thirteen flavonoids with anticancer properties and is especially effective against prostate, skin, colon, and bone cancer. It's a natural anti-inflammatory, is good brain food, reduces neurological damage after strokes, improves vision, and is a good source of iron. Plus it contains four natural ACE inhibitors to reduce blood pressure, and vitamin K for osteoporosis prevention.

2. **Kale:** This contains organosulfur compounds for cancer prevention. It improves detoxification, reduces cataracts due to the lutein and zeaxanthin that it contains, plus it's a great antioxidant with fiber, calcium, and cardiovascular protection.

3. **Broccoli:** This contains numerous agents such as sulforaphane and the indoles (indole-3-carbinole and DIM) that are protective against prostate, gastric, skin, and breast cancer. The flavonoids reduce cardiovascular disease and blood pressure. Broccoli contains compounds that are anti-inflammatory and antioxidant and support the immune system and the eyes.

4, 5. **Blueberries and blackberries:** Blueberries have the highest antioxidant capacity, making them highly protective for the cardiovascular system. They contain pterostilbene, which lowers cholesterol, and anthocyanins, which improve vision and brain function and guard against macular degeneration. The ellagic acid in them has anticancer activity. Blackberries are similar.

6. **Strawberries:** This fruit contains phenols such as anthocyanins and ellagitannins, which are potent antioxidants and anti-inflammatory agents; they're natural COX-2 inhibitors. Strawberries help improve brain function, reduce macular degeneration, and improve rheumatoid arthritis. The ellagitannin helps prevent colon cancer.

7. **Raspberries:** They contain ellagic acid, quercetin, kaempferol, and other flavonoids that are great antioxidants with anticancer properties; plus, they support eye and cardiovascular health.

8. **Cold-water fish (e.g., tuna, salmon, mackerel, cod, and herring):** Their omega-3 fats offer cardiovascular protection and reduce heart attacks, sudden death, and cardiac arrhythmias. The omega-3s are anti-inflammatory and improve brain function, memory, skin health, and kidney function. Plus they lower blood pressure and reduce triglycerides, cancer risk, and stroke risk.

9. **Whey protein:** This boosts the body's stores of glutathione, one of the most important antioxidants. Whey protein contains natural ACE inhibitors, which lower blood pressure and improve cardiovascular health. It also improves immune function.

10. **Wild game (venison, caribou):** Wild game is high-quality protein with a complete complement of amino acids, low saturated fat, no trans fat, and a higher content of polyunsaturated and especially omega-3 fats. It also contains natural ACE inhibitors, which reduce blood pressure, and compounds that improve skin, bone, and vascular health.

CHAPTER 3

BEANS AND LEGUMES

When I first introduced this section ten years ago, I had some hesitations about including them in a book on the world's healthiest foods. That I would have any hesitation at all may seem surprising to you, but at the time I was very influenced by the writing of professor Loren Cordain, Ph.D., an authority on ancestral diets and one of the original founders of the Paleo movement.

Cordain—and most of the Paleo gurus who came after him—shun beans because of their lectin content (more on that in a moment). But in the years since, I've come to believe that the lectins in beans are only a problem for about 10 percent of the population. For everyone else, beans are superfoods.

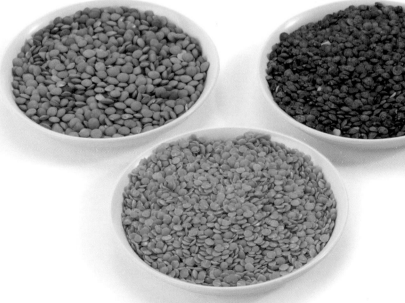

You'll read all about the positive aspects of beans in the coming entries: Beans are loaded with fiber, which has been associated with lower risk of heart disease, diabetes, obesity, and cancer. The exploding research on the microbiome and gut health in general has shown us that fiber does even more than we thought it did ten years ago. Fiber feeds the good bacteria in your gut, helping to keep your gut healthy while promoting the creation of important compounds in the gut like butyric acid.

Beans contain protein. They digest very slowly, providing sustained energy and making them an ideal food for those who need to avoid the blood-sugar roller coaster. And they're loaded with protective phytochemicals, antioxidants, and vitamins.

And Now the Bad News: Lectins Spell Trouble for Some

Lectins are substances contained in legumes and grains that originally evolved to fight off insect predators. But a portion of the lectin can bind with tissues in our body and create problems. Loren Cordain, Ph.D.—the aforementioned Paleo guru and a highly respected researcher at the University of Colorado—published a paper in the *British Journal of Nutrition* detailing a theory that dairy foods, legumes, grains, and yeast may be partly to blame for rheumatoid arthritis and other autoimmune diseases in genetically susceptible people, due in part to the lectin molecule.

According to Cordain, the lectins in food are known to increase intestinal permeability (also known as "leaky gut"). Lectins allow partially digested food proteins and remnants of gut bacteria to spill into the bloodstream. That's why Cordain calls lectins "cellular Trojan horses." They make the intestines easier to penetrate, impairing the immune system's ability to fight off food, and bacterial fragments that leak into the bloodstream. In his highly regarded book, *The Paleo Diet*, which is based on a lifetime of respected nutritional research into hunter-gatherer diets, Cordain lists all beans in his foods-to-avoid list.

Is this something the average person should be concerned about? I no longer believe it is. Obviously, beans have huge health benefits if you're not one of the people who responds badly to them. If you're one of the (admittedly small) group of people who has unexplained symptoms possibly related to food, it might be worthwhile to avoid beans till you figure out what's going on.

★ Beans

Beans are one of the best sources of fiber on the planet. And people in most industrialized societies consume much less fiber than they should. I've been singing the praises of fiber for as long as I've been writing and talking about nutrition. Fiber protects our health by slowing the entrance of food into the bloodstream and therefore helping to prevent blood sugar spikes. We now know that fiber also serves as food for the good microbes in your gut, and the importance of gut health (and the microbiome in general) is only now beginning to be appreciated. We do know that higher-fiber diets are associated with lower risks of cancer, heart disease, diabetes, and obesity.

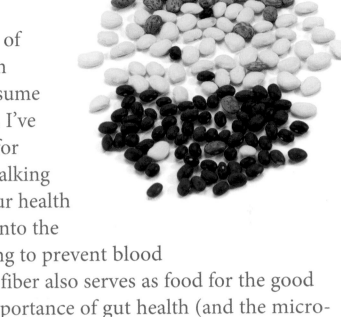

Consider this: Our Paleolithic ancestors got anywhere from 50 to 100 g of fiber a day in their diet. The National Cancer Institute—not exactly a hotbed of nutritional radicalism—recommends at least 25 g a day, as do the U.S. Dietary Guidelines. The position paper on dietary fiber and colon cancer of the American Gastroenterological Association states that "reasonable recommendations based on currently available data" argue for a recommended daily fiber intake of at least 30 to 35 g a day. In my book, *Smart Fat: Eat More Fat, Lose More Weight, Get Healthy Now*, I recommend that people consume at a minimum 30 grams of fiber a day.

Want to know the average daily intake in the United States?

Eleven grams.

Beans Provide the Fiber Missing from Our Diet

So, premise number one is that fiber is good. Premise number two is that we don't get nearly enough of it. Adding beans to your diet is a great way to correct that deficit. If for no other reason than their fiber content, beans deserve a place on your plate. Overall, a cup (172 g) of generic cooked beans will give you anywhere from 11 g (kidney beans) to an amazing 17 g (adzuki) per serving. That's phenomenal. There's no other food I know of that is as good a source of this important food component.

There's more good stuff, though most of it is related to the fiber content. Beans lower cholesterol, but if you've read my book *The Great Cholesterol Myth*, you know that I don't think that matters very much. Nonetheless, according to Patti Bazel Weil, R.D., nutrition educator at the University of Kentucky, a cup (172 g) of cooked beans a day can lower your total cholesterol by up to 10 percent in a mere six weeks. In fact, a school study showed that in only three weeks of eating ½ cup (weight will vary) of navy and pinto beans per day, the cholesterol of the male subjects was lowered by 19 percent.

Beans Are the Ultimate Blood Sugar Regulator

Beans—or at least the fiber in them—have major consequences for those with diabetes and blood sugar challenges. The soluble fiber in beans influences the rate by which glucose is absorbed. And a significant amount of research dating back to the 1970s has shown that large amounts of fiber in the diet improves hyperglycemia (high blood sugar). Low-glycemic diets were on the cutting edge of nutrition when I first wrote this book, but have since become well-recognized as being one of the healthiest dietary strategies around. They're routinely recommended—even by the nutrition and medical establishment—for diabetics, those with weight challenges, and those with metabolic syndrome; frankly, they should probably be recommended for everyone. And beans are the ultimate low-glycemic food. Their high fiber content means they raise blood sugar very, very slowly, and eating high-fiber foods like beans has been shown in several studies to improve glycemic control—the regulation of blood sugar and insulin.

Then there's cancer. Based on analysis of food questionnaires in the Nurses' Health Study II, researchers found a significant reduced frequency of breast cancer in those women who consumed a higher intake of common beans or lentils. What's more, it didn't take all that much to produce the result: Eating beans or lentils two (or more) times a week resulted in a 24 percent reduced risk!

It's reasonable to assume that some of the anti-cancer effect comes from other compounds in beans besides the fiber. One phytochemical that is found in beans—diosgenin—appears to inhibit cancer cells from multiplying. And phytochemicals in beans such as saponins, protease inhibitors, and phytic acid appear to protect cells from the type of genetic damage that can lead to cancer. In laboratory studies, saponins have shown the ability to inhibit the reproduction of cancer cells and slow the growth of tumors; protease inhibitors have shown the ability to slow the division of cancer cells; and phytic acid has shown the ability to significantly slow the progression of tumors. According to one study listed on the website of the American Institute for Cancer Research, men who consumed the most beans had a 38 percent lower risk of prostate cancer than men who consumed the least.

Why Red Beans Take the Cake

Finally, if that weren't enough, there's the vitamin content of beans. They're loaded with antioxidants. The USDA's ranking of foods by antioxidant capacity lists small dried red beans as having the highest antioxidant capacity per serving size of any food tested; in fact, of the four top-scoring foods, three were beans (red beans, red kidney beans, and pinto beans). Many bean varieties have a lot of folic acid (especially adzukis, black-eyed peas, lentils, and pinto beans), which have serious benefits for the heart; there's also magnesium, iron, zinc, and potassium and—especially in red kidney beans—an important enzyme-enhancing mineral called molybdenum.

Beans are also a good source of protein, typically containing 15 g per cup (172 g). And unlike most commercial, factory-farmed animal protein sources, they don't come with any steroids, hormones, or antibiotics.

Garbanzo Beans (chickpeas)

Chickpeas are beans with a complexion problem! Though other lentils and beans have a smooth-looking "face," chickpeas have bumps that, if you look closely, resemble a chick's beak (hence the name?). But looks aren't everything. The chickpea was one of the first cultivated crops, and it is one of the most popular legumes in the world.

Chickpeas are beans with a complexion problem! Though other lentils and beans have a smooth-looking "face," chickpeas have bumps that, if you look closely, resemble a chick's beak (hence the name?). But looks aren't everything. The chickpea was one of the first cultivated crops, and it is one of the most popular legumes in the world.

Chickpeas belong to the class of food called legumes or pulses, which also includes beans, lentils, and peas. Eating more legumes can reduce the risk of coronary heart disease. In a large study of almost 10,000 men and women in the United States, those who ate pulses four or more times a week had a 22 percent lower risk of coronary heart disease and an 11 percent lower risk of cardiovascular events than those who ate pulses less than once a week. This health benefit was independent of other health habits.

And speaking of fiber, garbanzo beans weigh in at a remarkable 12.5 g per cup (240 g). That makes it a fiber heavyweight in my book, right up there with lentils (16 g). Virtually every study that has looked at high-fiber diets has found some measure of health benefits, sometimes striking ones. The results of the European Prospective Investigation into Cancer and Nutrition (EPIC) study showed that Europeans who ate the most fiber had an almost 40 percent lower risk of colon cancer than those who ate the least. As much as I promoted fiber back when the first edition of this book came out, the latest research on the microbiome shows that fiber is even more important than we thought it was because it makes an important contribution to gut health. Garbanzo beans are a great way to add fiber to your diet.

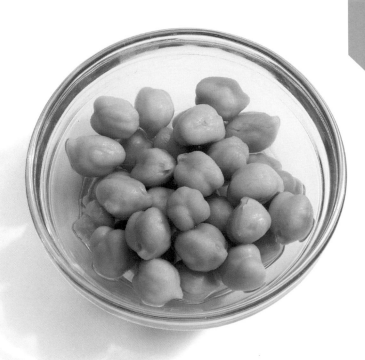

Garbanzos Curb Overeating

Fiber—particularly soluble fiber—can also lower blood cholesterol levels and slow the absorption of sugar, which is hugely important both for people with diabetes and for people with any blood sugar challenges (metabolic syndrome). Soluble fiber also serves as food for the good microbes in your gut. And a high-fiber diet will probably reduce the risk of developing type 2 diabetes. Legumes in general cause less of a rise in blood glucose than foods such as potatoes or almost any wheat-based food such as cereal.

Eating a high-fiber diet may also help with weight loss. High-fiber foods generally require more chewing time, giving your body extra time to register the fact that you're no longer hungry, so you're less likely to overeat. A high-fiber diet also tends to fill you up longer. And high-fiber diets tend to have more volume for fewer calories, which has been shown in research by Barbara Rolls, Ph.D., at Pennsylvania State University to be a boon to weight management. In my book, *Living Low Carb*, I suggested that the number-one supplement for weight loss was fiber, and well more than a decade later, I still stand by that statement!

Chickpeas also have calcium and magnesium in a great 1:1 ratio, a decent amount of folate, and a ton of heart-healthy potassium (477 mg per cup [240 g]!). They even contain the powerful antioxidant mineral selenium. All this, plus the vegetable equivalent of 2 ounces of protein!

Noted natural-foods expert Rebecca Wood warns that if your only contact with chickpeas has been at a salad bar, you're missing out on some serious flavor. She suggests simmering them till tender with garlic and toasted cumin seeds and then getting ready to enjoy one of the creamiest, tastiest beans on the planet. You can also cook, season, and roast them for a snack that replaces nuts and chips.

Green Peas

When I was a kid, these were my favorite vegetable. I used to melt butter over them, then salt them, and mix them with my mashed potatoes. I loved it. Go figure.

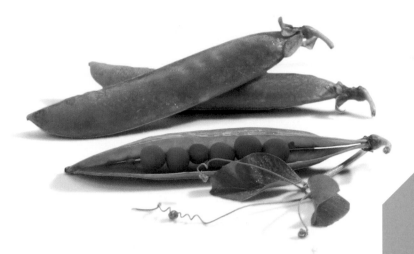

Peas are legumes that originated in western Asia. In Switzerland, traces of peas have been found near home-sites, where they were probably being eaten during the Bronze Age, more than 5,000 years ago. Traveling from Greece to India, the pea arrived in China during the seventh century, where it was named *ho tou*, or "foreign legume." Peas were popular during the Middle Ages in Europe, being easy to grow, inexpensive, hearty, and a source of protein.

There are probably more than 1,000 varieties of garden peas, the most common of which are the smooth peas you usually find frozen in the supermarket. Some varieties, like the snow pea (see page 77) have edible pods. Peas are available fresh in the pod, dried (either whole or split), and frozen. They're also available canned, but never in a million years would I recommend that you eat them. One reason they're such a dull green is that the health-promoting chlorophyll is destroyed by the heat of the canning process, along with most of the other nutrients. My opinion on canned vegetables in general is that they're next to useless.

Peas Are Packed with Vitamins A and K

Peas are a little high in sugar as legumes (or vegetables) go, but that's balanced by the fact that 100 g—a little more than ½ cup—of cooked peas has 5.5 g of fiber. Peas also have 42 percent of the Daily Value for vitamin A, and 5 g of vegetable protein. They're also low calorie (78 calories for 100 g). And 100 g of peas contains 30 percent of the Daily Value for vitamin K, an important vitamin that helps anchor calcium to the places in the bone where you need it to be, thus making this vitamin an essential part of a nutrition program for bone health.

Dried peas don't hold their shape as well as the fresh (or frozen) peas, and their taste is a little earthier than the sweeter fresh ones. They're best used in purees, soups, and dishes that need some thickening. Dried peas, being more concentrated and dense than the fresh variety (which are more than 70 percent water) are even higher in fiber—½ cup (112 g) of dried split peas has more than 8 g. Not many foods can make that claim.

THE REAL DEAL ON FIBER: IT'S MUCH MORE IMPORTANT THAN WE THOUGHT

When I was a kid, my grandmother was always trying to get me to eat a lot foods you had to chew a lot. "Gives you roughage," she'd say wisely. "Keeps you regular."

Well, that was then, this is now.

Our prune-eating grandmothers were onto something, but they had just scratched the tip of the iceberg. Research on fiber is exploding, and its résumé of health benefits now extends to weight loss, as well as cancer, diabetes, heart disease, and blood sugar management. Fiber is essential to the care and feeding of a healthy microbiome.

What's more, the old conventional wisdom about there being only two kinds of fiber (soluble and insoluble) was upended in the 1980s when two English researchers—Englyst and Cummings—discovered a third kind of fiber called resistant starch which, as of this writing in 2016, is currently the subject of an enormous amount of research interest. (More on this in a moment.)

So what is fiber? What does it do? Why do we need it? And why should we care? Let's start with weight loss.

Fiber's not expensive, it's not exotic, and it's certainly not sexy, but when it comes to weight loss, it works like a charm. More than a dozen clinical studies have used dietary fiber supplements for weight loss, most with positive outcomes. When you take the fiber supplement with water before meals, the water-soluble fiber binds to water in the stomach, making you feel full and less likely to overeat. It also suppresses hunger. Fiber supplements have also been shown to enhance blood sugar control and insulin effects. It has even been shown to reduce the number of calories that the body absorbs—adding up to about 3 to 18 pounds (1 to 4 kg) a year. And a study in the *New England Journal of Medicine* found that a diet with 50 g of fiber today lowered insulin levels in the blood. For the record, insulin's two common nicknames among health professionals are "the hunger hormone" and "the fat-storing hormone."

My co-author on the book, *Smart Fat*—Steven Masley, M.D.—followed patients at his south Florida clinic for ten years, tracking what they ate, how much exercise they did, what vitamins they took, and how much weight they lost. He found that fiber intake was one of three variables that predicted weight loss success better than anything else. (The other two were minutes spent exercising and vitamin D intake.) The study was presented as a poster at the 2015 annual meeting of the American College of Nutrition.

One of the most impressive studies of all followed 2,900 healthy subjects for ten years and looked at the relationship between fiber, cardiovascular disease, weight, and insulin. The results were spectacular. Fiber was inversely associated with insulin levels and weight, and low fiber intake turned out to be a better predictor of heart disease than saturated-fat consumption. That finding, which was once eyebrow-raising, is no longer surprising, as at least two major peer-reviewed meta-analyses published in major journals have found that saturated fat does not cause heart disease.

Remember, the benefits of fiber aren't limited to weight loss. High blood sugar and high insulin have now been implicated in a baker's dozen of unwanted degenerative disease, including heart disease. Even Alzheimer's is now being called "type 3 diabetes" because of the connection to insulin resistance, which has consequences not only for your waistline but for your brain as well.

Americans currently get a paltry amount of fiber in their diets, estimated at around 10 to 11 grams a day. That's not nearly enough. I don't usually agree with conventional recommendations from traditional health agencies, but in this case, they're on the right track: Current recommendations range from 25 g to 38 g a day (depending on age and sex), but in my opinion more is better. Our caveman ancestors got much more—50 to 100 grams daily, according to most research.

So let's talk about what fiber is, where it's found, and how to get more of it.

There are three kinds of fiber:

Insoluble fiber is what your grandmother was talking about when she said to eat roughage. It doesn't break down in the gut, so it acts as a bulking agent and is good for relieving constipation.

Soluble fiber does break down in the gut. It's specifically broken down by good bacteria which convert it into short-chain fatty acids (SCFAs), the most important of which is butyric acid (also known as butyrate).

Why is this so important? Because the cells that line the gut depend on butyrate for food. "Butyrate has been around in the mammalian gut for so long that the lining of our large intestine has evolved to use it as its primary source of energy," writes obesity researcher and neurobiologist Stephen Guyenet, Ph.D. "It also has potent anti-inflammatory and anticancer effects." Butyrate—or butyric acid—supplements are frequently used in inflammatory bowel diseases, such as ulcerative colitis and Crohn's disease. If you're not getting enough soluble fiber (and resistant starch, as we'll see in a moment), you're probably not making enough butyric acid.

Resistant starch is the third kind of fiber, so named because it literally resists breakdown (or digestion). And it's currently getting a lot of research attention. Instead of being broken down by enzymes, resistant starch makes its way directly through the small intestine and winds up in the colon, where—much like soluble fiber—it becomes food for good bacteria in the gut (sometimes called "probiotics"). Resistant starch is their favorite food, ever. In fact, gut bacteria create more butyric acid (butyrate) from resistant starch than they do from any other fiber. Butyric acid that comes from the metabolism of resistant starch is the number one source of butyric acid in the body.

Remember, butyric acid is pure joy to the cells that line your gut, and it keeps the cells healthy. Theoretically at least, that means less chance of leaky gut and all the myriad problems that can accompany it. A healthy, well-fed gut lining helps make for a healthy microbiome. That's one reason that soluble fiber and resistant fiber are both often known as prebiotics—they are food for the probiotics in your gut. All prebiotics are fiber, but not all fiber is prebiotic. The indigestible, insoluble kind your grandma called roughage, although important, is not prebiotic fiber because it can't be broken down and metabolized into short-chain fatty acids by the good bacteria in your gut. Prebiotics, on the other hand, are what keep your good bugs alive and thriving.

We now know how important a diverse and thriving microbiome is, and how important gut health is to overall health. That means ensuring the gut cells are well nourished with prebiotic fiber—and its metabolite, butyric acid. Feeding those cells resistant starch and soluble fiber is a good beginning! Resistant starch, in particular, even improves insulin sensitivity. Mark Sisson calls it "top-shelf food for your gut bugs."

Interesting factoid: In 1981, the *American Journal of Clinical Nutrition* published a paper by Thomas Almy, M.D., called "The Dietary Fiber Hypothesis." The Fiber Hypothesis, as it's now called, basically put forth the notion that high-fiber diets were protective against a potential host of diseases. But researchers recently pointed out that some of the low-risk African populations that gave rise to the fiber hypothesis in the first place didn't consume high-fiber diets; they did, however, consume diets high in resistant starch.

Food sources of soluble fiber include beans, oatmeal, Brussels sprouts, apples, nuts, blueberries, oranges, and flaxseeds. Food sources of insoluble fiber (known to grandma as roughage) include the seeds and skins of fruits (eat the peel!), avocados (especially Florida avocados), wheat bran, and brown rice. Food sources of resistant starch include white beans, chickpeas, lentils, rolled oats, peas, black beans, red beans, kidney beans, unripe bananas, and potato starch.

I'm a big believer in fiber supplements, simply because just about no one gets the ideal amount from food anymore. I'm a fan of Sunfiber, which is a soluble (prebiotic) fiber that can be added to a host of foods and beverages. It's used as an ingredient in many commercial fiber supplements, and available under the Sunfiber brand. I put a scoop of it in all my shakes—it's odorless and tasteless and mixes well. If you're looking specifically for resistant starch, try Bob's Red Mill Potato Starch, which my friend Mark Hyman, M.D., calls "the starch that makes you lean and healthy." Potato starch—unlike potatoes—won't raise blood sugar.

And yes, you most certainly can use both!

★ Lentils

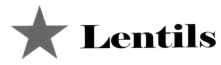

Lentils are small, disk-shaped legumes that grow on an annual bushlike plant. Lentils are native to central Asia. They're used throughout the Mediterranean region and the Middle East and are especially popular in India, where they're cooked to a puree called dahl, an amazing-tasting lentil curry. The crisp Indian crackers called pappadams are made with lentil flour. In the United States, lentils are often enjoyed in soup.

Lentils are dried as soon as they ripen and then sold that way. There are at least fifty varieties of lentils in addition to the brown variety most common in the West, with colors that range from yellow to red-orange to green. Lentils are distinguished from beans in that they don't contain sulfur and therefore don't produce gas. So anyone wanting the benefits of high fiber without the social unpleasantness associated with beans would do well to check out this cool little legume.

The history of lentils goes way back. The earliest archaeological dating of lentils is from the Paleolithic and Mesolithic layers of Franchthi Cave in Greece (13,000 to 9,500 years ago), and from the end-Mesolithic at Mureybit and Tell Abu Hureya in Syria, and about 8000 BCE in the Jericho area of Palestine. The ancient Greeks used lentils in a variety of ways, including breadmaking. Catholics who could not afford to buy fish during Lent ate lentils. The double

convex optical lens gets its name "lenticular" from the shape of the lentil.

Lentils Help Treat High Cholesterol and High Blood Sugar

The real claim to fame for lentils is the fact that they're so loaded with fiber, especially soluble fiber. Soluble fiber breaks down as it passes though the digestive tract, forming a gel. It also helps control blood sugar by delaying the emptying of the stomach and retarding the entry of sugar into the bloodstream. This is why high-fiber foods like lentils have such a low glycemic load. Because fiber slows the digestion of foods, it can help blunt the sudden spikes in blood sugar and insulin that can cause you to be hungry again an hour after eating a low-fiber meal. Those constant spikes in blood sugar and insulin can also contribute to diabetes and can make weight very hard to take off. High-fiber diets have been consistently associated with better glucose control for both diabetics and nondiabetics, and with better management of weight. High-fiber diets also are associated with lower risks for cancer and heart disease.

In recent years, a third type of fiber has gotten a lot of research attention—it's called resistant starch. (See page 96.) Lentils are a great source of resistant starch, which serves as food for the good bacteria in your gut. You get the most resistant starch when you cool the lentils—resistant starch is formed during the cooling process—but lentils have so much of it that even if you eat them warm (as most people do), they still have plenty.

A cup (198 g) of lentils contains a nice amount of protein—about 18 g. But best of all, that same cup contains a whopping 16 g of fiber. That's an awesome combination, and a rare one. Lentils are also a terrific source of folate and a good source of at least seven minerals. One cup provides 37 percent of the Daily Value for iron and 49 percent of the Daily Value for manganese, an important trace mineral that's essential for growth, reproduction, wound healing, peak brain function, and the proper metabolism of sugars, insulin, and cholesterol.

WORTH KNOWING

Unlike beans, lentils need no presoaking and are ready in 20 to 30 minutes. Brown and green lentils hold their shape well after cooking and are excellent for salads or other dishes where you want texture. Red lentils cook quicker and work best in purees and other dishes where softness is an advantage.

Unfortunately, the lentils used to make those delicious Indian dahls I mentioned earlier have had their outer skins removed, which lowers their nutritional value, especially the fiber content. They're still delicious, though, and they do still have some fiber left.

Tamarind

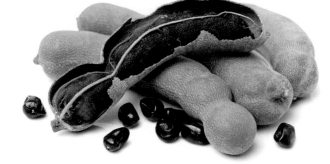

Put simply, tamarind is a fruit with benefits.

That fruit is also a legume. It comes from a tree known as *Tamarindus indica*, which is native to Africa, but grows in many other tropical regions in the Indian sub-continent, Pakistan, and Bangladesh. The tree produces pods that kind of look like edamame, only they're a light orange. Inside the pods are seeds, with a fibrous pulp around them. That pulp starts off sour but thickens into a kind of paste as it ripens, and the taste becomes more sweet-sour.

So what are the benefits I mentioned earlier? Let's start with its antimicrobial effect.

Research shows that extract of tamarind has antibacterial properties against at least seven different microbes, including E. coli and Staphylococcus aureus, the bacterium that causes staph infections. It's believed that the antibacterial effect of the plant is due to its lupeol content.

Tamarind and tamarind extract are used for abdominal pain, diarrhea, dysentery, some bacterial infections, parasites, wound healing, constipation, and inflammation (Kuru, 2014). And it's a rich source of phytochemicals and most of the essential amino acids. One research paper noted that tamarind has "a good potential to contribute to affordable local health care based on traditional medicine."

Tamarind is high in nutrients. A cup (120 g) of the pulp has magnesium, potassium, iron, vitamin B_1 (thiamine), B_2 (riboflavin), and niacin. Although it doesn't contain spectacularly high amounts of these nutrients, it does have a decent amount—28 percent of the RDI for magnesium, for example, and 34 percent of the RDI for vitamin B_1. (Of course, I think the RDIs for most nutrients are ridiculously low, but still.)

My colleague, Kris Gunnars of Authority Nutrition, notes that you can use the fruit to "add a sour note to savory dishes," using it, for example, instead of lemon. You can find the fruit in the form of raw pods (which you open to remove the pulp), a pressed block (the seeds and shell are removed, and the pulp is pressed into a block), or as a concentrate (a pulp that has been boiled down, and may have preservatives added).

Just be aware that tamarind is high in sugar. Gunnars suggests that the healthiest way to eat this fruit is either raw or as an ingredient in savory dishes.

THE EXPERTS' TOP TEN LISTS

Steven Masley, M.D., L.L.C.

Steven Masley, M.D., L.L.C., is the host of one of the most successful and popular PBS health shows of all time, *Thirty Days to a Younger Heart*. He's a physician, nutritionist, speaker, researcher, and a best-selling author.

I've worked closely with Steven— he was my coauthor on *Smart Fat: Eat More Fat, Lose More Weight, Get Healthy Now*, and he's one of the smartest M.D.s I know. He's a fellow of the American Heart Association *and* the American Academy of Family Physicians, plus he's also a fellow of the American College of Nutrition. (Fun fact: He's a trained chef, having spent a year studying at the Four Seasons.)

Having hung out with him for about a year while we were working on *Smart Fat*, I know that Steven routinely seeks out foods that have a documented benefit on heart and brain health.

1. **Green cruciferous vegetables (broccoli, kale, Brussel sprouts).** Eating 1 cup (weights vary) of green eafy vegetables each day can help extend life expectancy by eleven years. Green leafy veggies protect you from aging and are loaded with fiber, vitamin K, mixed folates, potassium, and healthy plant pigments. And the crucifers have compounds that improve detoxification and reduce your risk for cancer.

2. **Beets.** The pigments in beets improve circulation, helping exercise performance and sexual function.

3. **Wild salmon.** This is one of the best sources of the anti-inflammatory long-chain omega-3 fats, plus a terrific source of protein, potassium, and selenium.

4. **Extra-virgin olive oil.** It provides fantastic flavor to salads and a wide variety of dishes, plus helps lower your risk for heart attacks, strokes, and memory loss. Cook with it on medium or lower heat.

5. **Avocado/avocado oil.** Avocados are a rich source of fiber, monounsaturated oil, potassium, and they taste fantastic. Avocado oil has become my favorite cooking oil, for its delicate flavor, its healthy monounsaturated fat, and the fact that it tolerates medium-high heat without being damaged.

6. **Berries and cherries.** The anthocyanins (pigments) in berries and cherries block inflammation and oxidation, and both are a wonderful source of vitamins. They taste fantastic whether eaten raw, added to a smoothie, or used in a recipe. Consuming more berries will help prevent heart disease and protect against memory loss.

7. **Dark chocolate.** What's not to like about dark chocolate? It protects your arteries from plaque growth, protects against memory loss, and improves blood pressure control. It's delicious and packed with fiber and magnesium. Purchase varieties not loaded with sugar; look for bars with at least 74 percent cocoa.

8. **Red wine.** One to two servings of red wine with dinner improves blood sugar control, protects you from heart attack and stroke, improves cognitive function and prevents memory loss. It helps with digestion, kills harmful microbes, and makes dinner taste wonderful. The challenge is limiting it to one or two 4.5-ounce servings, and never drinking more than three per day; excessive alcohol intake of any type—including red wine—is harmful.

9. **Curry spices.** Curry spice lowers oxidation and inflammation, protects the brain from cognitive decline, and decreases the risk for cancer. The most studied component of curry spice is turmeric, which contains the active ingredient curcumin.

10. **Italian herb seasoning.** This combination of herbs is my favorite cooking seasoning. It adds fantastic flavor to almost anything I'm preparing and the combination of herbs lowers oxidation and inflammation.

CHAPTER 4

FRUIT

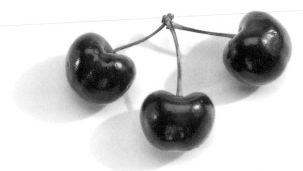

Let's be clear on one thing: There are no bad fruits.

Fruit has gotten a bad rap from some sections of the low-carb and Paleo community, but I think their assessment of fruit is generally too harsh. Sure there's sugar in fruit, but it's bound with fiber, phytonutrients, vitamins, minerals, flavonoids, and all kinds of other good compounds. Unless you're highly sensitive to sugar of any kind in any amount, most fruits won't present a problem for you and should be an integral (and delicious) part o a nutritious diet.

Selecting fruits for this book presented a problem that I didn't encounter in many of the other categories (except vegetables): an embarrassment of riches. The problem wasn't finding fruits that belong on the list, it was eliminating worthy contenders to get the list down to manageable proportions.

Of course, some fruits are just absolute superstars and there was never any question that even if there were to be only ten foods on the list, they'd make the cut. Apples and blueberries, for example. And guava. If this list were an all-star basketball team going to the Olympics, they'd be the Kobe Bryants. To continue the analogy, we also found some good utility players that, while terrific, wouldn't have made a short list of Olympic contenders. The star fruit, for example, is not quite as loaded with nutrients as some of the winners, plus it's harder to find and smaller in size. Star fruits went on the runners-up list.

Why Some Fruits Didn't Make the Cut

Sometimes the selection process had to do with convenience, and sometimes the decision considered whether the fruit was most commonly available. And, sometimes, things change. For example, pomegranate is a great fruit, but it takes a lot of work to eat it, and the edible part of the fruit is small. So when the first edition of this book came out, pomegranate seeds didn't make the cut, but the widely available pomegranate juice did. Since the publication of the first edition, that's no longer the case. Pomegranate seeds have become widely available at grocery stores such as Trader Joe's and Whole Foods. The work is done for you—they dig out all the edible, delicious seeds from the inedible pulp, and then package them in a little plastic container. They're expensive, but they're fantastic. I highly recommended them if you don't mind spending a little extra for the convenience of not having to dig the seeds out of the fruit.

Noni and acai berries also presented a couple of problems. The noni berry tastes terrible (but the juice does not—see page 290); plus, you can't find the berry itself anywhere but the tropics. The acai berry used to be only available in Brazil, but since the publication of this book you can now find them in the United States, and acai juice products can be found everywhere. The goji berry (see page 118) originally made its way to the United States in both berry and juice form. I decided to include the whole goji berry on the list because space was limited and the juice isn't as well known or widely available.

Although the mantra "eat more fruits and vegetables" has been repeated so often it's become a cliché, it's worth pointing out that fruits and vegetables as categories are quite distinct from a blood sugar point of view. If you forced me to choose one of the two categories, it would be no contest: Vegetables are the clear winner. That's because fruit—wonderful though it is—does have more sugar and has the potential to play havoc with both blood sugar and insulin. For this reason, there are dietary programs (for example, most low-carb programs) that don't allow fruit at all during the first few weeks. Almost all the nutrients found in fruits are obtainable in vegetables, and with substantially less impact on blood sugar.

High Blood Sugar? You Can Still Eat Fruit

Does this mean that people watching their weight or their blood sugar should avoid fruit? Not at all. But if you're in that category, fruit is not an unlimited item. Much has been written about the sugar impact of fruits, and if you're concerned about sugar, or if weight, diabetes, or metabolic syndrome are issues for you, it would be wise to read more about on the subject of glycemic index and glycemic load. (See the introduction to this book, page 8, for more information.)

If you're not overweight and don't have issues with blood sugar, there are no concerns about fruit at all. Eat it, juice it, consume it raw or cooked, just make it a part of your daily routine (along, of course, with tons of vegetables).

The ancient Greek aphorism "Know thyself" was inscribed in golden letters at the entrance to the Temple of Apollo at Delphi. It's as true now as it was then. Some people are more sensitive to sugar than others. That's just how it is. To quote Shakespeare, "To thine own self be true"—it's the key to making good choices in food as well as good choices in life.

Apples

"An apple a day keeps the doctor away" is a good example of one of those old clichés that actually turns out to be right. Researchers at Oxford University found out that eating even one medium-sized apple a day (or a handful of fresh strawberries) could slash heart disease risk by an impressive 40 percent.

Apples have certainly rehabilitated their image since first becoming known as the little fruit that brought down the Garden of Eden. Their résumé of health benefits could easily fill a book. Epidemiological studies have linked the consumption of apples with reduced risk of some cancers, cardiovascular disease, asthma, and diabetes. And that's just for openers.

Apples contain quercetin, a flavonoid that, in a 2001 Mayo Clinic study, helped prevent the growth of prostate cancer cells. Another study, at Cornell University, showed that phytochemicals in the skin of an apple inhibited the reproduction of colon cancer cells by 43 percent. And the National Cancer Institute reported that foods containing flavonoids may reduce the risk of lung cancer by as much as 50 percent.

Apples' Antioxidant Power

But wait, there's more!

Apples contain a host of phytochemicals, including quercetin, catechin, phloridzin, and chlorogenic acid. So what does that mean for you? Strong—really strong—antioxidant power. Since both cardiovascular disease and cancer are thought to be highly related to what's called oxidative stress (the damage done to cells and DNA by oxidation), the ability to fight off the destructive effects of that oxidation is a major weapon in the healing power of any food. Apples have that antioxidant power in spades. In fact, apples have the second highest level of antioxidant activity of any other commonly consumed fruit in the United States (beaten out only by cranberries).

Apples are also high in phenolic compounds, a huge class of biochemically active substances most of which belong to the flavonoid group. There are literally thousands of flavonoids, but all you really need to know about them is this: they are really, really good for you. And compared to every other fruit, apples have the highest portion of free phenolics. While that may sound like the phenolics just got out of prison, it means they're not attached to other compounds in the fruit, which in turn means they're more available for absorption into your bloodstream, where they can go to work providing you with all the amazing health benefits and cancer-fighting ability they have to offer.

FRUIT

Apple Eaters Enjoy a Lower Risk of Tumors, Lung Cancer, and Cardiovascular Problems

Now we already know from a zillion studies that eating more fruits and vegetables helps protect against a host of diseases. In data involving 34,467 women in the Nurses' Health Study, frequent consumption of fruit in general was found to be associated with a significant reduction in the risk of developing colorectal adenomas (benign tumors).

It's not often, however, that the individual fruits or vegetables are examined for their impact. But in the Nurses' Health Study and the Health Professionals Follow-up Study, women who consumed at least one serving per day of apples and pears had a reduced risk of lung cancer. In a study conducted in Hawaii, there was a 40 to 50 percent decreased risk in lung cancer in participants with the highest intake of apples, onions, and white grapefruit. Other studies have also shown a relationship between flavonoid intake—particularly quercetin—and the development of cancer. And in the Women's Health Study, the women ingesting the highest amounts of flavonoids had a 35 percent reduction in the risk of cardiovascular events.

Apple consumption has been inversely linked with asthma (the more apples, the less asthma). And apples may also be associated with a lower risk for diabetes. In a study in Finland, apple consumption was associated with a reduced risk of type 2 diabetes, and in a study in Brazil it was associated with weight loss.

Apples contain pectin, a valuable source of soluble fiber that can lower LDL cholesterol and help regulate blood sugar. Speaking of sugar: Yes, apples do have some sugar (fructose), but I wouldn't worry about it (unless you are a diabetic or have serious blood sugar challenges). The sugar in apples come wrapped with 5 g of fiber and a rich blend of nutrients, very different from the high-fructose corn syrup used to sweeten every junk food on the market. And one study, by Silvina Lotito, Ph.D. of the Linus Pauling Institute, suggests that the fructose in apples might even turn out to be responsible for some of the apple's health benefits.

Osteoporosis and Apples

Oh yes, one more thing. No one ever seems to mention this, but apples are one of the best dietary sources of boron. Boron is a mineral that has real bone-building properties, and it is an important part of an osteoporosis prevention program. An article in the *Journal of Applied Nutrition* by Rex E. Newnham, Ph.D., D.O., demonstrated a high probability that there's a connection between not having enough boron in your system and having symptoms of arthritis. This arthritis-boron connection was observed in various populations around the world. Boron also seems to be energizing.

My friend John Hernandez, M.D., director of the Center for Health and Integration in San Antonio, Texas, tells of a study in which drowsy college sophomores were given supplements of 3 mg of boron—all of a sudden, no more falling asleep in class. Sure, it's anecdotal evidence, but clinical experience should never be ignored just because it's not a randomized clinical trial. My nutrition mentor, the late great Robert Crayhon, used to say that the New York City fire department didn't have a single randomized trial to show that water puts out fire, but they observed that it worked!

WHAT ABOUT APPLE JUICE?

Nope. Sorry. Doesn't even come close to making the list of healthiest foods.

So if apples are great but apple juice stinks, why am I such a fan of juicing (see page 284)? Simple. I'm a fan of the kind of juices you make at home. Homemade juice isn't even close to the stuff you get in the supermarket. Home juicing gives you all those amazing vitamins, phytochemicals, live enzymes, and all the other good stuff in the apple (except, of course, the fiber, unless you use a high-speed blender such as the Vitamix). Plus, most juice recipes call for a mix of veggies and other fruits to go with the apples (for example, spinach).

Sure, homemade apple juice is still a little high in sugar, but I'm okay with that because of all the benefits you get. Not so with commercial apple juice in the bottle, which is nothing more than sugar water and apple flavoring. Sure, it may have a tiny amount of vitamins, but the sugar cost is way too high for a beverage that gives us few, if any, of the benefits of real apples. Store-bought apple juice, for the most part, is no better than soda. I'm convinced that a lot of the behavioral problems we see in kids would be modulated noticeably if we didn't fill them with sugar water all day long.

The Best Apple of All

By the way, when you eat (or juice) apples, don't forget the peel. Apple peels have been found to have potent antioxidant activity, and they can greatly inhibit the growth of liver cancer and colon cancer cells. Though almost all apples contain valuable phenols and antioxidants, the good old Red Delicious seems to frequently come out the winner when it comes to antioxidant power.

Apricots

An apricot is basically a tasty little low-calorie bundle of nutrients put together in a beautiful, sun-colored package. What's not to like?

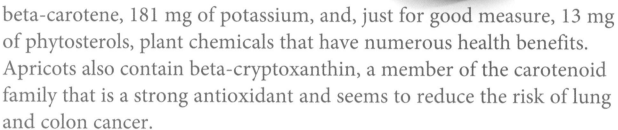

Two medium apricots have about 1½ g of fiber, 1,348 IUs of vitamin A, 766 IUs of beta-carotene, 181 mg of potassium, and, just for good measure, 13 mg of phytosterols, plant chemicals that have numerous health benefits. Apricots also contain beta-cryptoxanthin, a member of the carotenoid family that is a strong antioxidant and seems to reduce the risk of lung and colon cancer.

Some studies have demonstrated that beta-cryptoxanthin can reduce the risk of lung cancer by more than 30 percent, and other studies have shown that it reduces the risk for arthritis as well. To absorb the beta-cryptoxanthin, it's essential that your diet contains some fat, since, like other carotenoids, beta-cryptoxanthin is fat soluble. That makes a pretty strong argument for apricots and almonds as a healthy treat, don't you think?

The apricot originally hails from China, where it has been grown for more than 4,000 years. Legend has it that it was brought to the West by Alexander the Great. Most of the apricots in the United States are grown in California, but many varieties come from the Middle and Near East, especially Turkey. I remember that one of the first natural food stores I ever patronized was owned by a Turkish family who were especially proud of their imported, high-nutrient, fresh apricots.

What about Dried or Stewed Apricots?

Dried apricots are a favorite health food, and they are frequently found in trail mixes. They're a little high in sugar since they're so concentrated. Dried apricots are also higher in calories (½ cup [65 g] of dried apricots has 157 calories vs. 34 for two small whole apricots). And, for some strange reason, you lose the beta-cryptoxanthin in the dried version. But they're still a good source of beta-carotene and vitamin A.

Another option is stewed apricots (106 calories for ½ cup of stewed fruit, unsweetened). They're delicious, even higher in potassium and fiber, and still loaded with beta-carotene and vitamin A. No beta-cryptoxanthin, though—for that, you need to eat the whole fruit raw.

★ Avocados

Avocados are an amazing food. In 2016, when Steven Masley, M.D., and I published *Smart Fat: Eat More Fat, Lose More Weight, Get Healthy Now*, we put an avocado on the cover. It's the poster child for a healthy high-fat food.

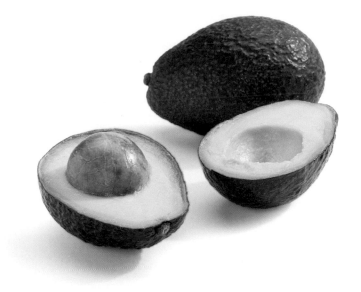

But the luscious avocado was not always held in high regard. Avocados were almost a casualty of the fat phobia that swept the nation back in the 1980s—and is sadly still very much with us. I'm counting the days until fat phobia dies a much-deserved death, and there are promising signs that it's starting to happen. That's very good news for those of us trying to redeem the reputation of this (and other) glorious high-fat foods that are, good for your health.

Why the Fat in Avocados Is Good for You

So yes, avocados are high in fat. But that fat is largely monounsaturated fat, specifically oleic acid, an omega-9 fat found in high amounts in olive oil and many nuts. Monounsaturated fat actually benefits your cholesterol profile. In research at the Instituto Mexicano del Seguro Social in Mexico, forty-five volunteers who ate avocados every day for a week experienced an average 17 percent drop in total blood cholesterol. More important, is the effect avocados had on specific kinds of cholesterol. In the study, both LDL and triglycerides went down, while HDL—which is mostly protective—went up.

Monounsaturated fat like the kind found in avocados has also been linked to a reduced risk of cancer and diabetes. Research published in the *Archives of Internal Medicine* and reprinted on the American Diabetes Association website demonstrated that people following a modified low-carb diet higher in monounsaturated fat lost more weight than a matched group of people following the standard National Cholesterol Education Program diet. And monounsaturated fats are a key component of the Mediterranean diet, which in every major study has been linked with lower rates of heart disease.

Great for Eyes, Heart, and Skin!

Avocados also contain lutein, a valuable member of the carotenoid family; it is a natural antioxidant, helps your eyes stay healthy, and helps maintain the health of your skin. According to David Herber, M.D., director of the Center for Human Nutrition at University of California in Los Angeles and one of my favorite nutritionists, "California avocados rank highest in lutein, which acts as an antioxidant, and beta-sitosterol, which blocks cholesterol absorption compared ounce-per-ounce to other fruits. These attributes make the avocado an important fruit to choose, along with other fruits and vegetables, to protect your heart."

Though there are a few grams of saturated fat in an avocado, it's precisely the kind of saturated fat I'm not the slightest bit afraid of. It's from a natural whole food, and quite different from the saturated fat you might find in an order of fries. It doesn't contain a large helping of toxins like steroids, antibiotics, and bovine growth hormone found in a factory-farmed animal. Good, healthy, natural saturated fat—whether it comes from grass-fed beef or from a delicious avocado—is finally making a comeback. One study in the prestigious *American Journal of Clinical Nutrition* showed that in postmenopausal women who consumed a reasonable 25-percent-fat diet, a greater amount of monounsaturated fat and a greater amount of saturated fat intake was associated with less progression of coronary atherosclerosis. High-glycemic carbs were associated with a greater progression. This finding lead to the publication of an editorial in the *American Journal of Clinical Nutrition* entitled, "Saturated Fat Prevents Coronary Artery Disease? An American Paradox."

I'll bet you didn't know that avocados are a great source of fiber. Don't feel bad—few people do. You'll get between 11 and 17 g of fiber per avocado!). Avocados are also a good source of potassium. And they contain folate, vitamin A, beta-carotene, and beta-cryptoxanthin, another healthy carotenoid. I frequently eat a whole avocado as a mini-meal right, out of the skin. Couple hundred calories, tons of heart-healthy fat, one-third to one-half of the day's fiber, plus it's filling and delicious. And next to zero effect on blood sugar.

WORTH KNOWING

There's a slight difference in the nutritional composition of California and Florida avocados. A California avocado has about 20 percent fewer calories (289 compared to 365 for the Florida variety), 13 percent less fat, and about 60 percent fewer carbohydrates. California avocados are also the only one of the two that is a significant source of lutein and zeaxanthin, two important carotenoids that are becoming the superstars of eye nutrition and are being studied for their ability to help prevent macular degeneration. On the other hand, Florida avocados have 20 percent more potassium, plus a bit more calcium and phosphorus. If you're still worried about calories, go with the California version, but either way you can't miss.

Bananas

Bananas aren't necessarily a nutritional heavyweight, but they're a healthy food. Their main claim to fame is potassium and fiber (more on the fiber part in a minute). And yes, they have a lot of potassium, but they're hardly the only food source of that important heart-healthy mineral. Calorie for calorie, foods like spinach and broccoli beat the pants off them. So does a cup of baked beans, navy beans, tomato juice, cantaloupe, or two medium kiwifruits.

The Importance of Potassium

Bananas are convenient and relatively low in calories (about 100 calories per banana). The fiber is also a big selling point. And even though other foods may contain just as much potassium, that doesn't mean the 422 mg of potassium per medium banana is anything to sneeze at. Let's not forget the major role potassium plays in the body, helping to maintain cell integrity, fluid and electrolyte balance, and, most important, a steady heartbeat!

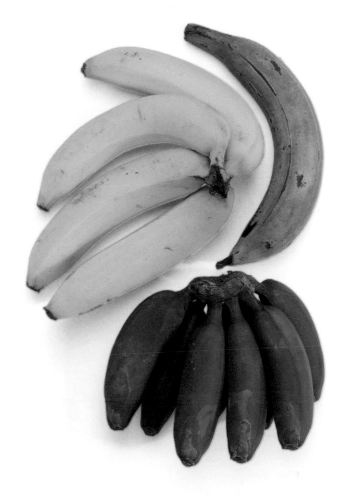

A drop in potassium levels can make you weak and tired, and low potassium is often connected to muscle cramps. Plus, many health professionals believe that potassium might both prevent and correct hypertension.

An interesting Swedish study on the risk of developing kidney cancer found that regular consumption of specific foods—bananas, root vegetables such as carrots and beets, salad greens, and cabbage—was linked to a 50 to 65 percent decrease in risk for kidney cancer. The study was published in the *International Journal of Cancer*. Women in the study who ate bananas four to six times a week had about half the risk of kidney cancer as those who didn't eat them.

The Fiber Connection: Bananas, Fructooligosaccharides and Resistant Starch

In the years since the original publication of this book, there's been an explosion of research on the microbiome, which is the name given to the huge population of non-human microbes that live in your gut and on your skin. Having a healthy balance of bacteria in your gut is now universally recognized as a vitally important component of human health, affecting everything from mood to weight. But those bacteria are living critters, and they need to eat. That's where fiber comes in.

Fiber comes in three forms—soluble, insoluble, and something called resistant starch. Bananas are high in a particular form of soluble fiber called *fructooligosaccharides*. Fructooligosaccharides (FOS) is especially important to us because it's a prebiotic—meaning it serves as a great food for the good bacteria (probiotics) in your gut. You want to keep the good bacteria in your gut healthy, happy and thriving, and one of the best ways to do that is to feed them a steady supply of prebiotics (like the FOS in bananas).

Unripe bananas are also a good source of resistant starch, which also serves as food for the good-guy microbes. But once the banana starts to ripen, the resistant starch turns into ordinary starch, and goodbye probiotic effect. An unripe banana is kind of the perfect food for gut bacteria, providing a combination of two of their favorite foods—prebiotic fructooligosaccharides and resistant starch.

In one study published in the *Journal of Agriculture and Food Chemistry*, bananas were hands down the most potent fruit source of fructooligosaccharides. The Jerusalem artichoke (see page 46) are the most potent source in the vegetable category, followed by onions. And bananas and rice have long been a folk remedy for digestive upset, especially diarrhea.

Not as High in Sugar as You Might Think

Bananas have gotten a bad rep as being a high-sugar food. That's partly true, but not nearly as bad as people think. The glycemic load of the average banana is 12. Glycemic load is the only measure that really counts when it comes to evaluating a food's effect on blood sugar. It's considered low if it's under 10, medium if it's 10 to 20, and high if it's higher than 20. The banana's rating of 12 puts it right in the low section of the medium category.

I think part of the problem with bananas was that they suffered from guilt by association with the typical 1980s low-fat breakfast that was once considered the epitome of a healthy meal—banana, crummy commercial cereal, skim milk, orange juice, and toast. And yes, we now know that combo is a nightmare from a blood sugar point of view.

But it wasn't really the banana that was the problem. Bananas, particularly those that aren't overripe, are not a problem for most people. And for what it's worth, bananas are considered a cleansing and rejuvenating food in yoga nutritional therapy.

WORTH KNOWING

The inner peel is rich in nutrients—either eat it directly, or scrape it and put it in your smoothie.

Black Currants

Black currant (also known as blackcurrant) is a shrub that produces pretty clusters of purplish berries during the summer. The berries are very tart, and they are usually combined with other fruits, or made into jams and jellies. They're rare in the United States.

Various medicines are made from the leaves and fruits of the plant, and especially from the oil from the seed, which contains gamma-linolenic acid (GLA), the same active ingredient in evening primrose oil. It's said to help ease inflammation. GLA was found to lower blood pressure and improve antioxidant status in an animal model, especially when combined in the diet with the two omega-3s found in fish oil—EPA and DHA.

In a published review of the health benefits of black currants, researchers noted "the potent anti-inflammatory, antioxidant, and antimicrobial effects of black currant constituents on a myriad of disease states." Several studies have focused on the therapeutic potential of black currants regarding hypertension and other cardiovascular-associated illnesses, neurodegenerative diseases, and diabetic neuropathy.

 # Blueberries

Mention blueberries around scientists, and you're sure to hear the name of James Joseph, Ph.D.

Joseph was lead scientist in the Laboratory of Neuroscience at the USDA Human Nutrition Research Center on Aging at Tufts University. His special interest was what we should eat if we want to keep our marbles intact as we grow older. And it's largely because of Joseph that blueberries now have a firmly established reputation as a memory-protecting food.

Blueberries Are Brain Food

In Joseph's lab, he had something he called the Rat Olympics. He tested motor function and memory function with mazes and assorted tests for muscle strength and coordination. Around middle age, rats start showing the same kinds of decline in performance that humans do. But what Joseph's studies show is that when you feed the lab animals extracts of blueberries, wonderful things start happening; or, more accurately, bad things don't happen.

Bad things meaning mental deterioration. And loss of coordination and balance. Gone. Those rats that chowed down on the blueberries behaved like young studs. In Joseph's lab, they'd found the Rat Fountain of Youth.

Blueberries contain compounds such as anthocyanin, which are antioxidant and anti-inflammatory. Inflammation and oxidative stress are involved in virtually every major killer disease: Alzheimer's, Parkinson's, diabetes, and heart disease, not to mention common conditions of aging such as arthritis. These compounds by themselves would be enough to land blueberries on anyone's list of superfoods. Blueberries do even more. They help neurons in the brain communicate with one another more effectively.

BLUEBERRIES KEEP YOUR MEMORY SHARP

"Old neurons are kind of like old married couples," said Joseph, who has since passed away. "They don't talk to each other so much anymore." Memory goes down, and the processing necessary for coordination and balance tend to decline. The technical term for this communication is signaling, and special compounds in blueberries called polyphenols turn on the signals. "Not only can you get one neuron to talk to another more efficiently, but you can enable the brain to grow new neurons," Joseph explained in an interview.

Blueberries are the ultimate memory food. Animal studies have demonstrated that daily consumption of blueberries dramatically slows impairments in motor coordination and memory that are the usual accompaniments of aging. What's more, they may help lower blood cholesterol and promote urinary health.

Bilberries, a close European cousin of the blueberry, have been shown to promote eye health and protect against glaucoma and cataract progression. In fact, wild blueberries are called "the vision fruit" in Japan, because they have very high concentrations of anthocyanins, natural antioxidants, and anti-inflammatories whose benefits include reducing eyestrain and improving night vision. And there are currently plans to study the ability of blueberries to prevent macular degeneration, a disease of the retina and the leading cause of blindness in people older than sixty-five.

Blueberries Are the Highest-Scoring Fruit of All Time

Then there are all those antioxidants and anti-inflammatory compounds, which help fight against cardiovascular disease. Back when the government was using a test known as the ORAC test (oxygen radical absorbance capacity) to measure antioxidant power in foods, blueberries were tested to have one of the highest ORAC values of any food in the world. The database of ORAC values was removed from the USDA Nutrient Data Laboratory website in 2012 due largely to the fact that food and dietary supplement companies were routinely misusing and misrepresenting ORAC scores to promote their products. Nonetheless, it's worth noting that the ORAC test showed blueberries to be the highest-scoring fruit of all time.

Blueberries are a great source of compound called pterostilbene. On a cellular level, it works much like resveratrol in regulating fatty acid metabolism and fats in the bloodstream—and it helps prevent the deposition of plaque in the arteries.

Need more reasons to eat blueberries? How about fighting cancer? A University of Illinois study tested different fruits for the presence of a flavonoid that inhibits a cancer-promoting enzyme. Of all the fruits tested, wild blueberries showed the greatest anticancer activity.

Fresh or Frozen, You Choose

Best of all, you can get all these amazing health benefits by just adding ½ cup (75 g) a day of wild or frozen blueberries to your diet. No studies have been done to date comparing fresh to frozen to canned berries, but virtually all forms of the fruit have essential anthocyanins and proanthocyanins, making them a genuine health bargain. In fact, all of Joseph's studies were done using frozen berries, which last time I looked, were relatively inexpensive and available in any grocery store freezer.

Throw them on a salad, in a blender with a protein powder, or best of all—my personal favorite—eat them frozen with a dollop of yogurt. The yogurt semi-freezes upon contacting the ice-cold blueberries, making the resulting blend the most delicious, healthy dessert you can imagine.

Cranberries

The only time most people come face to face with an actual cranberry is during Thanksgiving dinner, but there are a lot of reasons to get more familiar with this tart little red berry.

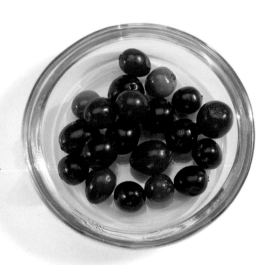

Cranberries are low in calories (44 per cup [110 g]), high in fiber, and low in sugar. But, like grapes, many of their real benefits aren't clear from the typical nutrition facts label.

Cranberries Really Do Prevent UTIs

Studies presented at the twenty-third national meeting of the American Chemical Society show that the ruby red berries have some of the most potent antioxidants of any common fruits studied. They possess anticancer properties, inhibit the growth of common foodborne pathogens, and contain antibacterial properties to aid in the prevention of urinary tract infections (UTIs).

Catherine Neto, Ph.D., assistant professor at the University of Massachusetts–Dartmouth, isolated several bioactive compounds from whole cranberries and found compounds in the berries that were toxic to a variety of cancer tumor cells. "The tumor cell lines that these compounds inhibited most in our assays included lung, cervical, prostate, breast, and leukemia," according to Neto.

Cranberries are high in phenols (also known as phenolic acids), plant chemicals known to be highly protective against a wide range of health problems and conditions. According to the *Journal of Agricultural and Food Chemistry*, cranberries had a higher phenol concentration than any of the twenty commonly eaten fruits studied: A ½ cup (55 g) contains 373 phenols per serving, more than red grapes, apples, strawberries, or blueberries.

What You Don't Know about Cranberries

It's widely known that cranberries help prevent UTIs. This is accomplished by preventing bacteria from sticking to the lining of the urinary tract (see also cranberry juice, page 282). More recently it has been discovered that the same properties help reduce bacterial adhesion to teeth, thus reducing the formation of dental plaque. Studies have also revealed that com-pounds in cranberries stop certain disease-causing bacteria from sticking to the stomach lining, thus helping to prevent ulcers.

Remember now, we're talking about actual, raw cranberries here. Once you dry and sweeten them they may still have a lot of the healthful phenolic compounds, but the calories jump into the stratosphere (from 44 per cup [110 g] to 370 per cup!) and so does the sugar. If that's not a problem for you—i.e., if you're an avid hiker about to go out for five hours—by all means throw them in the trail mix! If not, use the dried and sweetened kind sparingly.

Note: You can get raw, whole berries in the frozen section of the grocers. I find them a terrific addition to smoothies. If the tart taste is too much for you, sweeten with some xylitol, erythritol, stevia, or—if you're not too sensitive to the effects of sugar—a small amount of raw, unfiltered honey.

Elderberries

A couple of years ago, Mehmet Oz, M.D., posted an article called "The Brain Diet," in which he and neurologist Majid Fotuhi, M.D., Ph.D., talked about the superfoods you must include in your diet to help prevent Alzheimer's and boost your memory.

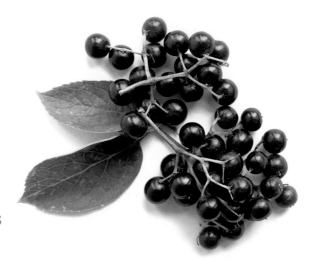

Ready for "Brain Superfood Number One"?

Elderberries.

These berries are nutritional and medicinal powerhouses.

So why aren't we all eating them?

Two reasons. One, they're impossible to find, and two, they taste horrible.

And you probably don't want to go picking them wild, even if you could find them (which you probably can't). Only the completely ripe, purple-blue (almost black) berries and flowers are edible. The unripe berries and seeds of the elder tree are poisonous. They contain glycosides—molecules consisting of a sugar and a non-sugar group—which release cyanide. Yup, that cyanide. Probably something you don't want to be consuming.

Fortunately, you can get the medicinal properties of elderberry in a tasty extract form known as Sambucol. It's available everywhere and it's terrific.

Sambucol came into being because of research by a world-renowned Israel virologist, Madeleine Mumcuoglu. Back in the 1980s, Mumcuoglu began studying the elderberry, which had been used in medicine for centuries. Elderberry wine, for example, was traditionally used both for influenza and the chills. Mumcuoglu discovered the key active ingredient in elderberry and found it to be effective against the flu virus. She first tested it during the southern Israeli flu epidemic of 1992–1993 and found that within twenty-four hours, 20 percent of patients taking it had dramatic improvements in fever, aches, pains, and coughing. By the second day, a whopping 74 percent improved, and by the third day, 90 percent. In the untreated placebo control group, only 16 percent felt better after two days, and most took nearly a week to report feeling better. Mumcuoglu created a company—Razei Bar—which now markets the product.

Sambucol has been widely studied. Its main claim to fame is that it shortens the length of time you're sidelined from the flu. In one study (Zakay-Rones, 2004), Sambucol relieved flu symptoms on an average of four days earlier. The researchers reported that "Elderberry extract seems to offer an efficient, safe, and cost-effective treatment for influenza."

In another study, Sambucol was shown to be effective against ten strains of influenza virus, and reduced the duration of flu symptoms to three to four days. That's impressive. If you've ever had the flu, you know you can easily be down for a week, and reducing that time by half would be awfully nice. The same study tested the effect of Sambucol products on a healthy immune system, specifically on the production of inflammatory cytokines, one of the immune system's best weapons. Production of inflammatory cytokines, including TNF-alpha, were significantly increased. "We conclude from this study that, in addition to its antiviral properties, Sambucol Elderberry Extract and its formulations activate the healthy immune system by increasing inflammatory cytokine production," wrote the authors. "Sambucol might therefore be beneficial to the immune system activation and in the inflammatory process in healthy individuals or in patients with various diseases."

I keep Sambucol in the house and use it at the first sign of cold or flu. It's the best way I know to get the medicinal properties of elderberries without having to traipse around North America or Europe in hopes of finding them in the wild. Plus you never have to worry about being poisoned!

Goji Berries

First things first. Goji berries are delicious. They're also expensive. But partisans claim they are one of the best foods on the planet. A deep-red, dried fruit about the size as a raisin with an unusual taste—sort of a cross between a cranberry and a cherry—goji berries have been used in Tibet for at least 1,700 years. They're used in Chinese medicine, and they're traditionally regarded by the people of Tibet and elsewhere as a longevity, strength-building, and sexual potency food of the highest order.

Do Goji Berries Really Cure Cancer?

These exotic berries and the juices made from them (goji, noni, acai) are incredibly healthy foods. The problem is foods that have been used in medical and healing traditions for thousands of years generally don't keep their reputation unless they actually deliver the goods.

Multilevel marketers discover these foods, and then you have a war in which everyone claims their product is the only "real" one. Fantastic health claims are made that range all over the map and compete for sheer silliness, and before you know it you're in marketing hell and don't know what to believe. I've seen websites that claim that goji berries cure cancer, guarantee you an extra twenty years of life, and make you a sexual superman. All of this is nonsense.

The goji berry is one of about eighty varieties of the Lycium berry (*Lycium barbarum*) that is indigenous to the Tibetan and Mongolian regions. A lot of published research exists on the Lycium berry, most of it positive, but none of it strong enough to support the claim that it cures cancer.

Marketing hype aside, this is a great food. Research shows that polysaccharides extracted from *Lycium barbarum* had a positive effect on insulin resistance in rats and a neuroprotective effect on animal cells. Polysaccharides extracted from the Lycium berry also demonstrate strong antioxidant properties. At least two studies showed they have a significant effect on the immune system. In one study, they reduced the weight of tumors; in at least two others, they protected animal cells from DNA damage.

When this book was first published in 2007, the goji berry wasn't listed in the USDA database. Ten years later, data is available and it shows that those early champions of the goji berry had good intuition! A quarter cup (26 g) of goji berries has 90 calories, 4 g of protein, and 4 g of dietary fiber. It also has a little bit of vitamins A and C and iron—and, very likely, many unidentified flavonoids or phytochemicals with (likely) antioxidant and anti-inflammatory properties.

I say likely because it's turned out to be the case with just about every other richly colored berry on the planet. So it's a good guess it's true for the goji as well.

Stay tuned another ten years, and I hope I'll be telling you I was right.

You can buy the juice if you don't mind paying astronomical rates and wading through a bunch of multilevel marketing hype. Personally, I buy the organic berries themselves in a package at the natural food supermarket. One of my favorite raw-food breakfasts is made of raw oats, almond slices, apple slices, flaked coconut, and goji berries. Moisten with some pomegranate juice and enjoy!

Golden berries

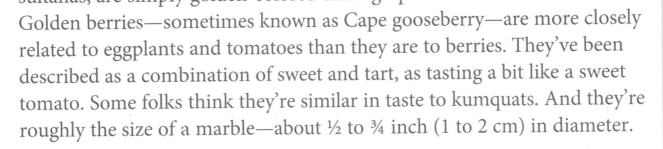

Golden berries look very much like golden raisins, but the resemblance is only superficial. Golden raisins, also known as sultanas, are simply golden-colored dried grapes. Golden berries—sometimes known as Cape gooseberry—are more closely related to eggplants and tomatoes than they are to berries. They've been described as a combination of sweet and tart, as tasting a bit like a sweet tomato. Some folks think they're similar in taste to kumquats. And they're roughly the size of a marble—about ½ to ¾ inch (1 to 2 cm) in diameter.

Scientifically known as *Physalis peruviana*, golden berries (goldenberries) are loaded with important plant compounds, one of which is the important flavonoid quercetin. Quercetin is one of the most powerful natural anti-inflammatories I know of. I consider it so important that I often recommend quercetin supplements as part of an anti-inflammatory regimen.

One 2013 study investigated the main compound derived from golden berries, a chemical with the totally weird and unpronounceable name of 4β-Hydroxywithanolide E. The researchers wanted to investigate its "antiproliferative effect on a human lung cancer cell line." They concluded that this natural compound found in golden berry was a potential chemotherapeutic agent against lung cancer.

Goldenberries have high levels of vitamin C, vitamin A and the vitamin B-complex (ibid). They're also one of the few food sources for a unique group of organic compounds called withanolides. Withanolides are both antioxidant and anti-inflammatory. (Withanolides are also found in the adaptogenic healing plant ashwaganda.) Not surprisingly, studies have demonstrated that golden berries do indeed have both anti-inflammatory and antioxidant properties.

Many health or natural food stores carry goldenberries in bulk or by the bag. You can also order them online.

Gooseberries and Amla

(Indian Gooseberries)

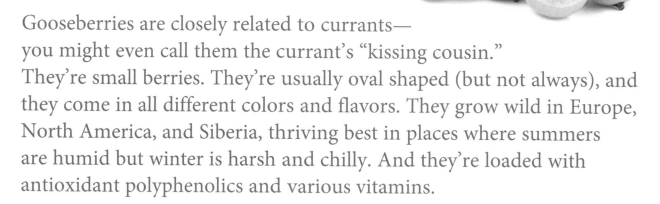

Gooseberries are closely related to currants—
you might even call them the currant's "kissing cousin."
They're small berries. They're usually oval shaped (but not always), and
they come in all different colors and flavors. They grow wild in Europe,
North America, and Siberia, thriving best in places where summers
are humid but winter is harsh and chilly. And they're loaded with
antioxidant polyphenolics and various vitamins.

Gooseberries contain small amounts of essential vitamins such as pyridoxine (vitamin B6), pantothenic acid (vitamin B5), folate, thiamin (vitamin B1), and vitamin A. Gooseberries also contain decent levels of minerals such as copper, calcium, phosphorus, manganese, magnesium, and potassium.

Many parts of the gooseberry plant are used to treat various diseases, but the most important part is the fruit—the actual berry. It's used either alone or in combination with other plants to treat many ailments such as the common cold and fever; as a diuretic, laxative, liver restoration; treatment of stomach issues; anti-pyretic; anti-inflammatory; hair tonic; to prevent peptic ulcer and dyspepsia, and as a digestive aid.

Indian gooseberries, also known as amla, are quite different from gooseberries even though they share a name. A study published in the *European Journal of Cancer Prevention* in 2011 referred to amla as "a wonder berry in the treatment and prevention of cancer" (Baliga, 2011). The researchers called amla (Indian gooseberry) "arguably the most important medicinal plant in the Indian traditional system of medicine, the Ayurveda." Some of its constituents—like ellagic acid—have long been studied for their anticancer activity, and studies show that amla possess neuroprotective, liver-protective, kidney-protective, gastroprotective, and cardioprotective properties.

Amla berries are extremely high in antioxidants and vitamin C—but they are also very acidic and bitter tasting. They do have significantly high amounts of phenolic phytochemicals, especially flavones and anthocyanins. Many of these compounds have been found to have anticancer, anti-inflammatory, and antiaging benefits, and they also seem to offer some measure of protection against neurological diseases. Amla also contains other antioxidant compounds like tannins (emblicanin, punigluconin and pedunculagin) as well as the vitamin C (445 mg for about 4 ounces [115 g] of amla!)

Mulberries

Mulberries look like the offspring of a blackberry and a raspberry. They've been used in Chinese herbal medicine for thousands of years, primarily to treat heart disease, diabetes, anemia, and arthritis. They have a high total phenolic content— i.e., they're loaded with plant compounds such as anthocyanins and chlorogenic acids, which have multiple health benefits (Isabelle, 2008).

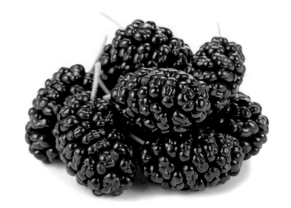

There are twenty-four species of mulberry trees. Most commonly grown are black, white, and red. The black ones appear to have more antioxidant power (Ercisli, 2007). They're low in calories (60 per cup [140 g]), and are often consumed dried (such as raisins). They're an excellent source of vitamin C and iron, and a good source of vitamin K₁, potassium, and vitamin E.

They're also rich in plant compounds called *anthocyanins*, which are responsible for their color and have a number of proven health benefits. For one thing, anthocyanins inhibit the oxidation of LDL cholesterol. When cholesterol is oxidized (damaged), that's the time we need to worry about it, so anything that slows down that damage is a good thing indeed.

Mulberries contain an interesting compound called *DNJ* (1-deoxynojirimycin), which inhibits an enzyme that breaks down carbs, and is therefore considered to be beneficial against diabetes because it slows down the rise in blood sugar that happens after meals.

Polyphenols—such as those in mulberries—have great potential for cardiovascular disease. They also reduce oxidative stress, which is a component of many diseases, including (but not limited to) cancer.

Mulberries are sweet and delicious and packed with nutrition. They have quite a range of potential benefits.

Raspberries

Raspberries deserve a place of honor on the healthy foods list if for no other reason than the fact that they are a high-fiber powerhouse. For a measly 64 calories a cup (125 g), they provide—get this—8 g of dietary fiber, making them calorie for calorie one of the most high-fiber foods on the planet.

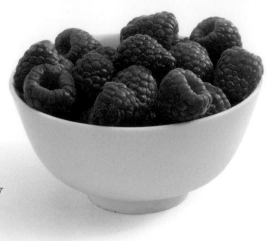

But the benefits of raspberries hardly stop with the fiber. Raspberries have calcium, magnesium, phosphorus, potassium, vitamin C, and bone-building vitamin K. And, if you're watching your carbs, only about 7 g of "net" carbs (the kind that count) per cup. But that's just what shows up on the nutrition facts label. There's way more to this picture than meets the eye.

Raspberries' Ellagic Acid Fights Cancer Cells with No Damage to Healthy Cells

Raspberries are one of the best sources on the planet of ellagic acid. Ellagic acid, also found in cherries and strawberries, has been shown in animal research and in laboratory models to inhibit the growth of tumors caused by certain carcinogens. A publication by the American Cancer Society called *The American Cancer Society's Guide to Complementary and Alternative Cancer Methods* says that ellagic acid is a promising natural supplement because it causes apoptosis (cell death) of cancer cells in the lab, with no change to healthy, normal cells.

Here's how it works: Healthy cells have a normal life cycle of approximately 120 days before they die. This process is called apoptosis (natural cell death). The body replaces the dying cells with healthy cells,

and life goes on. But with cancer cells, no such luck. Instead of dying, they multiply by division, making two, then four, then eight cancer cells (and so on). In lab tests, ellagic acid caused the cancer cells to go through the normal apoptosis process without doing damage to healthy cells. (Remember, chemotherapy and radiation cause the death of cancer cells also, but they leave some powerful side effects.)

No one is saying that ellagic acid cures cancer— but it's interesting and promising that it has shown such beneficial activity in the lab. Perhaps it will turn out to benefit humans as well. According to studies posted on the Memorial Sloan Kettering Cancer Center website, ellagic acid also has antiviral and antibacterial properties.

Raspberries Could Be a Natural Arthritis Treatment

Raspberries also contain anthocyanins. Anthocyanins have the ability to inhibit cyclooxygenase, a compound produced in the body in two or more forms, called COX-1 and COX-2. COX-2 is built only in special cells and is used for signaling pain and inflammation. (It was the ability of arthritis drugs like Vioxx and Celebrex to inhibit COX-2 that made them effective.)

Unfortunately, at least in the case of Vioxx, side effects were dangerous enough to cause it to be withdrawn from the market. Anthocyanins, on the other hand, have no such side effects. Research conducted at Michigan State University investigated a range of fruits and berries for the level and activity of anthocyanins found in each. The yield of pure anthocyanins in raspberries was the second highest of all the fruits tested. (Cherries were first, but not by much.) And anthocyanins also have significant antioxidant activity as well.

Raspberries are fragile. They'll turn to pulp if you hold them in your hand too long. So if you buy them fresh, handle carefully, and eat soon. You can also get them frozen, and they're great in shakes.

 # Strawberries

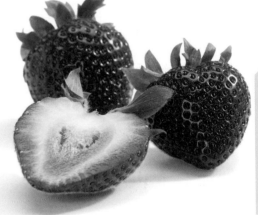

Strawberries, like all berries, are a real health bonanza. All berries—strawberries, blueberries, raspberries—contain chemicals found to protect cells against cervical and breast cancer. Researchers at Clemson University tested freeze-dried fruit extracts against two cultures of aggressive cervical cancer lines and two breast cancer cell lines. Extracts from strawberry and blueberry significantly decreased the growth of cervical and breast cancer cells.

In fact, preliminary data reported on the USDA website suggest that phytochemicals from strawberries and blueberries inhibit steps in tumor initiation. In addition, a study published in the *Journal of Agriculture and Food Chemistry* analyzed eight types of strawberries for their content of protective plant compounds like phenols and anthocyanins, as well as for their antioxidant capacity. All eight types of strawberries were able to significantly inhibit the proliferation of human liver cancer cells. And a number of other analyses have shown that strawberries have potent antioxidant action.

Strawberries also contain ellagic acid, which you may have read about in my discussion on cherries and raspberries. Research since 1968 has shown that ellagic acid has anticarcinogenic and antimutagenic activity. Ellagic acid is a naturally occurring phenolic compound in many plants, especially strawberries, raspberries, and blackberries. Ellagic acid has been shown in animal research and in laboratory models to inhibit the growth of tumors caused by certain carcinogens. *The American Cancer Society's Guide to Complementary and Alternative Cancer Methods* says that ellagic acid is a very promising natural supplement because it causes apoptosis (cell death) of cancer cells in the lab, with no change to healthy, normal cells.

Strawberry Compound May Improve Short-Term Memory

Compounds in strawberries may also protect your brain and memory. Researchers at Tufts University and the USDA published a study in the *Journal of Neuroscience* showing that animals that consumed an extract of blueberries, strawberries, and spinach every day had significant improvements in short-term memory. The rats that received the fruit and vegetable extracts learned faster than the other rats, and their motor skills improved significantly. This study was the first to show that fruits and vegetables actually reverse dysfunctions in behavior and nerve cells. The extracts also protected their little blood vessels against damage.

Strawberries also contain anthocyanins. Anthocyanins have the ability to inhibit cyclooxygenase, a compound produced in the body in two or more forms, called COX-1 and COX-2. COX-2 is built only in special cells and it is used for signaling pain and inflammation. It's COX-2 that we want to turn the volume down on if we want to inhibit pain. That's what arthritis drugs like Vioxx and Celebrex did—they inhibited COX-2, and that made them effective. Unfortunately, at least in the case of Vioxx, side effects were dangerous enough to cause it to be withdrawn from the market.

Anthocyanins, on the other hand, turn down the volume on COX-2 but have no nasty side effects. Though the anthocyanin content in strawberries isn't as high as that in cherries or raspberries, it's still significant. And anthocyanins have significant antioxidant activity as well.

A cup (170 g) of strawberries has only about 50 calories and delivers about 3 g of fiber. It has calcium, magnesium, phosphorus, and potassium, plus a very nice dose of vitamin C (about 85 mg).

WORTH KNOWING

Back when I first wrote this book, strawberries were on the Environmental Working Group's list of twelve fruits and vegetables most consistently contaminated with pesticides and other agricultural chemicals. In 2016, they were still on the list, and they had actually moved to the number one slot (meaning the worst of the worst as far as pesticide contamination). Put strawberries on your "buy organic" list.

Cantaloupe

All melons are high-volume foods. That means that for a given amount of weight, they contain a relatively high amount of water, fiber, and air—and a relatively low number of calories. Why should it matter? Consider this.

The Benefit of High-Volume Foods

Barbara Rolls, Ph.D., a nutrition researcher at Pennsylvania State University, has done a ton of research on appetite and appetite control. She has found that people ate about 3 pounds (1.4 kg) of food daily, regardless of whether the food was high calorie or low calorie. After about 3 pounds, people stopped eating. They'd eat nearly identical servings of food (by weight), whether it was watermelon (high volume) or cheesecake (low volume). Most important, the subjects in her studies felt just as full after the low-calorie meals as they did after the calorie-rich meals—as long as both meals contained the same volume of food.

Cantaloupe is a high-volume food. An entire large melon has only 277 calories, much less than most desserts, and more than most people can eat at one sitting. A typical serving is a wedge, or maybe half a melon. About 90 percent of the melon is water. As Rolls has shown in her research, study after research study, the water in the melon goes a long way toward filling you up. By the way, water in foods seems to do this more than water that you drink alongside foods. Melons and soups do a better job of appetite control than solid food plus a glass of water.

Cantaloupe Lowers the Risk of High Blood Pressure and Stroke

Cantaloupe's not a great food just because it's high-volume and low-calorie. It's also rich in potassium and vitamin A. One cup (156 g) of melon cubes provides 427 mg of potassium and a little calcium and magnesium). Many studies show that people who eat potassium-rich foods have lower rates of heart disease and stroke. Potassium is also a key component of healthy blood pressure.

According to the latest studies, people who regularly consume high-potassium foods have lower blood pressure than those who don't. A review of thirty-three studies examined the effect of potassium on blood pressure, and researchers discovered that participants who added 2,340 mg of potassium daily (from foods, supplements, or both) lowered their risk of developing high blood pressure by 25 percent. The reductions were ultimately greatest for people who already had high blood pressure. Another possible benefit of potassium: It may protect against stroke. People with high blood pressure who had a daily serving of potassium-rich foods (such as figs) decreased their risk of fatal stroke by 40 percent, according to one study.

Then there's vitamin A and beta-carotene, both of which are plentiful in cantaloupe. Though a lot of people know about vitamin A's role in vision and growth and bone development, what's not as well known is how terrific it is for the immune system. I consider it one of the best immune system boosters around.

Eat Cantaloupe to Ward Off a Cold

Vitamin A deficiency results in decreased resistance to infection. But you don't really have to have a deficiency to benefit from its effect on the immune system. There is some evidence that vitamin A can stimulate and otherwise favorably affect the immune system even in the absence of vitamin A deficiency. Whenever I feel a cold coming on, I take large doses of supplemental vitamin A for a few days, plus a few other things such as C, zinc, and N-acetyl-cysteine. It works. And some years ago, it was demonstrated that high-dose vitamin A can significantly protect against some of the immune-depressing effects of radiation and cancer chemotherapy.

Beta-carotene, a carotenoid that turns into vitamin A in the body, has protective health properties of its own. A cup (156 g) of cantaloupe cubes has more than 3,000 mcg of beta-carotene. Beta-carotene, in addition to being a great antioxidant that protects against cellular damage, may be protective against some forms of cancer in some populations; it may also play a role in protecting against heart disease. Though a large study a few years ago that looked at the effect on smokers of large supplemental dosages of synthetic beta-carotene had disappointing results, there is overwhelming epidemiologic evidence that those who consume three or more servings of fruits and vegetables daily have significantly lower risk of many forms of cancer and heart disease and that the protective association is particularly strong for dietary carotenoids, especially with respect to protection against lung cancer.

Cantaloupe also makes a great juice, and if your juicer can handle it, you don't need to remove the skin. You can mix cantaloupe and watermelon juices with sparkling water for an amazing summer cooler, or vary the recipe and add lemon juice and ginger.

 # Cherries

"The day when doctors say 'take 10 cherries and call me in the morning' may not be far off," said a *Newsweek* article. You might wonder what the writer was talking about if you looked cherries up in a food database. What's the big deal? Sure, they're relatively low in calories, and, like most fruits and vegetables they're a good source of potassium. And the sour ones have a nice amount of vitamin A. But the real benefits of cherries are not in plain sight, at least not if the only place you look is on the nutrition facts label. And when you understand the real benefits, suddenly the *Newsweek* reporter's comment starts to make a lot of sense.

Why? Because cherries are loaded with anti-inflammatory, antiaging, anticancer compounds that don't show up on your average nutrition facts label. The cancer-fighting agents in cherries include a flavonoid called quercetin, as well as ellagic acid and perillyl alcohol.

The Wonders of Quercetin and Ellagic Acid

Quercetin has been found by researchers to be a potent anticancer agent. It also exhibits significant anti-inflammatory activity, which is why quercetin is one of my favorite supplements for allergies and asthma.

Ellagic acid is a naturally occurring phenolic known to be both anticarcinogenic and antimutagenic.

Also found in red raspberries, ellagic acid has been shown in animal research and in laboratory models to inhibit the growth of tumors caused by certain carcinogens. *The American Cancer Society's Guide to Complementary and Alternative Cancer Methods* says that ellagic acid is a very promising natural supplement because it causes apoptosis (cell death) of cancer cells in the lab, with no change to healthy, normal cells. According to studies posted on the Memorial Sloan Kettering Cancer Center website, ellagic acid also has antiviral and antibacterial properties.

Perillyl Alcohol in Cherries May Inhibit Tumor Growth

Another compound in cherries is perillyl alcohol. Though the exact mechanism of its action is unknown, it appears that perillyl alcohol and its metabolites may inhibit tumor growth. In animal models, it exhibited this effect in pancreatic, stomach, colon, skin, and liver cancers. The Cleveland Clinic Taussig Cancer Center is currently running phase one of a multiple-dose trial of perillyl alcohol on healthy women with a history of breast cancer.

Cherries have been shown to lower levels of uric acid in the blood, which is one of the most common causes of gout pain. A study at the University of California–Davis showed that consuming a serving of cherries daily significantly lowered the blood uric acid levels of women by as much as 15 percent.

Even Cherry Juice Packs a Punch

The benefits of cherry juice are in compounds called anthocyanins, pigments that give cherries their bright red color and are believed to help the body relieve inflammation. These same anthocyanins may significantly reduce your risk for colon cancer, the third leading cancer in America.

Doctors and scientists believe that it's the anthocyanins in the cherries that cause the decrease in blood urates and the relief from gout pain.

Anthocyanins act like natural COX-2 inhibitors. COX stands for cyclooxygenase, which is produced in the body in two or more forms, called COX-1 and COX-2. COX-2 is used for signaling pain and inflammation. The popularity of arthritis drugs such as Vioxx and Celebrex was based on their unique ability to block only the pain and inflammation messages of COX-2 while leaving the noninflammatory COX-1 alone. Unfortunately, there were some really unpleasant side effects associated with Vioxx, and it was taken off the market. But anthocyanins produce a similar effect with none of the problems of drugs.

Cherries (and raspberries) have the highest yields of pure anthocyanins. In one study, the COX inhibitory activity of anthocyanins from cherries was comparable to those of ibuprofen and naproxen. And researchers feel that in addition to helping with pain and inflammation, consuming anthocyanins on a regular basis may help lower heart attack and stroke risk.

Your New Favorite Dessert

You can get the health benefits of cherries by eating the tart ones whole, or by juicing them. I have a favorite secret dessert that I'll share with you: I buy organic frozen red cherries and put them in my freezer. When I'm ready to eat them, I put them—direct from the freezer—into a little bowl with some raw milk or yogurt, which promptly semi-freezes on the cherries, forming a kind of ice milk. Stir it up, and the resulting mixture is like Cherry Garcia ice cream, only with a zillion times more health benefits. It's delicious, and it's my secret weapon against the dreaded Attack of the Ice Cream Craving (and I know you know what I'm talking about!).

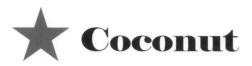 # Coconut

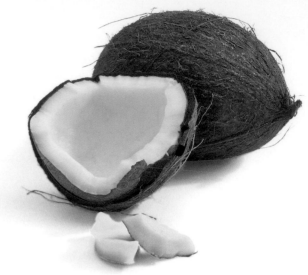

I really looked forward to writing this section, because I felt it would give me a chance to right one of the greatest nutritional misconceptions of all time: the idea that coconut is bad for you because it contains saturated fat.

Let me be very clear at the outset: Coconut and coconut oil are superfoods. Coconut—and its oil—is one of the most healthy, amazing things you can ingest.

Island Studies Prove the Value of Coconut

The good news on coconut started with research back in the 1960s and 1970s. It has long been observed that people from the Pacific Islands and Asia whose diets are very high in coconut oil are surprisingly free from cardiovascular disease, cancer, and other degenerative diseases. A long-term, multidisciplinary study was set up to examine the health of the people living in the small, idyllic coconut-eating islands of Tokelau and Pukapuka. And what it found was astonishing. Despite eating a high-fat diet (35 to 60 percent of their calories were from fat, mostly saturated fat from coconuts), the Pukapuka and Tokelau islanders were virtually free of atherosclerosis, heart disease, and colon cancer. Digestive problems were rare. The islanders were lean and healthy. There were no signs of kidney disease, and high blood cholesterol was unknown. Yet when these native people moved to the big cities, changed their diets, and gave up eating coconut oil in favor of the refined polyunsaturated vegetable oils that are believed to be healthier, their incidence of heart disease increased dramatically.

A ½ cup (47 g) of shredded coconut meat has almost 4 g of fiber, 142 mg of potassium, 13 mg of magnesium, less than 3 g of sugar, and—most important—13 g of the most heart-healthy, life-supporting fat on the planet (more on that in a moment).

Saturated Fat in Coconut Is Nothing to Fear

Since the original publication of this book, a lot has changed in the public perception of coconut and coconut oil. Before 2011, the year the *Dr. Oz* show debuted on television, Mehmet Oz, M.D., had a radio show on the Oprah Channel on SiriusXM. I appeared on that show for the full hour, and we discussed, among other things, coconut and coconut oil. Oz's writing partner, the distinguished physician and chief wellness officer of the esteemed Cleveland Clinic, Michael Roizen, M.D., was on the show with us, and I called coconut oil a superfood. Roizen basically said I was crazy—that coconut oil was terrible for you, it was highly inflammatory, and it contained saturated fat. I have (and had) great respect for Roizen, but he was dead wrong about this. I was gratified to see that a couple of years later, Oz himself listed coconut oil on his website as one of his favorite superfoods. (Google "Dr. Oz's Favorite Superfoods," and you can see for yourself.)

Still, in the eyes of many consumers, coconut suffers from a completely undeserved negative reputation. And how did coconut come to get this bad reputation? You guessed it—because it has fat. Not only does it have fat, it has saturated fat. And because of the mass hysteria and widespread misinformation about saturated fat in this country, most people think anything that has saturated fat should be avoided like the plague. Back in 1962, one writer observed that "the average American now fears saturated fat the way he once feared witches." I believe that's still true today, despite quite a lot of research disproving the notion that saturated fat has anything to do with heart disease.

The point here is this: amazing health foods such as eggs (with their yolks) and coconut have been absent from the American diet for no other reason than that people—including doctors—simply don't understand the full story when it comes to fat.

The human body needs fat. We can't exist without it. It's incorporated into our cell membranes. It's used as an energy source. It cushions and protects our organs. It makes certain critical vitamins—such as vitamins A and D—available to us. Some fats—like sterols—serve as the basic molecule for important hormones like the sex hormones. And fats are the precursors for a whole group of important compounds in the body known as prostaglandins that are vitally important for human health. (For more on the right way to incorporate fat into your diet, see my book with Steven Masley, M.D., *Smart Fat: Eat More Fat, Lose More Weight, Get Healthy Now*.)

Coconut's Medium-Chain Fatty Acids Are Easier to Metabolize

What we know as fats and oils are mostly made up of smaller compounds called fatty acids. These fatty acids—whether they're saturated or unsaturated—come in many different lengths. For convenience's sake, they're classified into three groups: short, medium, and long.

The saturated fats in coconut are mainly medium chain—they're also known as MCTs (medium-chain triglycerides). The physiology and biochemistry of medium-chain triglycerides are very different from their long-chain, saturated fat cousins. For one thing, they are easier to metabolize. For example, AIDS patients suffering from fat malabsorption and chronic diarrhea with weight loss were significantly benefited by a twelve-week regimen of medium-chain triglycerides. MCTs are also preferentially used for energy rather than stored as fat around your hips. Most important, they are mainly composed of a fat called lauric acid, which is antiviral and antimicrobial. According to no less a source than the *Physicians' Desk Reference*, there is preliminary evidence that MCTs may be helpful in some cancers and may have some positive effects on immunity.

Fifty percent of the fat in coconut is lauric acid. In the human body, lauric acid is formed into monolaurin, which is basically a bug killer: it's antiviral and antibacterial. The late Mary Enig, Ph.D., who was arguably one of the most distinguished lipid biochemists in the country, wrote eloquently on the antiviral and antibacterial effects of lauric acid and coconut in general, documenting its effects on a host of microbes and quoting study after study after study showing its immune-enhancing effects. She has also debunked the idea that the saturated fat in coconut has any adverse effects on the heart or on health in general. (Many of Enig's essays for the public are available online;

they're tough reading, but rigorously documented with strong science.)

Coconuts May Protect against STDs

Another 6 or 7 percent of the fatty acids in coconut fat are MCT called *capric acid*. Capric acid is formed in the human body into monocaprin, which has been shown to have antiviral effects. It is being tested for effects against herpes and antibacterial effects against chlamydia and other sexually transmitted bacteria.

Though some people believe MCTs can be helpful for weight control and athletic performance (because they are an easily metabolized source of calories that are not likely to be stored as fat), this use is controversial. One researcher estimated that people would have to eat more than 50 percent of their calories as MCTs to lose weight, though others have suggested that the

percentage is lower. What is not controversial at all is the use of MCTs therapeutically for cystic fibrosis, AIDS, cachexia (physical wasting secondary to cancer), and childhood epilepsy.

But you don't have to have any of those diseases to benefit from some healthy MCTs in your diet, the best food source of which is coconut and coconut oil. Remember the Pukapuka and Tokelau islanders: they ate a ton of coconut and very little processed food, and they had hardly any heart disease. In today's world, any food that tastes delicious and can enhance your immune system at the same time deserves a place in the honor roll of healthy foods.

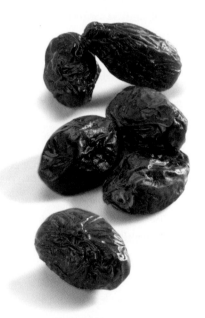

Dates

Dates are described as "nature's candy"—anyone who's ever tried them knows why. But dates aren't on this list because they are such an amazing source of nutrients you can't get anywhere else. No. They're on this list because well, let's face it, we love sweets, and if we're going to eat sweets, they might as well come in a package that does minimal harm and actually might do some good. Enter dates.

Full of Sugar, and Full of Nutrients

Dates are not a low-calorie food, nor are they a low-sugar food. A single large pitted date has a whopping 66 calories, not bad if you eat just one, which, unfortunately, almost nobody does. But that same single

date has calcium and magnesium in an almost perfect 1:1 ratio (15 mg to 14 mg), 1½ g of fiber, and more than 160 mg of heart-healthy potassium. There's even a smidgen of vitamin A, plus trace amounts of a half dozen other vitamins and minerals. You can't say that about a lot of commercial candy bars! The royalty of dates is the Medjool, which most people regard as the best-tasting variety.

And wait, there's more! In a comprehensive study published in the *Journal of the American College of Nutrition*, Harold Miller, Ph.D., and his colleagues analyzed the antioxidant content of cereals, fruits, and vegetables using a complicated scientific method that scores the foods in units called Trolox equivalents (TEs). The findings were surprising. Miller found that many popular vegetables tended to be relatively low in antioxidants. Of the fruits, his team found that red plums had the highest TE score (2200). Of the berries, blackberries won handily with 5500. And of the dried fruits, the winner was . . . dates! On the TE score, dates beat the nearest competitor (raisins) with a score of 6600!

Dates come in various states of dryness. The most common of the semidry dates is the Deglet Noor. Six Deglet Noor dates provide a reasonable 140 calories plus a very respectable 4 g of fiber, a bit of calcium, magnesium, and a nice 327 mg of potassium.

Who Should Avoid Eating Dates?

If you've got blood sugar issues, including metabolic syndrome or diabetes, or if you're trying to lose weight and control sugar, you might want to pass on this one. But if you're an athlete looking for a natural healthy food to provide sugar and calories or to help replace glycogen after a workout, dates might have a place in your kitchen. Chopped up and mixed with some higher-fat, lower-sugar foods like organic almonds and other nuts, they make the perfect trail mix for a long hike.

I rediscovered the joy of dates (and the joy of figs) when Michelle and I were vacationing in our beloved St. Martin, where—if enough of you buy this book and tell your friends—we may someday retire. (Just kidding about retiring.) We rented a house and made a lot of our own meals. There are tons of vendors along the roads selling delicious fresh fruits, and the markets have terrific cheeses, figs, and dates.

One of our go-to mini-meals was a plate of dates, figs, cheeses, and grapes, sometimes accompanied by apples. The dates are so sweet and delicious you can't believe they aren't candy, and the sweetness of the dates tempered with the flavor of tart or creamy cheeses and the juiciness of the grapes (or apples) is a food experience that's hard to beat, especially when you're eating it in a gorgeous tropical island.

WORTH TRYING: DATE MILK

A few pitted dates chopped up and blended into warm milk might just be the ultimate late-night comfort food. It may not be a low-carb, low-calorie, or low-anything food, but it tastes amazing.

FRUIT

Figs

I love figs. Fresh or dried, they're luscious, chewy, rich, textured, and sweet as honey. And, like dates, they might not be the single most nutritionally dense food on the planet, but they sure beat candy if you want some instant sugar in a nice nutritional package.

I recently rediscovered figs, when Michelle and I went on vacation to St. Martin. We rented a house, and we wanted to have as many healthy snacks and light meals around as possible so as not to have to eat out too often. (Restaurants on the French side of St. Martin are very expensive.) We discovered packaged local dried figs in the supermarket, took them home, and paired them with Brie and macadamia nuts. And now that's my new favorite snack!

Figs for Maximum Fiber

Besides tasting great and producing the famous leaves that covered key parts of Adam and Eve, figs have several claims to fame. First is fiber. The American Diabetes Association—with whom I rarely agree—is right on this one: When it comes to fiber, people should eat 25 g to 50 g a day. The National Academy of Sciences says 21 g to 38 g, depending on age and sex. Want to know what the average American takes in? A paltry 11 g. Research from Harvard University has shown that men with the highest dietary fiber intake (about 29 g a day) had a 40 percent reduction in heart attacks compared to men eating the least fiber. High-fiber diets are associated with better blood sugar control and with much better weight control. Six figs contain almost 5 g of fiber, making them a high-fiber food in my book.

Then there's calcium. That same six figs (about 125 calories) give you 82 mg of calcium (plus 34 mg of magnesium). That's more than three times the amount in a glass of orange juice.

You also get a whopping 473 mg of potassium, making figs a high-potassium food. A ton of studies show that people who eat potassium-rich foods have lower rates of heart disease and stroke. And potassium is a key ingredient in keeping blood pressure down. According to the latest studies, people who regularly consume high-potassium foods have lower blood pressure than those who don't. In a review of thirty-three studies that examined the effect of potassium on blood pressure, researchers discovered that participants who started out with normal blood pressure and then added 2,340 mg of potassium daily (from foods, supplements, or both) could lower their risk of developing high blood pressure by 25 percent. The reductions were ultimately greatest for people who already had high blood pressure.

Another possible benefit of potassium: It may protect against stroke. One study found that people with high blood pressure who had a daily serving of potassium-rich foods decreased their risk of fatal stroke by 40 percent.

Use Figs as Sweeteners

Here's a cool tip: Nutritionist Catrinel Stanciu notes that fig puree can be used as a sweetener or as a fat substitute in many recipes. You can make your own fig puree by combining 8 ounces (227 g) of figs with ¼ to ⅓ cup (60 to 80 ml) of water in a blender.

Grapefruit

Anyone who has ever tried to lose weight has likely heard of the Mayo Clinic Diet, which has been passed around for more years than I can remember and which always features grapefruit at every meal followed by some bastardized (and not very good) version of the Atkins Diet.

Only trouble is this: The diet has nothing to do with the Mayo Clinic, was never associated with the Mayo Clinic, and is not endorsed by the Mayo Clinic. Nevertheless, some version of the Mayo Clinic Diet (also known as the grapefruit diet) has been around forever, and so has the legend that grapefruit helps people lose weight. Nutritionists like me have been telling people for eons that that's simply not the case, but that grapefruit, being a whole food with enzymes and low calories and high volume, can certainly help fill you up and be part of any smart weight loss regimen.

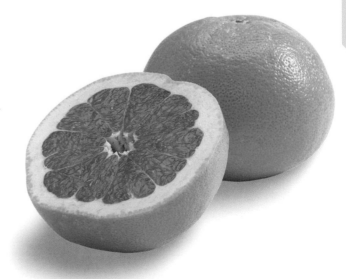

Grapefruit Diet May Be Credible After All

Now it turns out we may have spoken too soon. A study from the division of endocrinology of the department of nutrition and metabolic research at the Scripps Clinic in La Jolla, California, published in the *Journal of Medicinal Food*, shows clearly that the grapefruit legend may have some science to back it up! The researchers wanted to study the effect of grapefruit on weight and on insulin resistance, a central feature of metabolic syndrome (and often of diabetes). They took ninety-one obese patients and divided them into four groups. Group one got grapefruit capsules before meals, group two got grapefruit juice, group three got half a grapefruit, and group four got a placebo (nothing). The placebo group lost about ⅓ of a pound (150 g), the grapefruit capsule group lost 1.1 pounds (500 g), the grapefruit juice group lost 1.3 pounds (590 g), and the real grapefruit folks lost 1.5 pounds (680 g). Overall, only the fresh grapefruit group reached "statistical significance," but among those with metabolic syndrome, all three grapefruit groups lost significantly more weight. Insulin resistance was improved in everyone. The authors admitted that the mechanism isn't understood, but that it would be prudent to include fresh grapefruit in a weight loss diet.

Why Smokers Should Eat More Grapefruit

Meanwhile, even if you're not trying to lose weight, grapefruit's still a good food.

Researchers at Texas A&M University showed that freeze-dried grapefruit pulp, like whole grapefruit, reduced the incidence of early colon cancer lesions in an animal model of the disease. Grapefruit juice may help reduce the risk of cancer in smokers. In a controlled study involving forty-nine smokers, researchers at the University of Hawaii found that drinking three 6-ounce (256 ml) glasses of grapefruit juice a day reduced the activity of a liver enzyme called CYP1A2 that is thought to activate cancer-causing chemicals found in tobacco smoke.

It's reasonable to think that might be helpful for nonsmokers as well, because reducing the activity of an enzyme that activates cancer-causing chemicals is a good thing no matter where the chemicals come from! And speaking of cancer, grapefruits—depending on the species and harvest time—contain substances called limonoids, which inhibit the development of cancer in laboratory animals and in human breast cancer cells and reduce cholesterol. And red (and pink) grapefruit contains lycopene (see guava [page 138] and tomatoes [page 72]), a carotenoid that has been associated with reduced risk of prostate and other cancers.

Red or White?

Researchers in Israel found that a diet supplemented with red grapefruits was effective in lowering triglycerides, a blood fat that is a risk factor for heart disease. In this study, fifty-seven postoperative bypass patients with high triglycerides were divided into three groups. One group was given the standard heart-healthy diet, and the other two groups were given the identical diet but with the addition of either Israeli Jaffa red grapefruit or standard white grapefruit. Only the diet supplemented with the red grapefruit was effective in significantly lowering triglycerides. Those eating the red grapefruit also lowered their LDL ("bad" cholesterol) by 20 percent, more impressive given that all the subjects had previously failed to benefit from cholesterol-lowering drugs! "Red grapefruit is higher in antioxidants, which may explain the difference in health benefits," said study author Shela Gorinstein, Ph.D.

Potential weight loss, cholesterol-lowering, and anticancer benefits aside—and those are big benefits to put aside—grapefruit is a good low-calorie source of potassium and vitamin C. It even has a drop of calcium and magnesium, 20 mg of phytosterols, and a gram or two of fiber. The red and pink varieties also have vitamin A, beta-carotene, and the aforementioned cancer-fighting lycopene.

WORTH KNOWING

Don't take grapefruit juice with medicine. Why? It causes the medicine to stay in the bloodstream longer, which in some cases can boost the amount in your system to a dangerous high. Drugs that are affected include allergy medication (like Allegra), congestive heart failure medication (such as Digoxin), blood pressure medicines and/or calcium channel blockers (like Cozaar, Plendil, Procardia, and Sular), epilepsy drugs (such as Carbatrol and Tegretol), and cholesterol-lowering drugs (like Mevacor, Zocar, and Lipitor). There are probably tons more, so if your med isn't on that list, don't take a chance.

If you're curious as to why this happens, three compounds in grapefruit belonging to a class called furocoumarins inhibit a key enzyme, CYP3A4, that metabolizes and regulates certain drugs. Researchers are hoping to turn these enzyme blockers into a kind of super-pill that can be given with prescription drugs to increase their bioavailability. But until that day, do not mix and match prescription meds with grapefruit juice! Multiple studies have also suggested that grapefruit juice raises the risk of kidney stones.

FRUIT

Grapes

Grapes are one of my favorite desserts, but my secret is this: I freeze them. Don't knock it till you try it. They taste like little balls of sherbet, and they're the perfect munchy finger food for watching late-night reruns of *Seinfeld*.

Grapes are a whole pharmacy of healthful nutrients, many of which are potentially life extending. Take resveratrol. Resveratrol is a compound found in the skin of dark grapes and in the red wine that's made from them. Resveratrol is usually credited for the health-promoting properties of red wine.

Technically, resveratrol belongs to a class of compounds called phytoalexins, which are chemical substances produced by plants as a defense against attack by pathogenic microorganisms. But resveratrol doesn't just protect the plants that make it. In humans, high resveratrol intake is associated with a reduced incidence of cardiovascular disease and a reduced risk for cancer.

Scientists at the Illinois College of Pharmacy in Chicago found that resveratrol showed cancer-preventive activity in three major stages of tumor formation. Resveratrol also acted as an antimutagen, blocking other cell-changing agents from starting cancer. It's also a powerful antioxidant, helping to protect cells against DNA-damaging free radicals.

Grapes Can Add Years to Your Life

Resveratrol may be one of the best antiaging substances around. Research by David Sinclair, Ph.D., says the life span of all life forms tested so far—yeast cells, fruit flies, worms, and mice— have been dramatically lengthened by minute amounts of resveratrol. That's one of the reasons

resveratrol is touted (by me among others) as one of the best antiaging supplements you can take. But you don't have to take a supplement to get your daily dosage of this antiaging compound. Just make grapes a part of your diet! The skins of the dark (red, purple) grapes are the best source.

The benefits of grapes don't stop with resveratrol. Grape seeds and skins are also a huge source of a class of flavonoids called oligomeric proanthocyanidins, or OPCs. Proanthocyanidins are powerful antioxidants— several times more potent than vitamins C and E. They help protect against the effects of internal and environmental stresses (cigarette smoking, pollution). Additionally, studies have shown that OPCs may prevent cardiovascular disease by counteracting the

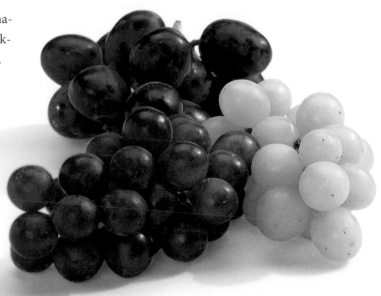

negative effects of high cholesterol on the heart and blood vessels. *Physicians' Desk Reference* states that grape seed proanthocyanidins may be "cardioprotective," a claim that was bolstered by a study from Spain showing that subjects who drank 100 ml of red grape juice every day for two weeks had significantly lowered LDL ("bad" cholesterol), increased HDL ("good" cholesterol), and decreased inflammatory markers.

And OPCs (proanthocyanidins) are terrific for allergies. According to Gina Nick, N.M.D., who has written in the alternative medicine newsletter *Townshend Letter*, on the use of OPCs for allergy symptom relief, OPCs found in grapes have a natural antihistamine effect.

Eat Grapes in Moderation

Many folks are concerned about the sugar in grapes, and yes, the carb count is moderately high if you're watching your carbs. But the glycemic index is moderate, and much more important, the glycemic load—the only measure of sugar impact you need to worry about—is moderately low (under 10). The trick is not to overeat them, which is sometimes difficult. One cup (150 g) contains 106 calories—and one cup disappears quick! Grapes have small amounts of calcium and magnesium, vitamins C, A, and K, and a

decent amount (294 mg) of potassium. I recommend eating them seeds and all. Too many amazing health-promoting compounds have been extracted from the seeds to throw them away.

A number of grape seed oil vendors have claimed that grape seed oil is high in OPCs (proanthocyanidins). However, independent studies have indicated that grape seed oil is the grape product with the lowest concentration of OPCs. I don't recommend grape seed oil in any case. According to natural-foods expert Rebecca Wood, the toxins of a plant (like the toxins in an animal) are concentrated in its fat, and a plant's fatty acids are concentrated in its seeds. Until someone makes an organic, unrefined grape seed oil free of the chemicals most commercial grapes are grown with, buying grape seed oil isn't advised.

WORTH KNOWING

The Environmental Working Group, a consumer advocate and protection nonprofit research organization, frequently puts grapes on its notorious "dirty dozen" list of twelve foods most contaminated with pesticides. It was on the list back in 2003 when I started working on the first edition of this book, and it's on the list in 2016 when I worked on the revised, 10th year anniversary edition. I suggest you buy organic.

FRUIT

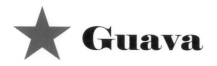 Guava

Guavas are fragrant, delicious tropical fruits that many Americans know only because they're frequently used in jellies. But these red-fleshed (and sometimes white-fleshed) fruits pack an amazing nutritional wallop. New government research demonstrates that guava may indeed deserve a place among the antioxidant elite. On one widely used test of antioxidant power called the ORAC test, guava beat out strawberries, spinach, and broccoli. Both the red and the white-fleshed types of guava scored in the top ten fruits and vegetables tested, but the red flesh had a higher antioxidant score.

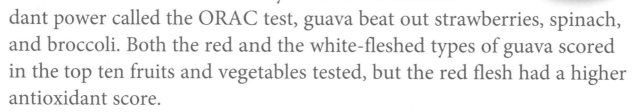

Let's start with the number-one-with-a-bullet reason why guava is such a superstar: lycopene.

Lycopene in Guava Fights Prostate and Breast Cancers

Guava has a higher concentration of the carotenoid lycopene than any other fruit or vegetable. Tomatoes are the main way Americans get their lycopene, but guavas are an even better source. A cup (165 g) of guava has 17 percent more lycopene than an equivalent amount of tomatoes. Why do we care? Consider this: In laboratory experiments, lycopene has been found to provide more protection against free radicals than any other member of the entire carotenoid family—and that includes beta-carotene!

And lycopene may save lives. It's an antioxidant that, once absorbed by the body, helps prevent and repair damaged cells. Antioxidants are the internal bodyguards that protect our cells from DNA-damaging free radicals. The degenerative effects of free radicals include—but are not limited to—cancer. Free radicals can also cause blockages in the arteries, joint deterioration, nervous system degradation, and aging.

There is promising research showing that lycopene is associated with significant reduction in prostate cancer. As far back as 1995, the *Journal of the National Cancer Institute* published the results of a study conducted by Harvard University researchers that looked at the eating habits of more than 47,000 men between the ages of forty and seventy-five. They found that the men eating ten servings or more a week of high-lycopene tomatoes, tomato sauce, tomato juice, and even pizza had 45 percent fewer prostate cancers than men who ate fewer than two servings a week. In another study, done a few years later at the

It's interesting to note that the leaves of the guava plant, though they are not eaten, have a huge history of medicinal uses. Guava leaves are in the *Dutch Pharmacopoeia* for the treatment of diarrhea, and the leaves are still used for diarrhea in Latin America, Central and West Africa, and Southeast Asia. In Peruvian herbal medicine systems today the plant is employed for diarrhea, gastroenteritis, gastric disorders, and menstrual pain. Indians through-out the Amazon make a leaf decoction—a tea made by boiling the leaves—and use it for mouth sores and bleeding gums. A decoction is also recommended as a gargle for sore throats, laryngitis, and swelling of the mouth, and is used externally for skin irritations and discharges. A Chinese study published in 2004 noted that the guava leaves contained "remarkably high phenolic content."

Karmanos Cancer Institute in Detroit, researchers gave lycopene supplements to thirty men who already had prostate cancer. Those given the lycopene supplements had smaller tumors and less spreading of the cancer. Best of all, the tumors in the participants who consumed lycopene supplements showed signs of regression and decreased malignancy.

Lycopene also inhibits the growth of breast cancer cells; in research, it has suppressed and delayed breast tumors in mice. And according to studies with Lithuanian and Swedish people, lower blood lycopene levels are also associated with increased risk of coronary heart disease.

Cooked or Uncooked, You Get All the Benefits of Guava

More lycopene is absorbed from cooked or processed tomatoes than from raw ones because their cell walls are tough and heat and processing breaks them down. According to my friend C. Leigh Broadhurst, Ph.D., of the USDA, the same isn't true of guavas, whose cell walls are much less tough. Unlike tomatoes, you'll get all the benefits of guava, the lycopene superstar, with or without cooking.

But it's not just lycopene that makes guava a superstar. It's also potassium. This fruit is a potassium heavyweight. One little cup (165 g) of guava cubes gives you a whopping 688 mg of potassium. Just for comparison, that's 63 percent more than a medium banana! A ton of studies show that people who eat potassium-rich foods have lower rates of heart disease and stroke. Potassium is also a key component of healthy blood pressure. According to the latest studies, people who regularly consume high-potassium foods have lower blood pressure than those who don't. A review of thirty-three studies examined the effect of potassium on blood pressure, and researchers discovered that participants who added 2,340 mg of potassium daily (from foods, supplements, or both) were able to lower their risk of developing high blood pressure by 25 percent. The reductions were ultimately greatest for people who already had high blood pressure. Another possible benefit of potassium: It may protect against stroke. One study found that people with high blood pressure who had a daily serving of potassium-rich foods (like figs) decreased their risk of fatal stroke by 40 percent.

Potassium Is Just the Beginning: Guava Is Also High in Fiber and Vitamin C

There's just no end to what this fruit has to offer. It's high in fiber. (In fact, if this fruit did nothing more

FRUIT

than offer the amount of fiber it does, it might make the top 150 list on that alone.) The same 1 cup (165 g) of fruit we've been talking about delivers almost 9 g of fiber, making it a high-fiber food in anyone's book. High-fiber diets have been associated with lower rates of cancer, heart disease, diabetes, and obesity, not to mention a healthier microbiome.

And if all that weren't enough, 1 cup (165 g) of guava delivers an amazing 376 mg of vitamin C, making it a heavyweight in that department as well. Plus it offers 81 mcg of folate, a decent amount of calcium and magnesium, and a significant amount of vitamin A (1,030 IUs) and beta-carotene (617 mcg). Fruit really doesn't get much better than this.

With all of these powerful nutrients, it is no wonder that a study from the Heart Research Laboratory in India demonstrated that people who ate five to nine guavas a day—about 2 to 3 cups (330 to 495 g)—for three months reduced their cholesterol levels by 10 percent, triglycerides by 8 percent, and blood pressure by 9.0/8.0 mm Hg, while boosting their "good" cholesterol (HDL) by 8 percent.

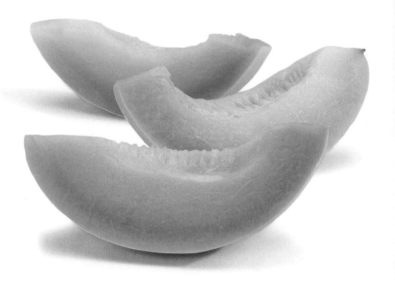

Honeydew

Honeydew melon may not be as loaded with vitamins and minerals as cantaloupe, but it's still a high-volume food that's both nutritious and potentially useful in a weight loss program.

Melons are high-volume foods. That means that for a given amount of weight, they contain a relatively high amount of water, fiber, and air (and a relatively low number of calories.)

Eat Honeydew to Control Your Appetite

Barbara Rolls, Ph.D., a nutrition researcher at Pennsylvania State University, has done a lot of research on appetite and appetite control. Rolls has found that people basically ate about 3 pounds (1.4 kg) of food a day, regardless of whether the food was high or low calorie. People stopped eating after consuming about 3 pounds (1.4 kg). They'd eat nearly identical servings of food (by weight), whether it was honeydew (high volume) or cheesecake (low volume). The subjects in her studies felt just as full after the low-calorie meals as they did after the calorie-rich meals—provided both meals contained the same volume of food.

Bottom line: Foods with high volume and low calories—that is, foods with a lot of water and fiber—are your best friend when it comes to weight loss.

Honeydew is truly a high-volume food. For goodness' sake, an entire half melon has only 180 calories, less than most desserts. A typical serving is a wedge, or maybe a quarter of a melon. About 90 percent of the melon is water. But, as Rolls has shown in research study after research study, that water in the melon goes a long way toward filling you up. And, by the way—water in foods seems to do this more than water that you drink alongside foods. Hence melons and soups do a better job of appetite control than solid food plus a glass of water. No one really knows why.

But honeydew's not a great food just because it's high-volume and low-calorie, though that certainly gives it points. It's also a potassium and vitamin A heavyweight. One little cup (165 g) of melon balls gives you a whopping 404 mg of potassium (not to mention a little calcium and magnesium and 31 mg of vitamin C). A ton of studies show that people who eat foods rich in potassium have lower rates of heart disease and stroke.

Potassium is also a key component of a healthy blood pressure. According to the latest studies, people who regularly consume high-potassium foods have lower blood pressure than those who don't. A review of thirty-three studies examined the effect of potassium on blood pressure, and researchers discovered that participants who added 2,340 mg of potassium daily (from foods, supplements, or both) could lower their risk of developing high blood pressure by 25 percent. The reductions were ultimately greatest for people who already had high blood pressure. Another possible benefit of potassium: It may protect against stroke. One study found that people with high blood pressure who had a daily serving of potassium-rich foods decreased their risk of fatal stroke by 40 percent.

Honeydew also makes an amazing juice. Like cantaloupe and watermelon, it can be combined with other melons and sparkling water for a terrific summer cooler. Try adding ginger and mint to the mix.

Note: Crenshaw and casaba melons are similar nutritionally to honeydew. All are high in potassium; all have a little calcium, magnesium, and vitamin C; and all are mostly water, low in calories, and utterly delicious.

Jackfruit

I wish I could tell you I discovered jackfruit the way my friend Chris Kilham (a.k.a the Medicine Hunter) would have, traipsing around the Brazilian rain forest with a machete searching for hidden sources of nutritional magic and medicine. But I found it in Whole Foods.

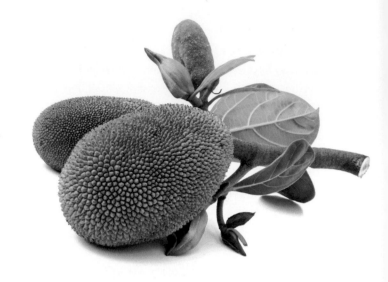

There it was sitting in a little plastic pouch, offering itself up as a new healthy snack and looking for all the world like dried papaya. I decided to try it, and I'm glad I did. The dried fruit sold in stores is chewy, sweet, fibrous, and delicious.

The fruit itself is huge. As in humongous. It's the largest tree-borne fruit in the entire world, and it can weigh as much as 100 pounds. And while the fruit has a lot of vitamin C, it contains hundreds and hundreds of nutrient-rich seeds that have a lot of protein, calcium, potassium and iron. The fruit itself comes from South and Southeast Asia—in fact, it's the national fruit in Bangladesh. And though you'll almost never find it in the United States, you can sometimes get whole jackfruit in places such as Chinatown in New York City. (And packaged jackfruit snack in places like Whole Foods!)

The unripe fruits are green but turn light brown, gaining a strong, sweet fruity smell as they ripen. Jackfruit is high in fiber, and the fruit has a fair amount of vitamin A, beta-carotene, and lutein, all of which play crucial roles in vision. It's also a good source of vitamin C, and is one of the rare fruits that are high in B-complex vitamins, especially B_6, niacin, riboflavin, and folic acid. It's also an excellent source of potassium, magnesium, manganese, and even iron. (Potassium is an important nutrient that helps control heart rate and blood pressure.)

Research shows that almost all parts of the jackfruit tree are used in preparations of many Ayurvedic and Unani medicines, and ripe fruits are eaten to prevent excessive bile formation, to strengthen the body, and to increase vitality. Medical practitioners in Sri Lanka and India use the leaves to treat diabetes. The roots, on the other hand, are useful for treating different types of skin diseases, asthma, and diarrhea. In Chinese medicine, jackfruit can potentially help with alcohol addiction.

Interesting factoid department: Though the jackfruit is prized in places like Bangladesh, it's avoided in India, even though it could bring food to millions of starving, malnourished Indian citizens. Up to 75 percent of jackfruit grown in India goes to waste, largely because it has a bad reputation in India as a "poor man's fruit." It grows everywhere and is not particularly valued, and most of it goes to rot.

Everywhere else in Southeast Asia, jackfruit is a booming business. It makes its way into curry, stir-fry, chips, ice cream, baking flour made from the seeds . . . and, as I recently found out, into tasty little snack packs of dried fruit sold at Whole Foods. If you can find it, it's worth trying. It's both delicious and nutritious, and it lends itself to all kinds of imaginative dishes.

 # Kiwifruit

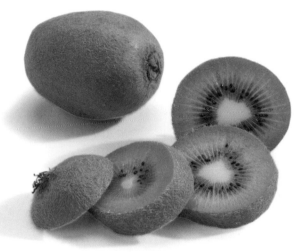

According to Dharma Singh Khalsa, M.D., the internationally acclaimed expert in integrative medicine and author of *Food as Medicine*, the kiwifruit is one of the most underrated healing foods. "Because of their rich array of disease-fighting antioxidants and phytonutrients, they are often prescribed in yoga nutritional therapy to help fight cancer and heart disease," he says.

Kiwis Have Twice the Vitamin C of Oranges

I'm not surprised. A study conducted at Rutgers University in New Brunswick, New Jersey, evaluated the nutritional value of twenty-seven different fruits to determine, ounce for ounce, which provides the most nutrition. The results? Kiwifruit, with an index of 16, was found to be the most nutrient dense of all fruits. Second place was papaya at 14, and third place was a tie between mango and orange, which both scored 11. Kiwi has the highest level of vitamin C, almost twice that of an orange, and it is also a decent source of magnesium. Two medium kiwifruits have almost 5 g of fiber. And kiwi—along with papaya and apricot—outranked bananas and oranges as the top low-sodium, high-potassium food!

Another study in the *Journal of Medicinal Food* examined nine different fruits and fruit juices and reported that eight of them—including kiwi—exhibited significant ability to reduce oxidative stress (damage from free radicals) in human plasma. This ability of kiwi to protect against cellular damage was confirmed in yet another study in *Carcinogenesis* that was even more promising: In this *Carcinogenesis* study, not only did the kiwifruit limit the amount of oxidative damage to DNA, but it also stimulated cellular repair of the damage that did occur! Even better, the effect of kiwifruit on DNA damage and repair was seen when it was simply added to a normal diet, and the effects were seen across a whole group of volunteers and in a very short time!

Kiwi Works as a Blood Thinner, with None of Aspirin's Side Effects

In research at the University of Oslo in Norway, kiwi has been shown to promote heart health by working as a blood thinner. This ability is important, considering how many people are told to take an aspirin a day for the same purpose. According to gastroenterologist and author of *Optimal Digestion,* Trent Nichols, M.D., daily aspirin can cause small breaks in the intestinal walls, contributing to all sorts of problems. In the Norway study, lead researcher Asim Duttaroy, Ph.D., noted that it was unlikely that kiwi would create any of the risk factors associated with aspirin such as stomach pain, excessive bruising, or bleeding. Kiwi also doesn't disrupt the effects of any other medication. Can you imagine how great it would be to find natural food substances and supplements that accomplish the same cardiovascular protections as some medicines do, without any of the side effects?

Kiwifruits look like little brown furry eggs. They are native to China, though they're now grown in Australia, New Zealand, and California. The little black seeds inside are edible, and the kiwi makes a great addition to fresh juice. If you juice them unpeeled, and with the seeds, they are rich in healthy enzymes.

Consumption of fresh fruits rich in vitamin C has been shown to be beneficial in protecting against respiratory symptoms associated with asthma and to help with wheezing symptoms in children. Kiwi has one of the highest vitamin C contents of any fruit.

WORTH KNOWING

The Environmental Working Group, a consumer advocate and protection nonprofit research organization, frequently names kiwifruit on its annual list of foods least contaminated with pesticides. The list is called the "Clean Fifteen" and can easily be found online. Kiwis made the list in 2003 when I first began work on this book, and were still on the list in 2017, the year I finished the revised edition. Nice to know!

Lemons/Limes

"When life gives you a lemon . . . squeeze it, mix with 6 ounces of water, and drink twice daily." That folk wisdom was first reported by Jethro Kloss in his classic book, *Back to Eden.*

He was on to something.

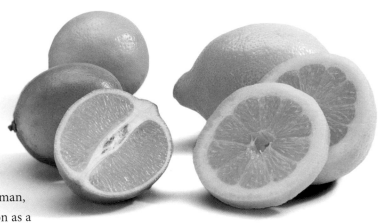

Lemons

Lemons have been used in folk remedies for as long as anyone can remember, and the health benefits are now being documented in the science lab. (I love when that happens!) Back when I was a musician, I remember all the singers drinking hot water and lemon for their throats. My good friend Ann Louise Gittleman, Ph.D., C.N.S., has long used hot water and lemon as a staple in all her dietary programs, largely for its positive effects on the liver, the bile, and digestion. And according to naturopathic physician Andrew Rubman, N.D., half of a lemon daily raises the level of citrate in the body, which may help in fighting kidney stones.

Note: Other citrus juices do not have this effect; grapefruit juice has the opposite effect and should be avoided if you're prone to kidney stones.

Lemon Peel and Hot Black Tea for Reduced Risk of Skin Cancer

Most of us know that lemons, like other citrus fruits, are a great source of vitamin C, a powerful antioxidant as well as an anti-inflammatory agent. For that reason alone, lemons would be a healthy fruit. But lemons also have been found to have two other compounds—a group of chemicals called limonoids, and specifically a compound called limonene, both of which have documented anticancer properties.

WORTH KNOWING

There are two basic types of lemons—acidic and sweet. While the acidic types, Eureka and Lisbons, are the most widely available, the sweet types are becoming increasingly more available, though they're used primarily as ornamental fruit. There's also a seasonal lemon known as a Meyer lemon that lots of people positively love. It's moderately acidic, but it doesn't have nearly the sour "kick" of regular lemons. In fact it's sweet. Meyer lemons are believed to be a cross between regular lemons and mandarin oranges. They generally show up in stores between December and May.

Limonene is found in the peel and has been shown in studies to be chemopreventive against mammary, liver, lung, and UV-induced skin cancer, and chemotherapeutic against mammary and pancreatic tumors. A study from the University of Arizona concluded that when citrus peel is consumed with hot black tea, the risk of skin cancer is reduced by 30 percent. (It's amazing how these traditional combinations—tea and lemon, for example—keep being validated by science, isn't it?). And it doesn't take much limonene to get the value. According to the researchers, consuming 1 tablespoon (6 g) a week of the grated peel is all you really need to make a significant difference. One good idea: When making lemonade, use the whole fruit, including the peel! And don't be afraid to make fresh juice with a juicer, using the whole fruit.

WORTH KNOWING

Citrus fruits are among the dozen or so most allergenic foods—not as high on the list as wheat and dairy, but they can pose a problem for some sensitive people.

Limes Saved Lives

Back in the days when the maritime explorers started penetrating the Indian and Pacific Oceans, huge numbers of crew members were being lost to scurvy. Vasco da Gama lost two-thirds of his crew to the disease while making his way to India in 1499. Magellan lost 80 percent of his crew while crossing the Pacific. The symptoms of scurvy weren't pretty: skin black as ink, ulcers, difficult respiration, teeth falling out, and perhaps most revolting of all, a strange mass of gum tissue sprouting out of the mouth. Not anything you'd want to have.

Now we know that scurvy was a vitamin deficiency disease, mainly of vitamin C, and sometimes compounded by an overdose of vitamin A from eating seals' livers. Only when Captain James Cook of England insisted on feeding his crew sauerkraut and lime juice to fight scurvy (based on studies done by physician James Lind in 1747) did the death rate begin to go down. But it was not until 1795 that lime juice rations were provided for all sailors in the Royal Navy, and to this day, British sailors are known as "limeys."

Limes don't differ a lot from lemons in their nutritional value. They're hardly a nutritional powerhouse, but they're a good source of vitamin C, add a nice tart taste to foods and drinks, and can be substituted for lemons in most dishes.

Mangoes

Mangoes are known as the "king of fruit," and it's easy to understand why: They're just plain delicious. They originated in Southeast Asia, where they have been grown for more than 4,000 years; legend has it that Buddha found tranquility in a mango grove.

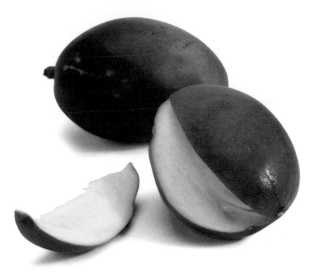

In India, the mango tree plays a sacred role: it's a symbol of love, and some believe the tree can grant wishes. Many Southeast Asian kings and nobles had their own mango groves, which were a source of great pride and status. That's where the custom of sending gifts of the choicest mangoes began.

Mangoes are a high-volume food, meaning they contain a high percentage of water, so you get a lot of food for a relatively few number of calories (135 for a whole mango). Mangoes have a lot of potassium, vitamin A, and beta-carotene, plus they have some vitamin C, vitamin K, calcium, phosphorus, and magnesium, as well as a smattering of other nutrients. They're believed to be a rich source of enzymes, making them ideal to use as a tenderizing agent and perfect for marinades. And one mango contains more than 3½ g of fiber.

Choosing the Best Mango

Picking out a mango to buy is pretty easy. The ripe ones have a full, fruity aroma coming from the stem end. When they're slightly soft to the touch and yield-

WORTH KNOWING

According to natural-foods expert Rebecca Wood, mangoes—along with poison ivy, poison oak, and poison sumac—all contain urushinol, a toxic resin that can cause contact dermatitis. The peel and the juice seem to be the problem rather than the flesh. It's possible—though not common—that eating mangos to excess could cause itching or skin eruptions. On a good note, the Environmental Working Group, a consumer advocate and protection nonprofit research organization, regularly includes mangoes on its "Clean Fifteen" list of foods least contaminated with pesticides. Nice to know!

ing to gentle pressure, they're considered ready to eat. The best way to ripen them is at room temperature, though you can hasten the process by putting them in a paper bag. Some folks put an apple in the bag with the mango because it further decreases the ripening time by creating more natural ethylene gas. They have the most flavor if you eat them at room temperature, though you can refrigerate them if you like.

Mangoes are another of the tropical fruits that got a bad reputation among the low-carb folks due to their sugar content. While it's true that a whole mango contains 30 g of natural sugar, and people with blood sugar concerns may have to watch their intake of fruit, mangoes don't actually have a very high glycemic load, weighing in at about 8 (under 10 is considered low, over 20 is considered high).

Mangosteen

(and Mangosteen Juice)

You won't find mangosteen growing in the United States. But in Southeast Asia, it's referred to as "the queen of fruits" and "the fruit of the gods." That's because on the islands of Southeast Asia—where it grows on a native evergreen tree it plays a central role in traditional medicine.

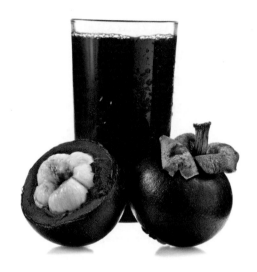

The rind of the fruit is rich in substances known as xanthones, which are naturally occurring plant chemicals. Xanthones—named for the Greek word for yellow—are a yellow pigment that can offer some protection against certain types of cancer. One review study on xanthones from mangosteen extracts noted that "Multiple lines of evidence from numerous in vitro and in vivo studies have confirmed that xanthones inhibit proliferation of a wide range of human tumor cell types."

The problem is that the xanthones are found primarily in the rind, which no one eats, but some of the higher quality mangosteen juices are made from both the fruit and the rind (the pericamp), so theoretically you should get some xanthones in the better juices.

Besides having anticancer effects, xanthones exhibit a wide range of biological activities—they're both anti-inflammatory and antibacterial.

Aside from the xanthones, mangosteen (the fruit) contains a good amount of B-complex vitamins as well as minerals such as copper, manganese, magnesium and potassium. But the real selling point of the fruit (and specifically, the fruit juices) are the xanthones.

That's an important point. The mangosteen fruit is still considered exotic in the United States, and they're not exactly easy to find nor particularly popular. But mangosteen juice products have made a big splash, largely because of aggressive marketing and an almost insatiable need for the next big thing.

There's no doubt that the scientific literature on xanthones is strong and promising, but that begs the question: how much xanthones make it into mangosteen juice products? Some juices may have a high-xanthones level, some may have a zero xanathones level. This doesn't mean they're bad. Mangosteen is a perfectly fine juice with a lot of good stuff in it, but it really doesn't have anything you can't get in other less exotic juices.

Tip: Look for mangosteen juice that's made from both the mangosteen fruit and the pericarp. (The pericarp is the rind, where all the xanthones hang out.)

Oranges

A few years ago, when the low-carb craze was sweeping the country, there were rumblings that an association of citrus growers was threatening to sue low-carb diet docs who were claiming that orange juice was not much more than sugar water. At the time, my book *Living Low Carb* was a bestseller, so Fox News asked me to be a talking head on one of their magazine shows, debating another talking head representing the orange growers.

On my way to the studio I picked up a well-known brand of "single serving" orange juice drink from the local 7-Eleven. Shortly after the "debate" began, I simply held the bottle up, and read the ingredients out loud. As I recall, the first two ingredients were water and sugar and the total carb (sugar) content was somewhere around 50 g. "But wait," said my opponent. "Look how much better it is than soda!" "Better than soda?" I said. "Yes. Does that make it 'good'? No. It makes it 'better than soda.'"

Game over.

Orange Juice Can't Compete with Whole Oranges

Don't get me wrong. Real, squeezed orange juice isn't all bad. In fact, the Harvard Nurses' Health Study, which included more than 87,000 people, showed a 25 percent lower risk of stroke in those who drank one glass of orange juice a day, though those results may have been due to other healthy habits of the juice drinkers. And many of the cancer-fighting limonoids (see below) are also present in the juice. But compared to the whole fruit, orange juice is a second-class citizen and contributes far too much sugar to our diet;

it doesn't hold a candle to the health benefits of the whole orange.

So no, I'm not much of a fan of orange juice, especially not "orange juice drinks" (translation: sugar water with chemically created orange flavor). I am, however, a huge fan of oranges, for a host of reasons of which vitamin C is only the first. Vitamin C, of course, is one of the premier antioxidants on the planet, maintaining the health of cells and helping to protect them against damage from destructive molecules known as free radicals, which are linked to cancer, DNA damage, and aging. But though the orange is famous for its vitamin C content (63.5 mg per medium fruit), it actually has more than 170 cancer-fighting phytochemicals and 60 flavonoids, making it a complete package of health-promoting goodness.

Orange Therapy

Oranges contain limonoids, phytochemicals abundant in citrus fruit that account for the scent of fresh lemon and orange peels. (Many of the plants used in traditional healing, such as the neem plant, are rich in limonoids.) Currently limonoids are under investigation for a wide variety of therapeutic effects such as antiviral, antifungal, antibacterial, antineoplastic, and antimalarial. In laboratory tests with animals and with human cells, citrus limonoids have been shown to help fight cancers of the mouth, skin, lung, breast, stomach, and colon. And a metabolic by-product of these limonoids called limonin remains in the bloodstream for up to twenty-four hours, helping to explain some of its ability to fight cancer cells. Early research has speculated that limonin may help lower cholesterol—Agricultural Research Service scientists are now investigating its cholesterol-lowering ability.

In addition to limonoids, oranges have other polyphenols that have been shown to have a wide range of benefits. Hesperidin, for example, is the predominant flavonoid in oranges; it strengthens the capillaries and has anti-inflammatory, antiallergic, vasoprotective, and anticarcinogenic actions. Hesperidin works together with vitamin C to protect the heart, combat cancer, and fight infection. Together, these two powerful antioxidants also reduce the risk of stroke, lower high blood pressure, reduce inflammation, and improve cholesterol profiles.

Oranges also contain additional heart-health promoters, including blood pressure–lowering potassium, cholesterol-lowering pectin fibers, and homocysteine-lowering folate. Plus, the heart is protected by the orange-yellow carotenoid beta-cryptoxanthin. Numerous studies have shown that citrus fruits lower the risk of many cancers. To top it off, oranges contain calcium to promote strong bones and teeth. One medium orange also contains a nice 3.4 g of fiber, another benefit of eating the fruit instead of just drinking the juice.

Don't Forget: Pulp Is Your Friend

The thing to remember is that a lot of these healthy compounds like the limonoids are found in the white stuff that surrounds the orange, or even in the peel. That's another reason I prefer eating (or juicing) the whole orange. If you do juice, remember that the pulp is your friend—don't throw it away. If you want to make orange juice and your juicer is one of those powerhouses that can handle it, throw the whole fruit in, peel and all. It'll be a little tart, but you can handle it. Or try throwing a little of the peel in just to get used to the flavor. Even a little is better than nothing!

Papaya

Papaya—along with pineapple—is one of the best sources of digestive enzymes. Papaya contains *papain*, an enzyme that helps break down or digest protein. Papain is often extracted from papaya and used in digestive enzyme supplements as well as in enzyme supplements that are used for pain (e.g., arthritis, sports injuries).

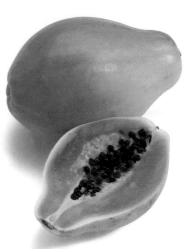

Papaya Enzymes Ease Digestion, Pain, and Inflammation

Papaya is a potassium heavyweight. One medium papaya has 781 mg of potassium and 119 calories, not to mention 5.5 mg of fiber. A cup (145 g) of cubed fruit has only 55 calories and still contains 360 mg of potassium, as well as 34 mg of calcium, 2.5 g of fiber, 86.5 mg of vitamin C, 53 mcg of folate, more than 1,500 IUs of vitamin A, 386 mcg of beta-carotene, and 105 mcg of the eye-protecting carotenoids lutein and zeaxanthin.

Figure there's a little more than 2 cups (290 g) of fruit in one medium papaya. And papaya could easily be considered an immune system–building fruit because vitamin C and vitamin A are both needed for the proper function of a healthy immune system.

Reduce Your Lung Cancer Risk by 30 Percent

Papaya is also a great source of the lesser-known cousin of beta-carotene, beta-cryptoxanthin. (One medium fruit contains 2,313 mcg.) Studies have shown that beta-cryptoxanthin can reduce the risk of lung cancer by more than 30 percent. Other studies have shown that it reduces the risk for rheumatoid arthritis as well (by 41 percent in one study). It also appears to have strong antioxidant properties.

There are about fifty varieties of papayas, many of which are inedible and not sold commercially, and they can range from 8 ounces (225 g) to—believe it or not—20 pounds (9 kg). Most common commercial varieties, such as the Hawaiian Solo, are on the small side. Papayas with reddish flesh have a taste that differs from that of the orange-fleshed types, which are sweeter.

If you buy papayas green and firm, they will probably not ripen, but you can use them in cooking (they can be cooked like winter squash). For eating raw, choose fruit that's free of black spots and skin damage. The spreading yellow color indicates that the fruit is softening and shows how far along it is in ripening. By the way, the black seeds inside are edible—they have a slightly bitter, peppery taste.

WORTH KNOWING

The Environmental Working Group ranked papaya seventh on its list of foods least contaminated with pesticides, known as the "Clean Fifteen."

Peaches

Peaches are my idea of a nice, generic fruit. Maybe they're not the nutritional superstar of the fruit community, but they sure meet all the requirements of a healthy food. Low calorie, 1½ grams of fiber, small but measurable amounts of calcium, magnesium, phosphorus, vitamins C and K, plus not insignificant amounts of vitamin A, beta-carotene, and potassium. And peaches contain a little beta-cryptoxanthin, a carotenoid with some anticancer and anti-inflammatory properties. They even have a smattering of lutein and zeaxanthin, the carotenoids now considered the superstars of eye nutrition.

Not bad for a mere 38 calories per medium-size fruit. And just for good measure, they have a low glycemic load—a measure of the impact a food has on your blood sugar.

The New Superbreed of Peaches

In coming years, peaches may even reach superstar status, if researchers at the Texas Agricultural Experiment Station have anything to say about it. "The trend is to develop varieties that have more health benefits, because the public is becoming more health conscious and making decisions based on that," said David Byrne, Ph.D., experiment station researcher who has been breeding peaches for about twenty years. "Twenty years ago, the [breeding] emphasis was on big and pretty. That's still important, but now we are looking at quality and trying to develop peaches with better health benefits." Peaches already rank high in some types of phytochemicals and have been shown to have good to excellent antioxidant activity, some antimicrobial activity, and good to excellent tumor growth inhibition activity.

Did I mention that they're also delicious?

The peach originated in China, and the peach tree was the Tree of Life to the ancient Chinese. Both peaches and nectarines have to be picked ripe—they don't ripen well after picking. You also have to be careful with them, as one small bruise and they'll go bad. Clingstone peaches are ones in which the pit clings to the flesh; freestone peaches are ones where the pit breaks free.

Pineapple

This delicious fruit not only looks healthy, but also it smells healthy. And most important, it is healthy. How can you miss?

Nutritionally, pineapple's claim to fame is the fact that it contains bromelain, a rich source of enzymes that has many health benefits, including aiding digestion, speeding wound healing, and reducing inflammation. According to integrative medicine expert Andrew Weil, M.D., bromelain is effective in treating bruises, sprains, and strains by reducing swelling, tenderness, and pain. It's also a natural blood thinner, as it prevents excessive blood platelet stickiness.

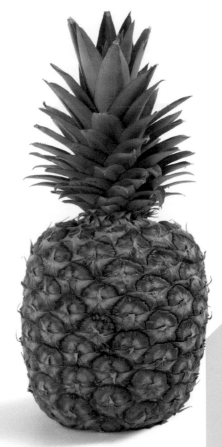

The Good Stuff Is in the Stem

Because it's a group of powerful digestive enzymes, bromelain can relieve indigestion. A member of the class of enzymes known as proteolytic enzymes, bromelain breaks down the amino acid bonds in protein. It's often extracted from pineapple and is a key ingredient in most over-the-counter digestive enzymes.

But—like many nutritive compounds found in our food—bromelaine may have multiple benefits, including some that are still being investigated. In research at the Queensland Institute of Medical Research in Australia, two molecules—CCS and CCZ—were extracted from bromelain and shown to have promise in fighting cancer growth. Lead researcher Tracey Mynott, Ph.D., said " . . . [W]e discovered that the CCS and CCZ proteins . . . could block growth of a broad range of tumor cells, including breast, lung, colon, ovarian, and melanoma."

Remember that most of the extracts studied come from the inedible pineapple stem, (see below, under Worth Knowing).

A cup (165 g) of cubed fresh pineapple has almost 100 percent of the Daily Value for manganese, an essential trace mineral needed for healthy skin, bone, and cartilage formation, as well as for glucose tolerance. Manganese also helps activate an important antioxidant enzyme called superoxide dismutase (SOD). Depending on the variety, pineapple also has between 25 and 50 mg of vitamin C, plus a smattering of other vitamins and minerals, including potassium. One cup (165 g) contains about 2 g of fiber. And pineapple's glycemic load—a measure of a food's impact on your blood sugar—is relatively low.

Most of the bromelain is found in the stems—not necessarily something you'd actually eat. The bromelaine found in most supplements is extracted mainly from the stem. But some bromelaine is found in the fruit as well. Want proof? Try making a gelatin dessert with fresh pineapple. It's the bromelain enzymes that prevent the gelatin from setting, leaving you with a runny mess—and proof that there is some bromelain in the fruit. That said, those who are using bromelain for specific health reasons—digestion, anti-inflammation, blood thinning—might want to take supplements to get more bromelain than is found in the average serving of pineapple.

Bromelain has shown therapeutic benefits in doses as small as 160 mg per day, but for most conditions the best results are seen at 750 to 1,000 mg per day in divided doses, usually between meals.

The Environmental Working Group, a consumer advocate and protection nonprofit research organization, frequently puts pineapples on its "Clean Fifteen" list of foods least contaminated with pesticides. Nice to know!

Prunes

Okay, honest answer: What's the first thing you think of when I say "prunes"? Half the people I know think of shuffleboard courts, retirement communities, and their ancient relatives sipping prune juice for regularity. But, truth be told, this is one delicious fruit, and one of the best and easiest ways to get soluble fiber into your diet. And don't underestimate the whole idea of regularity—though it's hardly sexy, regular healthy bowel movements are a very good indication of good digestion, and because the gut is ground zero for both the immune system and nutrient absorption, they're more important for ultimate well-being than you might think.

Prunes Are the Dried Version of European Plums

All prunes come from plums, but not every variety of plum can become a prune. Prunes are actually the dried version of European plums. But juicy plums can't morph into prunes—the fermentation will spoil them before they can dry.

You can thank the California gold rush for domestic dried plums (another term for prunes). Though plum trees have been cultivated since ancient times, they weren't introduced to North America till 1856, by a Frenchman. When he failed miserably at mining gold, he planted plum trees, covering California with more than 90,000 acres of orchards over the next thirty-five years.

Prunes are high in fiber, which is beneficial in reducing the risk of colorectal cancer. Fiber is also important in reducing the risk factors for cardiovascular disease, breast cancer, diabetes, and diverticular disease. High-fiber diets are usually much more successful for weight loss than low-fiber diets.

Prunes are also a good source of vitamin A, vitamin C, potassium, and iron. They contain large amounts of phenolics, the general name for a huge and diverse group of plant compounds with numerous health benefits. The phenolics in prunes have high antioxidant activity. The two types of phytonutrients (nutrients from plants) found in plums and prunes, neochlorogenic acid and chlorogenic acid, are effective antioxidants, particularly effective against a very destructive free radical called the superoxide anion radical, which can really wreak havoc on the cells in your body.

Prunes Boast More Antioxidants Than Any Other Fruit

The damage-preventing substances in prunes have been shown to help prevent damage to fats. Our cell membranes and brain cells are largely composed of fats, and preventing free radical damage to fats is a significant benefit. Cholesterol is also a kind of fat, and in fact, is only a real danger to us when it gets oxidized (or damaged by free radicals) in the body. So anything helping to prevent this oxidation would be a very good thing. In actuality, prunes have the highest oxygen radical absorbance capacity (ORAC) of any food tested, which means that the compounds in prunes, working as a group, deliver more of a protective antioxidant punch than any other food tested. Prunes actually topped the ORAC list with more than twice the antioxidant capacity as other high-scoring fruits such as blueberries and raisins.

FRUIT

Raisins

Raisins—like figs and dates—are known as nature's candy. According to natural-foods expert Rebecca Wood, if you were to take 4 pounds (1.8 kg) of grapes and remove most 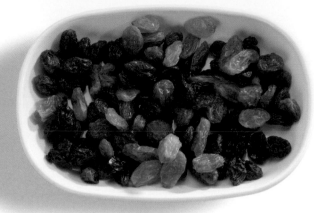 of the water, you'd be looking at 1 pound (455 g) of raisins. Wood also points out one of the good things about raisins is that their transformation from grapes takes place via an old-fashioned drying process called the sun (hence the term "sun-dried raisins"), although some companies do it by a mechanical process of oven drying.

One caution about raisins from a pesticide and contamination point of view—they're only as good as the grapes they come from. Since the raisins are basically concentrated grapes, they are believed to have the highest pesticide residue of any fruit. Which would be a good reason to go organic.

On the positive side, raisins are high in phenols, plant compounds that have repeatedly been shown to have antioxidant activity and to help prevent damage to cells in the body from destructive molecules called free radicals. University of Scranton scientists found that raisins (as well as prunes, dried apricots, and cranberries) scored higher in phenol content than their fresh counterparts.

In a study in the *Journal of the American College of Nutrition*, Harold Miller, Ph.D., and his colleagues analyzed the antioxidant content of cereals, fruits, and vegetables using a complicated scientific method that scores the foods in units called TEs (Trolox equivalents). The findings were surprising (Miller found that many popular vegetables tended to be relatively low in antioxidants). Of the fruits, his team found that red plums had the highest TE score (2200). Of the berries,

blackberries won with 5500. Of the dried fruits, dates were highest at 6600 followed by good old raisins, weighing in at a whopping 6400! That's a pretty darn high rating for antioxidant activity.

Raisins are also relatively high in boron, a mineral under scrutiny for the promotion of bone and joint health, particularly in women. In one study, twelve postmenopausal women were given a diet deficient in boron for 119 days, followed by a 48-day period in which they received 3-mg boron supplements daily. On the boron-deficient diet, the women experienced increased loss of both calcium and magnesium, but on the boron-supplemented diet the opposite was true. According to the *Physicians' Desk Reference*, "Boron appears to be a very important partner with calcium metabolism and as such should be expected to play an important role in the prevention of osteoporosis."

Raisins are also a source of the flavonoid myricetin, which may have anti-inflammatory activity. It may also inhibit beta-amyloid fibril formation, a key problem with Alzheimer's disease.

Watermelon

Watermelon owes its claim to fame as one of the world's healthiest foods to three facts: One, its high water content (more about that in a moment); two, its high content of lycopene; and three, its high levels of vitamin A and carotenoids, including the important but relatively unknown carotenoid beta-cryptoxanthin.

Watermelon Is Extra Filling, Helps with Weight Loss

The fact that watermelon is mostly water falls squarely under the heading of "duh" for most people, but that's a pretty important fact For years, Barbara Rolls, Ph.D., has been doing research at Pennsylvania State University on appetite, satiety, and weight loss. Her findings have been unequivocal: High-volume foods (defined as those that take up a lot of space for very few calories) are one of your best allies in the quest to lose weight. Watermelon is 92 percent water; it's the very definition of a high volume food.

Rolls has found that water as part of food has a very satisfying—and filling—effect. For example, soup made of vegetables and water will fill people up and cause them to eat fewer calories than the same amount of vegetables eaten along with a glass of water. "When you add water to a bowl of vegetables as in soup, the soup has greater satiety than when the vegetables are eaten alone with a glass of water," Rolls says. "When water is incorporated into food or shakes, satiety is increased and (people) ultimately eat less food."

The Big Myth About Watermelon

In the low-carb world, watermelon is considered "fruit non grata." It's not that it's not nutritious—you'll read about that in a moment. Rather, it's believed to be a very high-sugar fruit that you should stay away from if you're trying to control blood sugar. Anti-watermelon folks point to the high glycemic index of the fruit (around 76), meaning that it raises blood sugar a lot and does it quickly. When you're trying to control blood sugar and insulin—say you're trying to lose weight or you're just trying to get healthier—high blood sugar and high insulin are not something you want.

The truth is a little more complicated. The glycemic index is based on a "serving" of 50 grams of carbohydrate, not 50 grams of total weight. A 10-ball serving of watermelon is about 120 grams by weight, but it's mostly water. There's only 6 to 9 grams of carbohydrate in that serving. That's why the glycemic load of watermelon—a far more meaningful and relevant measure of a food's impact on blood sugar than glycemic index—is only about 4 (very low). The glycemic load takes into account portion size. So sure, if you ate 50 or 60 melon balls, you'd be closer to the amount of actual carbohydrate that was used in the study to determine glycemic index. But if you ate a normal, smallish portion of watermelon (i.e., the 10 balls), it would have minimal impact on your blood sugar.

The problem, of course, is, that it's very easy to eat that 50-ball portion. I've known people who could knock off half a melon at one sitting (including myself!) But if you can keep the portion small, then the glycemic impact of this fruit is nowhere near what people think it is.

That said, for people who are extremely sugar sensitive, have metabolic challenges (i.e. metabolic syndrome, prediabetes, obesity or diabetes) and need to watch their sugar very carefully, this is probably not as good a choice as berries.

Lycopene in Watermelon May Reduce Risk of Prostate Cancer

But water, low calories and a low glycemic load (for a reasonable portion!) aren't the only good things about watermelon. Watermelon is a great source of a carotenoid called lycopene, which in several studies has been shown to be associated with lower rates of prostate cancer. In one study, at the Karmanos Cancer Institute at Wayne State University, men facing surgery for prostate cancer were given 30 mg of lycopene for three weeks before undergoing surgery. The men who received the lycopene supplement had lower prostate-specific antigen (PSA) levels and less aggressive tumors than the nonsupplemented control group. Plus, their tumors were smaller.

Other studies have shown that people who eat lots of tomatoes and tomato products have less prostate cancer, a fact that has largely been attributed to the high lycopene content of tomatoes. And, in a review of seventy-two studies, one researcher reported fifty-seven associations between blood lycopene levels and reduced rates of cancer, thirty-five of which were statistically significant. The benefit was strongest for prostate, lung, and stomach cancers, although protective associations were also found for cancers of the pancreas, colon, rectum, esophagus, oral cavity, breast, and cervix.

Other researchers have pointed out that lycopene supplements may or may not give the desired effect. There's good reason to think these incredible plant compounds work best when found in their natural surroundings along with other food ingredients (like other carotenoids). That's another reason I like watermelon—it contains a nice supporting cast of other carotenoids and sources of vitamin A like beta-carotene and the less well-known beta-cryptoxanthin. In one study, beta-cryptoxanthin reduced the risk of lung cancer by 30 percent; in another study, it provided a 41 percent reduction in the risk of developing rheumatoid arthritis. And in rats, beta-cryptoxanthin has been found to have a bone-building effect.

High on Watermelon?

Interesting story: Medical doctor and yogi Dharma Singh Khalsa, M.D., sings the praises of watermelon as a detoxifier. Khalsa recounts a visit to Brazil in which he went on a watermelon fast: "After just three days I was very tuned in and meditating very deeply. This was one of the greatest highs I have ever experienced. When I boarded the plane for home, I was definitely in an altered state."

Watermelon: low calorie, high volume, filling, satisfying, thirst quenching, and with a nice dose of vitamin A and carotenoids, including cancer-fighting lycopene. Plus it's absolutely delicious. What's not to like?

Fruit Runners-Up

Bitter Melon

Bitter melon is actually not a melon, but a cucumber-shaped summer squash grown in tropical areas such as Africa, Asia, and South America. It's also known as balsam pear. By either name, it's a great source of fiber, vitamin A, vitamin C, folate, magnesium, potassium, zinc, and manganese. But its real claim to fame is its ability to lower blood sugar.

Historically, bitter melon has been used to treat a whole assortment of conditions ranging from common infections to diabetes. In China, India, Sri Lanka, and the West Indies, bitter melon is widely used for diabetics. It actually contains a number of compounds that have proven antidiabetic properties, including a compound known as charantin. According to the highly respected naturopathic physician Michael Murray, N.D., charantin is more potent than the drug Tolbutamide, which has been used to lower blood sugar levels in diabetics. There are at least two other groups of constituents in bitter melon besides charantin—insulinlike peptides and alkaloids—that are reputed to have blood sugar–lowering effects. It's not completely clear which of the three is most effective or if they all work together. Nonetheless, science has pretty much confirmed the blood sugar–lowering action of the fresh juice of the unripe bitter melon.

Usually, the bitter-flavored unripe fruit is used as a vegetable. It can be cooked a number of different ways, including stir-fried, steamed, and curried. Some enthusiasts recommend it as part of a vegetable curry with eggplants and onions. Cooking mellows its bitter flavor, which is due largely to the quinine content. Bitter melon is sold by many Asian grocery stores and is sometimes available frozen.

WORTH KNOWING

Experts recommend that bitter melon be eaten moderately—if at all—during pregnancy.

Pears

Fiber and potassium in a delicious package for about 100 calories—the same description that might apply to a banana applies equally well to a pear. One medium pear has a really hefty 5 g of fiber, plus about 200 mg of potassium; a smattering of other minerals such as calcium, phosphorus, and magnesium; 13 mg of phytosterols; and 75 mcg of eye-supporting lutein and zeaxanthin. Anjou, Bartlett, Bosc, and all the other varieties—including Asian pears—are pretty similar nutritionally.

When I was in New York hanging out with my friend the nationally known nutritionist and antiaging specialist Oz Garcia, Ph.D., he'd always make us detox drinks in a base of pear juice. While there's no strong scientific evidence for this, many natural healers recommend pears and pear juice because they believe they're less likely than other fruits to provoke any kind of allergenic response. I can't prove that to you, but it seems to be the conventional wisdom. One of my favorite juice recipes is celery, pear, and ginger (see page 286).

If for no other reason, pears are a great food because of their high fiber content.

Persimmons

Here's an interesting little factoid about persimmons that you might not know—assuming you knew anything about them in the first place, which not a lot of people do! The original "energy bar," used by explorers and Native Americans, was something called pemmican. Pemmican is a huge favorite of the Paleo crowd—it's basically dried meat (jerky) mixed with wild nuts and berries and pressed into a bar. It is quite tasty, by the way, especially when it's made with grass-fed beef. And one of the main fruits used in pemmican is persimmon.

You can buy persimmons in the grocery store, and they come in two basic flavors: astringent and nonastringent. It's important to know which one you're getting. The astringent kind needs to be soft and ripe before eating, or else it tastes horrible. The reason for this is the presence of tannins, a group of chemicals that are also in red wine and tea. Once the fruit ripens and gets soft, the tannins become inert and the taste is no longer astringent. A cool way to ripen it quickly is to leave it in the freezer overnight and then allow it to thaw in the morning. If you've accidentally tasted one of these "before its time," you might think this is the worst fruit on the planet, but give it another shot once it's soft. Without the bitter tannins, it's a whole different experience. The nonastringent kind, on the other hand, can be eaten firm or soft. Both kinds look like the plastic fruit you used to see on your grandmother's dining room table, but they taste a lot better (unless, of course, you're eating the astringent kind before it softens).

There are two basic varieties of persimmon: Hachiya (also called Japanese persimmon) and Fuyu. Hachiya is the most widely available persimmon in the United States, but it's astringent, so remember to let it ripen. Fuyu are nonastringent, so you can eat them firm or soft. There's also Sharon fruit (also called Israeli persimmon), which is round and sweet, and like Fuyu, can be eaten anytime.

PERSIMMON MAY LOWER BLOOD FATS

There are a couple of interesting studies on persimmons that are worth mentioning, even though they were done on rats. In one, a team of researchers led by Shela Gorinstein from Hebrew University of Jerusalem supplemented the diet of two groups of rats with added cholesterol. One group of rats was also fed supplemental persimmon. Now normally, when you feed rats cholesterol, their blood fats rise—but in the group fed the persimmon, the blood fats rose a lot less than expected. In fact, the rats with the persimmon-supplemented diet had much lower "bad" (LDL) cholesterol, triglycerides, and lipid peroxides (a measure of cellular damage caused by free radicals) than the rats that didn't get the persimmon. The researchers concluded that persimmon possesses hypolipidemic properties (the ability to lower blood fats) as well as being a potent antioxidant (having the ability to protect against free radicals).

Both the persimmon pulp and the peel are good sources of fiber. A study published in *Phytotherapy Research* concluded that persimmon peel extract has potential therapeutic value as an antitumor agent. And persimmons have a number of carotenoids and polyphenols that have been shown to have health benefits. The fruit also contains potassium, magnesium, manganese, and iron.

Finally, an interesting study done in South Korea found that polyphenols isolated from the persimmon leaf had an antiwrinkle effect when applied to human skin. I'm not sure you get those same benefits by eating the fruit, but, as my grandmother used to say, "It couldn't hurt."

Quince

What if it wasn't the apple that Eve used to tempt Adam?

Believe it or not, some historians think it might have been a quince. In fact, some people believe that a quince—not an apple—was the fruit that's mentioned in the Song of Solomon. This makes sense, because the quince was actually cultivated before the apple and probably reached Palestine by 100 B.C.E.

While all that makes for nice folklore, the quince of today is hardly tempting to look at, and it is almost never eaten raw, especially in the United States where its tannin content gives it a very astringent, tart taste. (In western Asia and tropical countries, the fruit is softer and juicier.) So quince is one of the few fruits that's almost always eaten cooked. But stewed or baked, it's a whole different story: Cooking brings out its unique flavor and makes it a really nice addition to various meat recipes or sweet dishes. It also makes a terrific fruit sauce, similar in texture to applesauce.

Quince is high in pectin, a kind of soluble fiber that lowers cholesterol and also delays the absorption of glucose (sugar) into the bloodstream. A single quince has more than 1½ g of fiber, plus 181 mg of potassium and 13 mg of vitamin C. While it's not exactly a nutritional superstar, it's a nice addition to your menu of healthy fruits to experiment with. The quince has a really powerful aroma, and if you leave it at room temperature, you'll smell it for weeks. In ancient times they were used as room fresheners.

Star Fruit (Carambola)

This exotic-looking golden-yellow fruit, a native of Indonesia, is unique because each crosswise slice is a perfectly shaped star. The major producers include Taiwan, Malaysia, Guyana, India, Philippines, Australia, Israel, and the United States (Florida and Hawaii).

WORTH KNOWING

In the 1990s, a sweeter variety called the apple quince was developed, which can be eaten raw. Another unique version, the passé-crassane, is actually a pear-quince hybrid that was developed in Normandy. It is particularly useful in cooking because of its firm, grainy flesh, but it is also tasty eaten raw. And if you're into making healthy jellies, jams, and preserves, the pectin content of quince makes it a perfect choice.

Two types of star fruit are grown, tart and sweet. Tart varieties typically have narrowly spaced ribs, while sweet varieties tend to have thick, fleshy ribs. The tastes between the two are not as distinct as you might think, because the tart variety still has some sweetness. The sweet star fruit can be eaten right out of your hand, used as a dessert, or thrown into a salad. The tart kind is a great substitute for lemon or lime. Truly a tropical fruit, it's readily available from July through February, at least in the United States.

Star fruit is a good source of vitamin C (45 mg per cup [132 g]), potassium (176 mg per cup), and fiber. According to natural-foods expert Rebecca Wood, star fruit is cooling and astringent, clears excess heat, and is very good for diarrhea. It's also low in calories.

According to research published in *Food Chemistry* and in the *Journal of Chromatography*, star fruit is a very good source of natural antioxidants. The major antioxidants present in the fruit's extract are proanthocyanidins, most notably one called epicatechin, an antioxidant more commonly associated with green tea and red wine. That puts this lovely little fruit in very good company indeed.

FRUIT

THE EXPERTS' TOP TEN LISTS

Barry Sears, Ph.D.

Barry Sears is the creator of the Zone Diet, and he is considered one of the leading authorities in the world on the hormonal response to food. He has written eleven books on his Zone technology, including the *New York Times'* number-one best seller *The Zone*. A superb scientist and biochemist by training, Sears is resident of the nonprofit Inflammation Research Foundation that is conducting worldwide research on the role of diet in controlling chronic disease. His website, www.drsears.com, is consistently interesting and informative.

Sears was the impetus for my move from personal fitness training into nutrition. His theories and research about the hormonal impact of food—revolutionary back in 1995 and now accepted as conventional wisdom—moved me away from the high-carb, low-fat dogma of the 1980s and inspired me to go back to school for nutrition. He and I don't agree on everything—egg yolks and soy being two examples—but I consider him one of the brightest and most dedicated people in the field.

1. **Wild salmon:** This is great source of omega-3 fatty acids coupled with great taste.
2. **Chicken breast:** This is standard low-fat protein that goes with everything.
3. **Egg whites:** These are a convenient source of low-fat protein that can be added to any meal to balance carbohydrates. A great snack is a couple of hard-boiled eggs in which the egg yolk has been removed and replaced with hummus.
4. **Broccoli/cauliflower:** Both are rich in fiber, vitamins, and minerals, with the least amount of carbohydrates. Cooking cauliflower, then mashing it up and baking, makes a great substitute for mashed potatoes.
5. **Spinach:** This powerhouse of vitamins and minerals can be sautéed with olive oil for a healthy carbohydrate source.
6. **Red peppers:** There is no better way to add color to a plate than red peppers. They're loaded with antioxidants and protective phytochemicals, not to mention fiber.
7. **Barley/oatmeal:** These two great grains are rich in soluble fiber that slows the entry of any carbohydrate into the bloodstream.
8. **Black beans:** These provide another great source of soluble fiber.
9. **Berries:** This is the best dessert known. They're rich in antioxidants, and they taste great, too.
10. **Extra-virgin olive oil:** This is number one favorite fat, as it contains powerful antioxidants known as *polyphenols*. Making a béarnaise or hollandaise sauce with olive oil instead of butter is a great way to make any vegetable taste better.

CHAPTER 5

NUTS AND SEEDS

The old saying "an apple a day keeps the doctor away" is as true as it ever was, but we might have to expand the prescription to include a handful of nuts. People who eat nuts regularly are less likely to have heart attacks or to die from heart disease than those who don't. Some of the largest and most important long-term studies such as the Nurses' Health Study, the Iowa Women's Health Study, and the Adventist Study, have shown a consistent 30 to 50 percent lower risk of heart attacks or heart disease associated with eating nuts several times a week.

Walter Willett, M.D., Dr. P.H., professor of epidemiology and nutrition at Harvard's School of Public Health and a professor of medicine at Harvard Medical School, and arguably the most distinguished nutrition researcher of our time, suggests that there may be several mechanisms at work here. One of them may be the fact that nuts contain arginine. Arginine is an amino acid that is touted for its role in protecting the inner lining of the arterial walls, making them more pliable and less susceptible to atherogenesis.

Arginine is also needed to make an important molecule called nitric oxide, which helps relax constricted blood vessels and ease blood flow. In addition, nuts are a great source of numerous phytonutrients—bioactive chemicals found in plants. These compounds have powerful health benefits, not the least of which are their antioxidant activity, which is linked to the prevention of coronary heart disease.

Nuts Are Full of Good Fat

One of the mechanisms that's almost certainly responsible for the health benefits of nuts is their fat. When this book was first written, the notion that fat might have significant health benefits was considered delusional. Ten years later, not so much. In the intervening

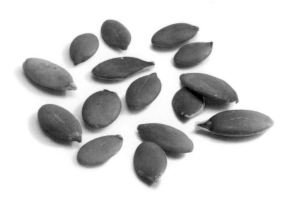

years there have been a spate of popular books touting the benefits of high-fat diets, including one which I coauthored—*Smart Fat* (with Steven Masley, M.D.). As far as the fat in nuts goes, the jury isn't even out anymore: it's all good!

Most of the fat in nuts is monounsaturated (more about that in a moment). Some is polyunsaturated, and, in the case of walnuts (see page 183), a significant amount of it is a specific type of polyunsaturated fat known as omega-3, whose health benefits are legion. Omega-3s have been the subject of more research than almost any food component I know of, with the possible exception of vitamin C. Some of the fat in nuts is saturated, and as you may have guessed by now, this does not concern me in the least.

Monounsaturated fat, also known as omega-9, is the main type of fat in nuts. That's the same fat that's predominant in the Mediterranean diet, which has been shown in virtually every research study to be associated with lower levels of heart disease and cancer, not to mention longer life spans. In the famous Lyon Diet Heart Study, people who had a heart attack between 1988 and 1992 were counseled either to follow the standard post–heart attack dietary advice (reduce saturated fat) or to follow the Mediterranean diet which contains a high percentage of monounsaturated fat. After about four years of follow-up, the people on the Mediterranean diet experienced 70 percent less heart disease (about three times the reduction in risk achieved by statin drugs!). Not only that, but their overall risk of death was 45 percent lower.

In 2015, researchers designed an interesting study in which people ate a basic Mediterranean-style diet but supplemented the diet with either extra nuts or extra olive oil. Those eating the Mediterranean diet plus olive oil had a relatively lower risk of breast cancer. Both groups—the Mediterranean diet plus nuts and the Mediterranean diet plus olive oil—had significantly improved cognitive function. (The study was published in *JAMA Internal Medicine* in 2015.)

Choosing the Right Nut

So which nuts are best? There's no perfect answer to that question. My personal answer is they're all good. Almonds, hazelnuts, pecans, walnuts, macadamia nuts, and pistachio nuts all alter the composition of the blood in ways that would be expected to reduce the risk of coronary disease. And it doesn't take a ton of them to give you the health benefits found in the research. One 1-ounce (28 g) serving a day—or 5 ounces (140 g) a week from a variety of nuts—ought to do it. It's possible you'd get benefits with even less.

Melissa Stevens, M.S., R.D., L.D., the nutrition program coordinator for preventive cardiology and rehabilitative services at the Cleveland Clinic, has come up with some quick, easy tips for adding nuts to your diet. Here are some of my favorites:

- Add cashews or peanuts to a stir-fry
- Toss roasted pine nuts into a marinara sauce
- Add slivered almonds to yogurt
- Toss walnuts into a spinach and strawberry salad
- Create your own homemade trail mix (I suggest nuts, dates, raisins, and oats.)

And of course, there's the snack that I've been recommending for two decades: natural peanut or almond butter smeared on an apple or a few sticks of celery. It's old school, but you really can't beat it!

★ Almonds/ Almond Butter

Almonds are our oldest cultivated nut and one of the great foods of all time. And to think, not so long ago they were avoided by health-conscious consumers because of their fat content. We've come a long way, baby!

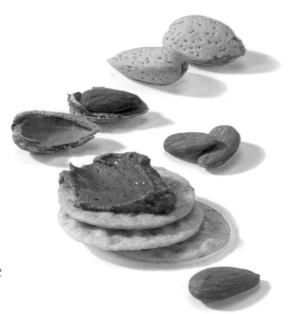

Eaten in Moderation, Almonds Help with Weight Loss

Let's get the "almonds are fattening" thing out of the way right at the start. Epidemiologic studies such as the Nurses' Health Study, the Adventist Health Study, and the Physicians' Follow-up Study universally show that those who eat the most nuts also tend to have the lowest body mass indexes (a measure of overweight). Nuts are most definitely not fattening.

Sure, almonds have fat and calories, and you can't eat two tons of them at a time and expect to lose weight, but there is a massive amount of research showing that fat (and protein) are highly satiating, and that almonds eaten in moderation can actually help with weight loss. One study compared two groups of dieters eating the same number of calories; one group ate 520 of their calories from almonds and lost more weight. Preliminary research is indicating that almond cell walls may partially limit the amount of dietary fat available for digestion or absorption, so it's possible that a small portion of the calories from almonds are not fully absorbed. In any case, research is quite clear that replacing a given amount of calories in the diet with an equal number of calories from almonds does not equal weight gain. Quite the opposite.

Almonds Rich with Heart-Healthy Benefits

Research shows that almonds may help lower cholesterol, but if you've read my book, *The Great Cholesterol Myth*, you know I don't think that's terribly important. Far more important than the fact that they may lower cholesterol is the fact that almonds are rich in monounsaturated fat, which has heart-health benefits well beyond the reduction of cholesterol. About 70 percent of the fat in almonds is monounsaturated fat, which is anti-inflammatory. That matters, because inflammation is a part of every disease of aging that we know of.

Monounsaturated fat is the main fat in the Mediterranean diet, which has been shown in virtually every research study to be associated with lower levels of heart disease and cancer, not to mention longer life spans.

One of the best studies on the Mediterranean diet was the famous Lyon Diet Heart Study. In this study, people who had already had one heart attack were put into two groups. One was counseled to follow the standard post–heart attack dietary advice (reduce saturated fat and cholesterol). The other was counseled to follow the Mediterranean diet. After about four years of follow-up, the people on the Mediterranean diet experienced 70 percent less heart disease (about three times the reduction in risk achieved by statin drugs!). Not only that, but their overall risk of death was 45 percent lower. These astonishing results were obtained despite the fact that there wasn't much change in their cholesterol levels, showing that cholesterol may not have as much to do with heart disease as we've previously believed (the premise of our 2012 book, *The Great Cholesterol Myth*). The Lyon study results were so impressive that the study had to be stopped early for ethical reasons—all participants were given the advice to follow the Mediterranean diet, with its generous amount of monounsaturated fat, the same kind found in almonds.

Almonds Safe for Diabetics

Almonds also contain about 6 g of protein in an ounce (28 g), not to mention a hefty 3 g of dietary fiber. And almonds are rich in calcium—1 ounce contains 80 mg. They also contain phosphorus and vitamin E and are an excellent source of magnesium. They contain virtually no carbohydrates, making them a perfect food for diabetics and those with blood sugar issues.

One ounce of almonds (or a smear of almond butter) together with a piece of fruit like an apple makes a great snack and is one of my five favorite pre-workout snacks. The almond butter also goes great smeared on a few sticks of celery. Total calories for either snack is reasonable (about 250), and the nutrient density is terrific.

WORTH KNOWING

You can make a great "milk" out of almonds and water. Throw a few tablespoons of organic almonds into a blender with a cup (235 ml) of bottled water, and you're good to go. If you need it sweeter, use some raw unfiltered honey, or some powdered xylitol, Stevia or erythritol.

Brazil Nuts

Brazil nuts have the highest selenium content of any food I know of, and for this reason alone belong among the world's healthiest foods. Selenium is an essential trace element that, in tons of research, has been shown to have a protective effect against cancer. According to the *Physicians' Desk Reference*, it's "antioxidant, immunomodulatory, anticarcinogenic, and anti-atherogenic," which translated into English means that it protects the cells, boosts the immune system, helps fight cancer, and helps prevent heart disease. Not exactly an undistinguished résumé.

Why Americans Need Brazil Nuts

Unless we're taking selenium supplements or eating Brazil nuts, we most likely get selenium from fish or from plants and the animals that graze on them (beef, chicken). How much we get depends on the soil in which the plants were grown (and how much fish we eat). In countries with selenium-poor soil—and consequently low selenium intake—all kinds of health problems have been noted, including higher rates of cancer. As far back as 1984, the government of Finland started adding selenium to fertilizers as a way of improving the selenium intake of its citizens. High plains areas such as northern Nebraska and the Dakotas have selenium-rich soil because it was derived from volcanic deposits. Most of the rest of the country is not so lucky. In any case, many Americans don't eat nearly enough plant foods anyway, and it's reasonable to assume that many people don't get nearly enough to get the protective benefits of this mineral.

Low intakes of selenium are associated with increased incidence of prostate, lung, colorectal, gastric, and skin cancers. And it's essential for healthy immune function. It also seems to be responsible for maintaining the structure of sperm, at least if you're a mouse. But it's probably so in humans as well: infertile men have low selenium levels.

Selenium also helps antagonize the effects of a number of toxic metals. Some of these toxic metals, such as cadmium, are found in cigarette smoke and other places, and they are carcinogenic. Others, like mercury, are just plain bad news. Selenium seems to bind with some of these bad guys, creating inactive complexes and helping to rid the system of them.

The thyroid is dependent on selenium to function properly. Selenium is a component of the enzyme that helps convert T4 (thyroxine), the less-active thyroid hormone, to the active one, T3 (triiodothyronine). If you're on conventional thyroid medication like Synthroid, which is pure T4, you need selenium to convert it. Sub-optimal levels of selenium may impair thyroid function.

The Important Connection between Mercury and Selenium

People often fear eating seafood—one of the best foods on Earth because of concerns about mercury. And there's no doubt about it—mercury is a nasty compound, a neurotoxin, and something you definitely want to avoid, particularly if you're pregnant. But here's a very interesting factoid: Selenium has a major role in preventing mercury toxicity, and the research on that has existed since 1967!

A number of studies have shown the power of selenium to counteract the effects of mercury exposure (Strain, 2015). Some researchers believe that mercury is toxic partly because it binds to selenium and renders it ineffective. So even if you had normal selenium levels, a lot of mercury exposure could put you at risk. But fish is pretty high in selenium, which may in fact, counter some of the negatives associated with mercury.

The Republic of Seychelles turns out to be the perfect place to examine any potential impact of persistent low level mercury exposure because the folks there consume about ten times more fish than we do in the US and Europe. That's why the Seychelles Child Development Study was started in the 1980s—to study the impact of fish consumption and mercury exposure on childhood development.

Yet numerous analyses have shown that even the children of mothers who ate, on average, twelve meals of fish each week during pregnancy, there was no evidence of a correlation between mercury exposure from fish and any neurological impairment.

None.

Why? Probably because of selenium. An impressive amount of research by Nicholas Ralston, Ph.D., and his colleagues at the University of North Dakota has demonstrated that selenium protects against mercury toxicity and when a food—such as fish—has more selenium than it does mercury, it poses no neurological or developmental risk. The Seychelle islanders eat an awful lot of selenium-rich fish.

Brazil Nuts Are the Best Source of Selenium

Without a doubt, Brazil nuts are the best source of selenium. One ounce (six to eight kernels) has a whopping 544 mcg. The next best sources are clams, oysters, tuna, turkey, and beef, but none comes close to Brazil nuts. Brazil nuts also have protein, calcium, and 2 g of fiber per ounce, and they are a good source of heart-healthy monounsaturated fat.

Cashews

I love cashews. Who doesn't? They got a bad rap for a short time during low-carb mania because their carb content is higher than any other nut, but for all but the most inveterate carb-gram counters this shouldn't be a deterrent from enjoying this delicious food.

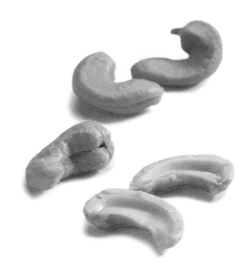

Frequent Nut Eaters Have Fewer Heart Attacks

The benefits of cashew nuts—besides how good they make you feel when you eat them—are similar to the benefits you get when you eat nuts in general. People who eat nuts regularly are less likely to have heart attacks or to die from heart disease than those who don't. Some of the largest and most important long-term studies, such as the Nurses' Health Study, the Iowa Women's Health Study, and the Adventist Study, have shown a consistent 30 to 50 percent lower risk of heart attacks or heart disease associated with eating nuts several times a week.

About half the fat in cashews is heart-healthy monounsaturated fat, the key fat found in the Mediterranean diet, which has been shown in virtually every research study to be associated with lower levels of heart disease and cancer, not to mention longer life spans. Compared with carbohydrates, for example, monounsaturated fat has a positive effect on blood lipids. In the Lyon Diet Heart Study, people following the Mediterranean diet, with its high level of monounsaturated fat (the same kind that's in cashews) experienced 70 percent less heart disease risk than is achieved by taking statin drugs.

Monounsaturated fat is also anti-inflammatory, which is a very good thing indeed.

Cashews Are Low in Calories, Rich in Healthy Minerals

Cashews are slightly lower in calories than other nuts. They're also slightly higher in carbs. Like other nuts they are mineral rich (magnesium, calcium, phosphorus, potassium, copper, and selenium) and full of protein (5 g per ounce of nuts). They also have about 1 g of fiber per ounce (28 g).

And here's some really interesting trivia for you: Raw cashews aren't really raw. The nut meat has an outer protective layer that itself contains a rather nasty, caustic oil that is highly irritating to the skin—not surprising because cashews are a member of the poison ivy family. The oil is removed by heating the nuts in an inclined, perforated, rotating drum. (You can't heat them in a shallow pan because the oil spurts and causes blisters.) Once they're rid of the oil, the harvesters spray the nuts with water to cool them. The ones closer to the heat source tend to get scorched and are sold at a cheaper price as a lower-grade nut, though they're just as tasty and nutritious. (Grade 1 nuts are white; grade 2 are lightly scorched.)

Chia Seeds

Chia seeds have become popular largely on the strength of their omega-3 content. They're one of a handful of plant foods (flaxseeds and hemp seeds are other examples) that contain omega-3 fat, though it's worth noting that it's not the same omega-3 fat found in fish. The omega-3s found in fish and animal foods such as grass-fed beef are EPA (eicosapentaenoic acid) and DHA (docosahexaenoic acid) while the plant-based omega-3s in chia seeds are ALA (alpha-linolenic acid).

Chia seeds are small black seeds that come from a plant called *Salvia hispanica*, which grows in South America. Though they're famous for their omega-3 content, they offer a lot more than that. A 1-ounce (28 g) serving of chia seeds has an astonishingly high 11 g of fiber. That same ounce also has double digit percentages of the RDA for calcium (18 percent), manganese (30 percent), magnesium (30 percent) and phosphorus (27 percent).

I think the RDAs or RDIs for most nutrients are woefully inadequate—particularly magnesium—but chia seeds still offer a lot of nutrition for a modest number of calories (137 calories per ounce [28 g] with only 1 gram of carbohydrate that isn't fiber.

They are also high in antioxidants, which is a good thing because those very antioxidants protect the fat in the seeds from going rancid. What's more they contain 4 grams of protein per ounce (28 g), and a good balance of essential amino acids. The combination of protein and fiber is excellent for weight loss.

Research has found improvements in health markers from a diet that mixed chia seeds with a few other ingredients, but the study that's most impressive is one that specifically investigated the effects of chia seeds on diabetes and cardiovascular risk factors. In this 2007 study, researchers randomly assigned diabetic patients on conventional medications to one of two groups. One group was supplemented with 37 g a day of chia seeds (about 1⅓ ounces), while the other group was supplemented with an equivalent amount of wheat bran. (The subjects continued with their conventional diabetes meds during the study.)

The folks who were supplemented with chia seeds reduced their systolic blood pressure, their hs-CRP (a systemic marker for inflammation) and decreased their hemoglobin A1C (a standard metric for diagnosing diabetes). Researchers concluded that long-term supplementation with chia seeds reduces blood pressure and other factors "safely beyond conventional therapy while maintaining good glycemic and lipid control in people with well-controlled type 2 diabetes."

Barlean's makes two chia seed products that I really like. One is organic chia seed, the other is a wildly popular flax-chia-coconut mix, which imparts a great texture and flavor to all kinds of dishes. I sprinkle one or the other on my famous antiaging dish, Dr. Jonny's Berries and Cherries: Frozen blueberries, frozen dark cherries, full-fat yogurt, a splash of pomegranate juice, almonds, coconut flakes, and a light sprinkling of either Barlean's chia seeds or the flax-chia-coconut mix. Both products are available on Amazon and at Thrive Market.

Hazelnuts (filberts)

Poor hazelnuts. Nobody loves them, at least not enough to invite them to the A-list parties in Hollywood. Sure, you'll find a few hanging out in the nut bowl, but you know they're just there because the supermarket stuck them in the variety pack. This is a shame, because they're so good for you.

Hazelnuts Help with High Cholesterol and Benign Prostatic Hyperplasia

Hazelnuts—like pecans—contain beta-sitosterol, a plant sterol that has been found to have two very important properties: One, it lowers cholesterol. Two, it lessens the symptoms of benign prostatic hyperplasia (BPH). BPH is the annoying condition every man over forty is familiar with, as it causes multiple trips to the bathroom at night. It's harmless, but it's a nuisance. A study in *The Lancet* showed that men with this condition who were given 20 mg of beta-sitosterol three times a day showed significant improvements in urinary difficulties. Of course, that's way more beta-sitosterol than is in one serving of filberts, but still, it's nice to know it's in there.

Hazelnuts also contain potassium, magnesium, phosphorus, and some vitamin E. And 1 ounce (28 g) contains almost 3 g of fiber. Hazelnuts add a rich, crisp texture and a smooth, mellow flavor to prepared foods.

Hazelnuts Go Hollywood

Hazelnuts got a nice public relations boost when they were discussed on Oprah. Mehmet Oz, M.D., told a national TV audience that hazelnuts are a source of omega-3 fatty acids during a show segment called "Inside Secrets to Make You Younger and Healthier." Now maybe they'll get invited to those Hollywood parties.

Macadamia Nuts

Because he died before I even began writing this book, I didn't get a chance to ask Robert Atkins, M.D., to submit a list of his top ten favorite healthy foods. But if he had, I'm pretty darn sure macadamia nuts would have been on his list. Here's what he said about them in *Health Revelations*, November 1996: "I've always looked for a food that could serve as a meal in itself—nutritionally complete and safe as a snack. All you need to do is keep a jar of macadamia nuts handy. I snack on them whenever a meal is late . . . I simply will not board an airplane without them."

Now I wouldn't go so far as to say that macadamia nuts are the perfect food, but they sure are a good one. The oil in macadamia nuts is more than 80 percent monounsaturated, higher than any other nut (olive oil is about 75 percent monounsaturated). Monounsaturated fat is the main fat in the Mediterranean diet, which has been shown in virtually every research study to be associated with lower levels of heart disease and cancer, not to mention longer life spans. In the Lyon Diet Heart Study, those following a Mediterranean diet, with its high intake of monounsaturated fat, experienced three times the reduction in risk for heart disease than that achieved by statin drugs, and they had an overall risk of death that was 45 percent lower. There's not much question that monounsaturated fat—such as the kind found in macadamia nuts—is awfully good for you.

Macadamia Nuts Can Help Lower Cholesterol and Promote Prostate Health

These nuts contain calcium, phosphorus, and magnesium (for strong bones and teeth), heart-healthy potassium, plus a couple of grams of fiber per ounce (28 g). Macadamia nuts also contain a small amount of selenium, a trace mineral with significant anticancer properties. And they contain phytosterols, including beta-sitosterol, which has been shown to help lower cholesterol and to promote prostate health, possibly by its anti-inflammatory activity.

Macadamia nuts are very high in calories—about 204 per ounce (28 g)—so if you're trying to lose weight, don't just go munching on them out of the jar. Instead, substitute an ounce of the nuts two or three times a week for an equivalent number of calories from other sources.

Peanuts/ Peanut Butter

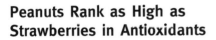

As former peanut farmer President Jimmy Carter would be the first to tell you, peanuts aren't nuts. They're actually legumes—like beans and peas—and they grow underground. But because their nutritional properties so resemble nuts—plus they look like nuts—plus everyone calls them nuts—I figured the nut section of the book is where you'd look for them.

Peanuts Rank as High as Strawberries in Antioxidants

Peanuts are surprisingly high in antioxidants. In a study published in the *Journal of Food Chemistry*, researchers at the University of Florida's Institute of Food and Agricultural Sciences found that peanuts rivaled many fruits for antioxidant content. "When it comes to antioxidant content, peanuts are right up there with strawberries," said Steve Talcott, one of the researchers. "We expected a fairly high antioxidant content in peanuts, but we were a bit shocked to find they're as rich in antioxidants as many kinds of fruit."

Researchers at the University of Florida also found that peanuts contain a high concentration of a polyphenol called p-coumaric acid. P-coumaric acid has been studied for its antioxidant abilities and its potential as an anticancer agent, though much more research is needed to determine the ideal dose. One research paper in the *American Journal of Physiology-Cell Physiology* showed that p-coumaric acid worked as a powerful antioxidant in rats, significantly inhibiting the oxidation of their LDL ("bad") cholesterol. And another study (in *Pharmacological Research*) concluded that it might be worthy to "consider the usefulness of p-coumaric acid as adjuvant therapy in cancer management." Of course, you have to remember that the amount of p-coumaric acid concentrates given in research is way more than found in a handful of peanuts—still, it's nice to know that these healthy compounds are found in the food in the first place. And best of all, research has shown that roasting can increase the level of p-coumaric acid, boosting their overall antioxidant content by as much as 22 percent.

Eating Peanuts May Stave Off Heart Disease

Don't get me wrong—peanuts are not blueberries or kale, or any of the other superpowers in the antioxidant world. But they're about equal in antioxidants to blackberries or strawberries. It's not just the obscure, newly discovered compounds such as p-coumaric acid that make peanuts a good food. Researchers at Purdue University investigated the impact of peanut consumption on total diet quality. "We found that including peanuts in the diet significantly increased magnesium, folate, fiber, copper, vitamin E, and arginine consumption, all of which play a role in the prevention of heart disease," said Richard Mattes, M.P.H., Ph.D., one of the principal investigators. The study was published in the *Journal of the American College of Nutrition* under the impressive title "Eating Peanuts Improves Cardiovascular Risk Factors in Healthy Adults." Their findings were consistent with a previous study at Penn State University that found a 13 percent decrease in triglyceride levels when participants consumed a diet with peanuts and peanut butter, compared to the average American diet. Peanuts are also high in niacin, a B vitamin important for keeping the digestive system, skin, and nerves healthy. Niacin is also critical to releasing energy from carbohydrates and helping to control blood sugar levels.

About half of the fat in peanuts comes from monounsaturated fat—the same kind that's so plentiful in the Mediterranean diet, which has been shown in virtually every research study to be associated with lower levels of heart disease and cancer, not to mention longer life spans. In the Lyon Diet Heart Study, people following the Mediterranean diet had 70 percent less heart disease risk than is achieved by taking statin drugs.

Note: A new peanut has been developed called a "high-oleic" peanut. This is good news—oleic acid is the official name of the monounsaturated fat that all the shouting is about. The new high-oleic peanut has been engineered to have about 80 percent of its fat (instead of 50 percent) from oleic acid, thus boosting the monounsaturated fat content even higher.

WORTH KNOWING

In just about any natural food store these days, you'll find a little grinder machine that sits in the produce section. You throw peanuts into the sieve and put a little plastic container underneath, flip the switch, and out comes the richest, most delicious, oily, thick peanut butter you can imagine. That's real peanut butter with nothing added—no sugar, no trans fat, no flavorings or colorings—just peanuts, with all the benefits described above. You can also buy ready-made jars of peanut butter like that in health food stores, usually labeled natural, and sometimes also organic. Do not confuse the real kind with the household brands that are crammed with sugar and frequently have trans fats. There should be no sugar in your peanut butter (other than the tiny amount in the peanuts), and there should certainly be no partially hydrogenated oil (translation: trans fats) in the ingredient list. (You'd be surprised how many famous brands of commercial peanut butter have those ingredients. Avoid them and grind your own.)

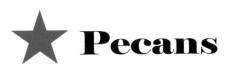

★ Pecans

Pecans deserve their reputation as a health food largely because of their monounsaturated fat content. Monounsaturated fat is the same kind of heart-healthy fat that you find in olive oil. Pecans are also loaded with nutrients like potassium, vitamin E, phytosterols, and beta-sitosterol, a plant compound that has been found to lower cholesterol. And one portion of pecans has almost 3 g of fiber, more than the average slice of bread with none of the negatives.

Three studies from Harvard University, two of which appeared in the *Journal of the American Medical Association*, all confirmed that nuts such as pecans belong in a healthy diet. One of the studies found that eating nuts may help lower the risk of type 2 diabetes. Another concluded that one of three strategies to effectively prevent coronary heart disease was a diet high in fruits, vegetables, nuts, and whole grains and low in refined grains. When I was in school, we were told to remember the good nuts by the acronym PAW: pecans, almonds, and walnuts. Actually there are others, but it's still a good acronym.

Pecans are indigenous to the United States and are grown mainly in Texas, Louisiana, Mississippi, and Georgia. There are more than 300 varieties. It's a good idea to eat them really fresh (within three weeks of harvesting), because they can go rancid pretty quickly because of the very thing that makes them healthy: their high oil content. Buying them in the shell ups the odds that they won't be rancid, because shelled ones can go south pretty quickly. You might want to keep them in the fridge or frozen in an airtight container, where they can keep for up to a year.

Portion Control Is Crucial When Eating Nuts

Nuts are one of those foods where portion control really makes a difference. They're amazingly healthy, but they're high in calories. A 1-ounce (28 g) portion is 196 calories, and nuts are very easy to overeat. I don't worry at all about the fat content—it's all good fat, and besides, if your calories are where they should be, who cares? The high fat content doesn't make the slightest bit of difference. But I have seen people go through bags of these babies. Remember: A portion equals twenty pecan halves. If you can't be trusted with the family-size bag, count out a portion and step away from the nuts.

NUTS AND SEEDS

Pistachio Nuts

If pistachio nuts had a public relations agent, she would have been mighty happy with the results of a study in the *Journal of Agriculture and Food Chemistry*. The study was the most comprehensive analysis of nut and seed varieties to date— it examined twenty-seven different products. Though pistachio nuts did not have the highest phytosterol content of all (that distinction went to sesame seeds and wheat germ), they did have the highest phytosterol content of any product generally considered a snack food (270 mg per 100 g). "Given the many possible mechanisms of action of phytosterols on cholesterol metabolism, it is important to have quantitative estimates of total phytosterol content," reported the team of researchers from Virginia Polytechnic Institute and State University. The main phytosterol identified in all the nut and seed samples was beta-sitosterol, which is known not only for lowering cholesterol but also for supporting prostate health.

Pistachio Nuts Give the Immune System a Boost

Unsalted pistachios have a very high potassium-to-sodium ratio, which helps normalize blood pressure and maintain water balance in the body. Pistachio nuts also contain the powerful antioxidant vitamin E, which boosts the immune system. Best of all, the vitamin E in pistachio nuts is mostly the gamma-tocopherol form, which may have even more health benefits than the more common alpha-tocopherol form found in most supplements. Pistachios also contain magnesium and phosphorus and trace amounts of other minerals and vitamins, as well as phytosterols. Extracts from the pistachio kernel have shown significant antiviral activity.

And they're so delicious.

Note: Some pistachio growers and importers dye the nut red, which exposes the kernels to chemical dyes. You're better off with the plain kind.

Pumpkin Seeds (pepitas)

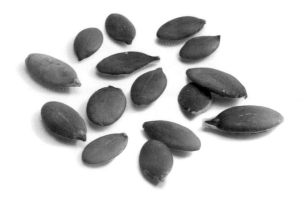

It's hard to pick up a vitamin supplement geared to men these days—especially a prostate support formula—without seeing pumpkin seed extract in the list of ingredients. That's because pumpkin seeds contain beta-sitosterol, a phytosterol that has some benefit in treating BPH (benign prostate hyperplasia). BPH is the annoying condition that causes men over forty to have to go to the bathroom several times a night. It's not dangerous—but it's annoying as hell.

Study Debunks Myth about Pumpkin Seeds

But here's the irony: Pumpkin seeds don't actually contain all that much beta-sitosterol. Researchers at the department of biochemistry and chemistry at Virginia Polytechnic Institute and State University tested twenty-seven nut and seed products commonly consumed in the United States. Pumpkin seeds were relatively low in beta-sitosterol (only 13 g per 100 g of seeds). But that doesn't mean pumpkin seeds don't have a role in prostate health. They may work synergistically with other botanicals like saw palmetto, as a couple of studies have demonstrated. And pumpkin seeds contain chemicals called cucurbitacins, which are believed to interfere with the production of a metabolic by-product of testosterone known as DHT (dihydrotestosterone). DHT is partly responsible for both hair loss and benign prostate hyperplasia. Men want to keep their DHT as low as possible—believe me, I know.

Prostate health aside, these delicious seeds pack a great nutritional wallop. In the Virginia Polytech research, published in the *Journal of Agriculture and Food Chemistry* in 2005, pumpkin seeds had a high phytosterol content (265 mg per 100 g), second only to pistachio and sunflower kernels in the subgroup of foods commonly consumed as snacks. Plant sterols have multiple health benefits, not the least of which is lowering cholesterol.

Pumpkin seeds are a rich source of minerals, especially magnesium, potassium, and phosphorus. Interestingly, the roasted kind have far more protein, at least according to the USDA food database. (They also have a lot more calories.) The roasted kind also have way more magnesium, phosphorus, and potassium, as well as more zinc, fiber, and cancer-fighting selenium. Both have a nice amount of manganese, an important trace mineral that's essential for growth, reproduction, wound healing, peak brain function, and the proper metabolism of sugars, insulin, and cholesterol. Ultimately, both the raw (dried) and the roasted are nutrient dense.

Oils and Spices Can Multiply the Health Benefits of Pumpkin Seeds

You can roast your own pumpkin seeds really easily and combine them with great oils and spices to multiply their health benefits even further. Try melting some organic butter—or macadamia nut or olive oil—then tossing in the pumpkin seeds and spreading them on a single layer on a baking sheet. Season 'em with turmeric, garlic, or cayenne pepper, and bake them till they're crisp. You can also add pumpkin seeds to trail mix, sautéed vegetables, and salads, not to mention my favorite—oatmeal.

Sacha Inchi Nuts

I first heard about sacha inchi when I was doing a story on protein powders. I've long been a fan of whey protein, but my editor wanted to be sure that I covered some vegetarian protein powders as well. That led me to investigate some of the more popular choices such as soy protein, pea protein, brown rice protein, hemp protein, and one that I had never heard of before—sacha inchi.

Sacha inchi is relatively new to the American market, but it's been around for thousands of years. Also known as the Inca peanut, it's the seed of a plant native to Peru that's been a food source for three thousand years in the Amazon rain forest. The seeds produce a fruit that's pretty much inedible—but the seeds themselves taste great when they're lightly roasted.

The plant itself—*Plukenetia volubilis*—is a rain forest vine that has star-shaped pods containing seeds that, when roasted, have been compared to dark roasted peanuts with a slightly woody flavor. The oil derived from the "nuts"—let's just agree to call them nuts even though, as mentioned, they're technically a seed—has traditionally been used for skin care and for treating wounds, insect bites and skin infection.

Besides being a terrific snack food, sacha inchi nuts have become a popular source of vegetarian protein, especially in combination with other vegetarian protein sources like rice, pea, or hemp. The seeds go through solvent-free and cold-pressed processing to remove most of the oil, leaving a kind of protein meal that is then ground into a powder, according to the food industry website NutraIngredients. It's said to be highly digestible, and it contains all nine essential amino acids.

One of the things that distinguishes sacha inchi as a protein powder is that it's very high in omega-3 fatty acids. Remember that the omega-3s found in plant foods such as sacha inchi (and in flax, chia, and hemp seeds) are different from the two omega-3s found in animal foods such as salmon and grass-fed beef. The plant-based omega-3 found in sacha inchi (and the other seeds mentioned above) is called alpha-linolenic acid (ALA); the omega-3s found in animal foods like salmon (or fish oil) are eicosapentaenoic acid (EPA) and docosahexaenoic acid (DHA).

Both EPA and DHA have been widely studied and are considered the superstars of the omega-3 family. But ALA has benefits of its own. People who eat a diet high in alpha-linolenic acid are less likely to have a fatal heart attack. Other population studies show that as people eat more foods with alpha-linolenic acid, heart disease deaths go down.

Sacha inchi nuts are also high in fiber, and so is sacha inchi protein powder. Each 1 ounce (28 g) serving contains 4 to 6 g of fiber (depending on manufacturer), which isn't bad, especially considering that protein powder typically has no fiber at all.

I wish there were more research on sacha inchi, or more information that didn't come from the manufacturers. But all the available evidence points to the conclusion that this is a healthy food, whether in the roasted nut version or the supplemental protein powder version.

As they say in politics, sacha inchi "checks a lot of boxes." It's completely plant-based, and suitable for vegans and vegetarians. It has a healthy dose of plant-based omega-3 fat, and it has a decent amount of fiber. Plus it's non-GMO, gluten-free, and (often) organically grown.

As my grandmother used to say, "What's not to like?"

Sesame Seeds/ Sesame Butter/Tahini

The sesame seed is truly ancient. In fact, sesame is the oldest known plant grown for its seeds and oil, and it is especially valued in Eastern, Mediterranean, and African cultures. The sesame seed pod bursts open when it reaches maturity, the origin of the famous phrase "Open sesame!" from *The Arabian Nights*.

In popular health food books, and on countless Internet sites, there is much confusion over the names of the healthful phenolic compounds found in sesame seeds and their oil. It's understandable, and you'll see why in a minute. The seeds contain 50 to 60 percent of a fatty oil that is characterized by two members of the lignan family: sesamin and sesamolin. When the seeds are refined (as in the making of sesame oil), two other phenolic antioxidants—sesamol and sesaminol— are formed.

Sesame Seeds Can Help Burn Fat

You don't need to know all the technical names and metabolites of the lignan family to understand that these plant chemicals are very good for you indeed. Sesame seed lignans—including the aforementioned sesamin and sesaminol—enhance vitamin E's absorption and availability, improve lipid profiles, and help normalize blood pressure. Animal studies show that sesame lignans enhance the burning of fat by increasing the activity of several liver enzymes that actually break down fatty acids. That research did not escape the notice of the manufacturers of bodybuilding supplements, which immediately began offering sesamin supplements for fat loss all over the Internet. Do they work? No idea.

Sesame lignans also help reduce cholesterol. In a study published in the *Journal of Lipid Research*, sesamin lowered both serum (blood) and liver cholesterol levels. The researchers suggested that sesamin deserves further study as a "possible hypocholesterolemic agent of natural origin." Of course cholesterol is becoming less and less of a target in the quest to lower heart disease, and this result may not seem as important as it once did, but there it is. In a study in the *Journal of Nutrition*, 50 g of sesame seed powder taken daily for five weeks by twenty-four healthy postmenopausal women improved total cholesterol, LDL ("bad") cholesterol, cholesterol ratio, and antioxidant status. The researchers noted some improvements in sex hormone status as well and suggested a benefit of sesame for postmenopausal women.

Sesame Seeds Rank Highest in Cholesterol-Lowering Phytosterols

It's hardly surprising that sesame seeds help reduce cholesterol because they are so rich in cholesterol-lowering phytosterols. How rich? Get this: A team of researchers from Virginia Polytechnic Institute and State University tested twenty-seven different nut and seed products. Sesame seeds (and wheat germ) had the highest phytosterol content of all the products tested: 400 mg per 100 g. The main phytosterol identified in all the nut and seed samples was beta-sitosterol, which is known not only for lowering cholesterol but also for supporting prostate health.

The Calcium Controversy

Sesame seeds are very high in calcium, but there is some controversy over how useful that calcium is to the body because much of it is bound to oxalic acid, making it less bioavailable. Hulling (the process of removing the outer skin) removes the oxalic acid, but it also removes most of the calcium, plus the fiber and a lot of the potassium and iron. In certain parts of Japan, whole sesame seeds are an essential part of the diet and are prepared as a condiment known as *gomasio*, made by toasting whole sesame seeds with unrefined sea salt at high temperatures. Toasting the

whole sesame seeds at these high temperatures may improve the assimilation of calcium by getting rid of the oxalates.

Calcium aside, sesame seeds are also a rich source of minerals, fiber, and protein. Two tablespoons (16 g) of seeds contain iron, magnesium, phosphorus, potassium, and manganese, 35 percent of the Daily Value for copper, 2 g of fiber, and 3 g of protein—more protein than any other nut or seed.

You can really enhance their nutty flavor by toasting them in a dry skillet over medium heat until they're golden brown. They come in shades of black, brown, and yellow as well as the more common beige variety. The black seeds have a stronger flavor. Sesame butter is a great alternative to peanut butter and it is usually made of whole roasted sesame seeds. Tahini is made from hulled sesame seeds and is therefore a more refined product, though still delicious. It is an essential part of hummus, a Middle Eastern appetizer made of ground chickpeas, garlic, and tahini. It is also found in baba ghanoush, which has a base of roasted eggplant seasoned with tahini, lemon juice, garlic, and salt.

NUTS AND SEEDS

Sunflower Seeds

According to research by Katherine Phillips, Ph.D., in the department of biochemistry at Virginia Tech, the sunflower kernel is rich in a number of components that have been shown to protect against disease and to act as antioxidants and anticarcinogens; thus, the kernel can be considered a functional food. Functional foods are generally defined as foods that provide benefits beyond basic nutrition. Pretty good for something that was once considered only useful as birdfeed!

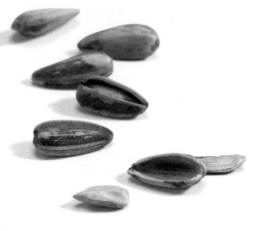

Snack on Sunflower Seeds to Lower Your Cholesterol

Sunflower seeds contain a wide variety of nutrients and protective plant compounds known as phytosterols. Phytosterols are well known for their ability to lower cholesterol and provide other health benefits. "Given the many possible mechanisms of action of phytosterols on cholesterol metabolism, it is important to have quantitative estimates of total phytosterol content," reported a team of researchers from Virginia Polytechnic Institute and State University, who tested twenty-seven different nut and seed products for phytosterol content. The results would have made the sunflower association very happy. Of all the products tested that are typically consumed as snacks, sunflower kernels were one of the two richest sources of phytosterols (the other was pistachio nuts). The main phytosterol identified in all the nut and seed samples was beta-sitosterol, which is known for lowering cholesterol and for supporting prostate health.

Sunflower seeds contain a potent antioxidant team of selenium and vitamin E to fight cancer and heart disease. Vitamin E is one of the most powerful antioxidants in the body, and ¼ cup serving of dried sunflower seed kernels provides more than 40 percent of the recommended Daily Value (yes, I personally think the Daily Value is too low, but still). Better yet, that same ¼ cup provides 30 percent of the Daily Value for selenium, a vitally important cancer-fighting trace mineral that works synergistically with vitamin E.

WORTH KNOWING

Though I'm a big fan of sunflower seeds (with or without the shell), I'm not a big fan of sunflower oil, which you might notice, is not listed in this book. It's way too high in proinflammatory omega-6s, with nothing much else to recommend it.

Sunflower seed kernels are also rich in protein and fiber, with ¼ cup (36 g) providing more than 8 g of protein and almost 4 g of fiber, not to mention 248 mg of potassium, 127 mg of magnesium, 254 mg of phosphorus, more than 2 mg of iron, plus manganese, copper, and zinc.

Sunflower Seeds May Lower Risk of Heart Disease

These little kernels are also a source of betaine (also known as trimethylglycine [TMG]), which may help lower homocysteine, a risk factor for heart disease. And they have a higher arginine content than almonds, hazelnuts, or pecans. Arginine is an amino acid that is touted for its role in protecting the inner lining of the arterial walls, making them more pliable and less susceptible to atherogenesis. It's also needed to make a very important molecule called nitric oxide, which helps relax constricted blood vessels and ease blood flow.

I've been known to eat the whole seed, hull and all. They're great to chew on, and take longer to consume—plus, who knows what beneficial compounds might be in the shell that haven't been discovered yet.

Also, it lets me share my stash with the birds, who don't seem to mind which version I feed them.

 # Walnuts

The "doctrine of signatures" is a concept in herbalism that's been around for centuries and is based on the idea that God marked everything God created with a sign (signature). The signature was an indication of the item's purpose. According to the doctrine of signatures, because the walnut looks just like a human brain, its purpose is to support that organ. This just might be one case of modern science supporting centuries-old wisdom, because walnuts— like fish—are truly brain food. Read on.

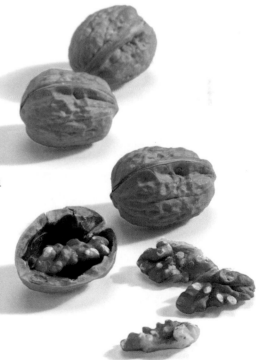

Can Eating Walnuts Improve Your Mood?

Walnuts contain the highest amounts of omega-3 fats of any other nuts. In addition to the other remarkable things omega-3s do for you, like help lower triglycerides and reduce plaque formation, they also support brain function on a number of levels. One of those levels has to do with mood and feeling.

There are compelling population studies linking the consumption of large amounts of fish (omega-3 fatty acids) to low rates of depression. Controlled clinical trials of omega-3s in depression are under way at any number of research centers. There is biochemical evidence of low levels of omega-3s in depressed patients (as well as a number of other behavioral and cognitive disorders and conditions). Here's why it makes sense: Fats in the diet are incorporated into cell membranes. Omega-3s are soft and fluid and give the cells enough "give" to allow them to communicate with each other, facilitating the movement of feel-good neurotransmitters like dopamine and serotonin in and out of the cells, and helping to support memory and thinking as well. Omega-3s truly are "brain food," and walnuts are rich in them.

Why Walnuts Make a Great Kid Snack

Several studies have demonstrated greater attention, reduction in behavioral problems, and less ADD-like behaviors in schoolkids when they're given omega-3s. Because it's hard to get kids to eat fish, let alone carry it to school in their lunchbox, walnuts are a really smart idea for a kid snack.

And walnuts may also be a great tool for weight management. According to experts at Loma Linda University, eating a few walnuts (say four to six halves) before meals decreases levels of hunger and may cause people to eat less at meals. "Walnuts help alleviate hunger and are naturally nutrient dense, meaning you consume many essential nutrients for a

relatively small percentage of daily calories," said Joan Sabate, M.D., M.P.H., Dr.P.H., chair of the department of nutrition.

Just don't add walnuts to an already high-calorie diet and expect to lose weight. As long as you replace some calories from your regular diet with an approximately equal number of calories from walnuts, you'll do fine. The nuts may even work as a natural appetite controller in addition to providing all those nutrients.

Walnuts Aid in Growth, Reproduction, and Brain Functioning

Walnuts, like most nuts, are nutrient rich, especially in minerals. They have protein, fiber, calcium, magnesium, phosphorus, and potassium, plus about half the Daily Value for manganese, an important trace mineral that's essential for growth, reproduction, wound healing, peak brain function, and the proper metabolism of sugars, insulin, and cholesterol.

Natural-foods expert Rebecca Wood cautions that you should purchase walnuts in the shell and crack them just before use. If you choose to purchase shelled whole walnut halves, make sure their flesh is white rather than yellow because the yellow indicates rancidity. Wood also points out that organic walnuts have darker brown shells, and their color will vary depending on how much sun the branch they grew on was exposed to.

There are two common kinds of walnuts—the English (most of which ironically come from California) and the black walnut, which is native to North America. They differ slightly in their nutritional profile—the English has slightly less protein and slightly more fat. Both are great.

THE EXPERTS' TOP TEN LISTS

Daniel Amen, M.D.

Daniel Amen has been called "the most popular psychiatrist in America" by the *Washington Post*. He's double board certified, has written more *New York Times* best-selling books than I could list in this paragraph (including *Change Your Brain, Change Your Life, The Brain Warrior's Way, Healing ADD,* and *Memory Rescue*), and had more hit PBS specials than anyone I know. He's also the founder and CEO of Amen Clinics, where they have the world's largest database of functional brain scans relating to behavior, totaling nearly 100,000 scans on patients from 111 countries. It was Daniel, in fact, who once told me "the prettiest looking brains I've seen are on gingko biloba."

I've known Daniel and his extraordinary wife, Tana, for about a decade, and he's my go-to guy for all things brain related. I've thanked him in the acknowledgments sections of most of the books I've written. He offered this list of top 11 foods for "bright minds." (Fun fact: Daniel once told me that from a brain point of view, the healthiest, most life-extending, brain-protecting sport in the world is Ping-Pong.)

1. **Cayenne pepper**—I like this for its enhancing effect on blood flow.

2. **Cloves**—These are healthy for their antioxidant power, which is beneficial especially for aging populations.

3. **Wild salmon**—Its omega-3 fatty acids and ability to fight inflammation are among its health and nutritional benefits.

4. **Turmeric**—This spice helps decrease the formation of beta amyloid plaque in the brain.

5. **Shrimp**—It boosts acetylcholine, an important neurotransmitter, which is beneficial for head trauma.

6. **Brassica vegetables**—This family of vegetables, including cauliflower, cabbage, broccoli, and Brussels sprouts, stimulates the body to make important detoxification enzymes.

7. **Saffron**—Saffron has been shown to ease depression symptoms.

8. **Garlic**—Garlic has many health benefits, including its ability to boost immunity.

9. **Eggs**—I recommend eggs for their cholesterol*.

10. **Lentils**—These legumes are rich in fiber.

11. **Tart cherries**—They increase levels of melatonin and have been shown to improve the quality of sleep.

*No, that is not a misprint. Daniel was an early endorser of my book, *The Great Cholesterol Myth* (coauthored with Stephen Sinatra, M.D.), and has known for a long time that conventional medicine is wrong on cholesterol and fat. He includes eggs on his list precisely because they contain cholesterol, a vitally important nutrient for brain health, not to mention hormone production and vitamin D.

NUTS AND SEEDS

CHAPTER 6

SOY FOODS

What about soy?

"Wait a minute," I can almost hear you saying. "In a book on the world's healthiest foods, you barely mention soy. What gives? Is there a misprint?" No misprint, and full disclosure: I'm not a big fan of soy.

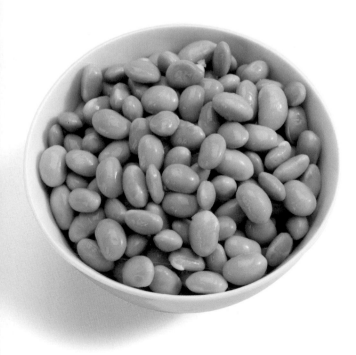

There was a huge controversy in the nutrition community over soy when I first wrote this book, and it's still going on. The pro-soy PR effort has been so strong that many people simply take for granted that anything with soy in it is a health food. You hardly hear about the many scientists, nutritionists, and researchers who have grave doubts about soy for a variety of reasons.

Meanwhile, for their part, the anti-soy contingent can be a bit strident and angry and sometimes tends to overstate the negatives associated with soy. That said, I think the reputation of soy as a health food is pretty overblown.

The Bad News about Soy

Soy contains large amounts of natural toxins or antinutrients, chief among them potent enzyme inhibitors that block the action of enzymes needed for protein digestion. (Of course, these same protease inhibitors are believed by some to have a cancer-protective effect, hence part of the controversy.)

Soybeans also contain haemagglutinin, a clot-promoting substance that causes red blood cells to clump together. They also contain goitrogens—substances that suppress thyroid function. And soy has one of the highest phytate levels of any grain or legume studied. (Phytates block the absorption of minerals; fermentation reduces them.)

Soy is often touted for its phytoestrogens, but whether that's a good thing or a not-so-good thing depends on many factors—such as sex and age, for example. As long ago as 2005, the Israeli Health Ministry issued a health advisory that strongly recommended that the consumption of soy foods be limited for young children and adults and that soy formula be avoided altogether by infants. And an article on soy protein infant formula in the *Journal of Pediatrics, Gastroenterology and Nutrition* suggested that soy protein formula had no nutritional advantage over cows' milk protein and that the "high concentrations of phytate, aluminum and phytoestrogens (isoflavones) . . . might have untoward effects."

FDA Reconsidering Its Position on Soy

The universal acceptance of all things soy may be showing signs of cracking, even among the establishment organizations. As of April 2006, the American Heart Association's (AHA) Nutrition Committee no longer recommended eating soy to lower cholesterol. In fact, the long-held belief that cholesterol is of prime importance in heart disease is beginning to show signs of weakening. Most of soy's health claims were based on its supposed ability to lower cholesterol. As more sophisticated ways of measuring heart disease risk come to be used, cholesterol is fading in importance, making the case for soy even weaker.

Even as the first edition of this book went to press, the FDA was reviewing its policy on soy health claims, and that review is still going on to this day. On June 30, 2016, the FDA stated on its website that it was "completing its evaluation of the totality of the current scientific evidence regarding the relationship between soy protein and coronary heart disease." But the disenchantment with soy has been going on for a long time, at least among health professionals. A decade ago, an article appeared in the *Harvard Women's Health Watch* with the title "Soy: Not So Miraculous?" Almost a decade later, in 2014, the Weston A. Price Foundation filed a lawsuit against the FDA, challenging the it on allowing health claims to be made about soy protein's effect on coronary heart disease. (That case is not expected to be heard until after this book was published.)

The soy associated with the Asian diet is a whole different animal from the soy we've been sold in America as a health food. Asians typically eat naturally fermented soy foods like tempeh and miso and old-fashioned fermented soy sauce—and they eat way less of it than you might imagine. It's also far from clear that the health benefits they get from their diet are attributable to eating soy rather than the fish and sea vegetables they consume regularly. In any case, there's no evidence that the soy they eat over there is exactly the same as the soy we eat over here. Last time I was in China, I didn't see a lot of soy ice cream, chips, milks, meat substitutes, and other processed foods. What I did see was some edamame served as an appetizer before a meal of fish, vegetables, a small amount of rice, and fruit.

The Real Deal on Soy

Let me be clear: In a world of french fries, fast food, trans fats, and high-fructose corn syrup, I hardly think a few servings of soy protein is the worst thing in the world. We have bigger battles to fight in the food arena. But I also don't think soy products are among the healthiest foods on the planet, for all the previous reasons mentioned.

I believe:

1. Fermented soy products such as miso and tempeh—fermented the old-fashioned way, the way they are in Asia—are healthy foods, as are most traditionally fermented foods (e.g., sauerkraut). Fermented foods (including fermented soy products such as tempeh) are great sources of prebiotics and probiotics.

2. One serving of a high-quality soy protein powder a day is not going to kill you, and it may even be good for some people.

3. Most soy products—e.g., soy chips, soy milk, soy ice cream, tofu ice cream, soy burgers, soy cheese, soy lattes, and all the rest—are junk food and no healthier than the foods they replace.

4. I would not feed soy formula to infants and small children unless there were absolutely no other choice, and there usually is.

5. I would not make soy my only source of protein under any circumstances. (Vegetarians take note.)

6. I do not recommend supplements of soy isoflavones. Period.

You don't have to look very hard to find pro-soy info but you might have to dig a little to get to hear the other side. I suggest that anyone interested in the soy controversy start by Googling "Mary Enig" and reading her extensive writing on soy, including "The Ploy of Soy" and "Soy Alert: Tragedy and Hype." For a more easy and entertaining—but no less scientifically documented—read the essential book, *The Whole Soy Story: The Dark Side of America's Health Food*, by Kaayla Daniel, Ph.D. (Daniel was a doctoral student under Enig.)

By the way, it's interesting that of all the experts I surveyed for their top ten favorite health foods in this book and in the original edition, not a single one chose soy. Just saying.

Edamame (green soybeans)

As you might have guessed by a cursory glance through this book, I'm not a huge fan of soy (to read why so few soy foods are included in this book, see page 186). One soy food I do like well enough to include it in the top 150 foods is edamame.

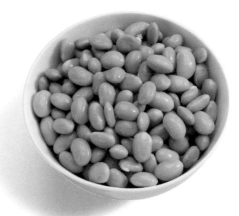

Edamame is the Japanese word for green vegetable soybeans. In Asia, they're finger food—the Japanese eat them as a snack with beer, much as Americans eat peanuts. And as snack foods go, they're great. They're young, they're sweet, and they're not very "beany" or bitter. They also have lower amounts of the compounds in soybeans that I'm not crazy about—protease inhibitors, trypsin inhibitors, and phytates.

And they're not terribly processed. Typically, edamame are boiled or steamed in the pod for 20 minutes, then chilled and salted. They are served at sushi restaurants as an appetizer, or they're quick frozen and packaged and shipped to your grocer. When the first edition of this book came out, there were only a couple of special stores like Trader Joe's that carried frozen edamame, but not anymore. You can find edamame in groceries across the country.

Edamame Makes a Healthy Snack Alternative

If you're comparing edamame to one of the cancer-fighting *Brassica* such as cabbage or broccoli, or to one of the fiber heavyweights like raspberries or lentils, it's not going to look like a nutritional superstar. But no one builds a meal around edamame. What it really is is a highly nutritious, high-protein vegetarian snack food. If they were to replace potato chips during football season, you'd probably see a quantum improvement in the health of the average sports fan. About 3½ ounces (100 g) of the edible portion (the actual beans) provides more than 12 g of protein, 4 g of fiber, 145 mg of calcium, 60 mg of magnesium, 111 mcg of folate, plus just for good measure, a tiny bit of vitamins A and C. It's also a potassium heavyweight, providing more than 500 mg per 100 g. Granted, not many people consume that much in a sitting, but still.

Research in the *Journal of Agriculture and Food Chemistry* found that edamame had a fair amount of both soy isoflavones and carotenoids. Cooked edamame have a sweet, nutty flavor and are traditionally eaten as a vegetable in stir-fries in China and Korea. As a snack, the seeds are usually squeezed directly into the mouth with the fingers.

Fermented Soy

(tempeh and miso)

Two soy products I like for their health benefits are tempeh and miso. Tempeh is actually a traditional Indonesian food, made from the controlled fermentation of cooked whole soybeans. It's usually fermented with a Rhizopus mold (also known as a tempeh starter), which binds the soybeans into a compact white cake. Tempeh fermentation produces natural antibiotic agents that are believed to increase the body's resistance to infections.

Tempeh May Ease Symptoms of Menopause

Tempeh contains phytochemicals such as isoflavones and saponins. The fermentation leaves the soy isoflavones intact. In research on soy protein, there is some evidence that the isoflavones may be responsible for helping to ease menopause symptoms. Soy protein and isoflavones such as those found in tempeh may possibly reduce the risk of heart disease and some cancers. Tempeh also contains saponins, health-promoting components of vegetables and legumes with strong biological activity, including acting as natural antibiotics. There is some suspicion that saponins may have cancer-protective or cancer-fighting activity. Saponins protect soybeans from predators and insects, but according to research from Keith Singletary, Ph.D., they may also help protect people from colon cancer.

Tempeh has a nutty mushroom flavor, and it can be sliced and sautéed till the surface is golden brown. It can also be used in soups, salads, and sandwiches. Any recipe that works with mushrooms will work with tempeh as well.

Miso

Miso is a soybean paste that has been a mainstay of Japanese cooking since the seventh century. It's made by mixing cooked soybeans with salt, a grain, and a fermenting agent called koji. There are many varieties of miso; hacho miso is made only from soybeans, and natto miso is made from ginger and soybeans. Most of the others are made from soybeans and a grain.

Despite my reservations about soy in general, there are benefits of some soy protein in the diet, and miso is one way to get soy protein in your diet from a healthy traditional food. A ¼ cup (64 g) of pure miso contains 8 g of soy protein. It also contains almost 5 mcg of the cancer-fighting mineral selenium, plus 144 mg of potassium, 109 mg of phosphorus, and a small amount of calcium and magnesium. And ¼ cup (64 g) of miso contains a respectable 3.7 g of fiber to boot. It does, however, contain 2,500 mg of sodium in ¼ cup. Most Westerners are likely to get miso in the form of miso soup, which also usually contains vegetables, making it a nice, low-calorie, healthy start to a meal.

Natto

Natto is a traditional Japanese food and definitely an acquired taste. It's made from soybeans fermented by the *Bacillus natto*, which result in a soybean that's sticky and can be rather . . . well, strong smelling. That's one reason it's not exactly an American favorite. Nonetheless, natto—also known as "vegetable cheese"—has been consumed safely for thousands of years.

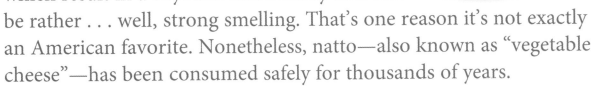

Its claim to fame is its richness in an enzyme called nattokinase. Nattokinase is a fibrinolytic enzyme that can help reduce and prevent clots. My coauthor on *The Great Cholesterol Myth*—cardiologist Stephen Sinatra, M.D.,—is a great fan of nattokinase for just that reason, and he has written about the value of nattokinase supplements for lowering blood pressure naturally.

Here's how it works: The body produces a number of substances that assist in blood clotting, one of which is called fibrin. Fibrin is like a web of sticky fibers that your body produces to form a structure that stops excess bleeding. You need fibrin for healthy blood thickness, but too much can impede blood flow and elevate blood pressure. One enzyme in the body, plasmin, dissolves and breaks down fibrin, but plasmin declines with age. Nattokinase, the enzyme in natto, is very structurally similar to plasmin and can directly break down fibrin, helping to prevent clots and keep blood flowing smoothly. That's why natto is such a "circulation-friendly" food.

Study Shows That Natto Contributes to Healthy Blood Flow

Nattokinase has been the subject of a number of studies, including two human trials. In one of them, twelve healthy Japanese volunteers were given 200 g of natto before breakfast. The amount of time it took to dissolve a blood clot dropped by 48 percent, and their ability to dissolve clots remained for 2 to 8 hours.

Some highly regarded vitamin companies began marketing nattokinase as a supplement, and some cutting-edge nutritionists recommend it as an alternative to blood-thinning medications and to help guard against strokes. (Note: Don't try this at home, folks. If you're going to wean off a medication, do it under the supervision of your licensed health professional.)

Nattokinase does help keep clotting factors in a nice, healthy range, but note that the actual food, natto, also contains vitamin K. Vitamin K is great for healthy bones, but it can interfere with Coumadin and other blood-clotting medications. This is no problem if you're eating natto for its circulatory benefits, but it is a potential problem if you're on meds. Some vitamin companies remove the vitamin K from their nattokinase supplements.

Natto Works Wonders for the Skin

I'm including natto in the list of the world's healthiest foods because it really is—but there's not much danger that too many people are going to start eating it. Most people hate the softness of the fermented soybeans, not to mention the stickiness and the smell. Even many Japanese don't like it. But if you can stand it, it not only supports good circulation, but it also makes your skin glow. The very same compound that makes it sticky—polyglutamic acid—also increases the natural moisturizing factor in skin.

THE EXPERTS' TOP TEN LISTS

Alan Christianson, N.M.D.

Alan Christianson is a naturopathic medical doctor (N.M.D.) specializing in natural endocrinology with a focus on thyroid disorders and adrenal functioning. He trains physicians internationally on thyroid disease, adrenal stress, and hormone replacement and has been featured on numerous media outlets, including *Dr. Oz*, *The Today Show*, *CNN*, *The Doctors*, *Women's World*, and *Shape* magazine. He's the *New York Times'* bestselling author of *The Adrenal Reset Diet*, *The Complete Idiot's Guide to Thyroid Disease*, and *Healing Hashimoto's—A Savvy Patient's Guide*.

Alan's one of the most athletic doctors I know—there are videos of him doing some of the most hair-raising mountain biking I've ever seen—and his personal story of overcoming significant health challenges is inspiring.

Alan frequently talks about food in terms of its potential to upset hormonal balancing acts. Here are his ten favorite foods and why he likes them.

1. **Sardines:** Sardines are a great source of clean seafood loaded with EPA and DHA (the two long-chain omega-3 fatty acids found in fish), plus, when you eat them with the edible bones, calcium and magnesium!

2. **Potatoes:** Potatoes are a reliable source of potassium and resistant starch.

3. **Adzuki beans:** These are one of the densest food sources of magnesium, and the beans themselves are a kidney tonic.

4. **Buckwheat:** I like this low-glycemic grain for the citrus bioflavonoids, especially rutin and hesperidin.

5. **Beet greens:** These greens are high in potassium and are an effective way to get vitamin K.

6. **Wild rice:** This grain is a good source of fiber, antioxidants, and vitamin B_6.

7. **Shiitake mushrooms:** They deserve their reputation as a tonic for the immune system because they're loaded with immunotonic polysaccharides.

8. **Flax seeds:** Besides being full of plant-based omega-3 (ALA), flax seeds have saponins and lectins; flax lignans have been shown to have anti-cancer activity, and the fiber in them has been shown to help lower blood sugar.

9. **Broccoli sprouts:** They contain cancer-fighting indoles and sulforaphanes.

10. **Oysters:** These contain selenium, zinc, protein, DHA, and vitamin B12. They have no nervous system, so might be acceptable to some ethical vegans.

CHAPTER 7

DAIRY

Let me be clear where I stand on the whole milk thing: I'm not a fan.

Let me explain. I'm a huge fan of raw, organic, unpasteurized, nonhomogenized milk from grass-fed cows that graze on pastures in small farms devoted to sustainable agriculture. In fact, I think milk—raw, whole milk from the cows I've just described—is one of the best whole foods in the world. But I can't say the same about the milk we find in the typical supermarket.

I realize this goes against generations of amazingly effective public relations campaigns from the dairy industry, including the Got Milk? ones with beautiful, healthy-looking, sexy, milk-mustachioed models smiling and against the warnings about how we will all get osteoporosis if we don't drink a quart (946 ml) of the stuff a day (not true). But this book is about facts, not about spin. And though there are many ways to read the facts on milk—it's a complex subject involving not only food but agribusiness, economics, and politics as well as nutrition—my job is to give you my reading of those facts. My reading is this: Cow's milk is a great food if you're a baby cow, and even if you're a human—provided it comes direct from grass-fed cows untreated with antibiotics, steroids, and hormones, and is raw, unpasteurized, and unhomogenized—but even calves probably wouldn't touch the stuff we get in supermarkets.

It's been well documented that the dairy industry spends a substantial amount of money on advertising and lobbying, and it's done a great job of convincing the public that homogenized, pasteurized milk from factory-farmed cows is a healthy product. And the dairy industry doesn't like competition. It fought tooth and nail to prevent small farms from putting the words "hormone-free" or "no rBgh" (recombinant bovine growth hormone) on their milk for the transparently self-serving reason that they didn't want the public to be confused and think that hormone-free milk was in some way better than regular milk. (It is.)

The industry also fought against the term *soy milk*. And it fought—successfully in most cases—against the sale of raw, unpasteurized milk. Thanks to its efforts, you can only buy raw unpasteurized milk in thirteen states, and even in those where you can legally buy it—such as California, where I live—grocers told me off the record that there's tremendous pressure on them not to sell it. My local Whole Foods in Woodland Hills yielded to pressure, whereas my local Sprouts Farmers Market—two blocks down the street—did not. So much for conscious capitalism.

The dairy industry's claim of wanting to protect the public from the dangers of raw milk seem self-serving. According to data from a 2007 CDC-FoodNet survey, reproduced on the website Food Renegade, about 9 million people drink raw milk. Want to know how many reports of raw milk causing people to get sick?

Forty-two.

Again, this book isn't the place to debate the politics of milk. But understand that just as factory-farmed meat has hormones, antibiotics, and all sorts of other undesirable compounds, so does the milk that comes from those factory-farmed animals. I'm not at all convinced that homogenization—which alters the fat content—and pasteurization—which kills an awful lot of good stuff—is necessary for healthy people. Personally, cold, raw, full-fat, unpasteurized, and unhomogenized milk is one of my favorite drinks, and I drink it daily. I suggest doing your own research and deciding if it's for you (or not). If you do want to try it, it's available through farm collectives even in states where you can't buy it in the grocery.

Modern Efficiency Leads to Nutritional Deficiency

In the modern factory farm—which is truly a farm in name only—cows are milk-and-beef production machines that exist to turn corn and grain (their main source of food) into milk and meat as quickly as possible. Given that the natural food of cows is grass, the resultant situation is no less than a biological absurdity, akin to keeping lions alive on a diet of chocolate chip cookies. As Michael Pollan wrote of the situation in his wonderful book *The Omnivore's Dilemma*, " . . . animals exquisitely adapted by natural selection to live on grass must be adapted by us—at considerable cost to their health, to the health of the land, and ultimately to the health of their eaters—to live on corn, for no other reason than it offers the cheapest calories around."

"Considerable cost" is putting it mildly. A concentrated diet of corn can give a cow acidosis, which can lead to a general weakening of the immune system that leaves the animal vulnerable to a host of horrible diseases. Cattle rarely manage to live on these diets for more than 150 days. Between 15 and 30 percent of them are found at slaughter to have abscessed livers. Some estimates are considerably higher.

In addition, with intensive production schedules (they don't call them factory farms for nothing), it's common for modern dairy cows to produce many times the number of pounds of milk they would produce in nature. Growth hormones and unnatural milking schedules cause dairy cows' udders to become painful, heavy, and infected. To prevent this, factory-farmed cows are routinely given large doses of antibiotics, the residue of which, along with that of the steroids and growth hormones they are given, invariably wind up in the milk and meat they produce.

If you think all those hormones don't have any impact on your health, consider this: A study in the prestigious *Journal of the American Academy of Dermatology* in February 2005 demonstrated a significant positive association between milk drinking and teenage acne. The researchers suggested that the most likely explanation was the presence of hormones and "bioactive molecules" in the milk.

The Truth about Pasteurization and Homogenization

So if hormones, steroids, and antibiotics weren't enough—and they are—the resultant milk is then pasteurized and homogenized. Both procedures destroy vitally important health-giving compounds in the milk. As Joe Mercola, D.O., accurately points out, "Pasteurizing milk destroys enzymes, diminishes vitamins, denatures fragile milk proteins, destroys vitamins B_{12} and B_6, kills beneficial bacteria and promotes pathogens."

Milk and Cancer?

There have been more than a few studies linking dairy consumption—especially milk—with increased risk for prostate cancer, and these studies go back at least fifteen years. One study in the May 2005 *American Journal of Clinical Nutrition* concluded that "Dairy consumption may increase prostate cancer risk through a calcium-related pathway" and that " . . . the mechanisms by which dairy and calcium might increase prostate cancer risk should be clarified and confirmed." On April 4, 2000, the Harvard School of Public Health issued a press release titled *Higher Intake of Dairy Products May be Linked to Prostate Cancer Risk*. And in October 2001, a paper called "Dairy Products, Calcium, and Prostate Cancer Risk in the Physicians' Health Study" appeared in the *American Journal of Clinical Nutrition*. Its conclusion:

"These results support the hypothesis that dairy products and calcium are associated with a greater risk of prostate cancer."

Connection between Milk and Ovarian Cancer Still in Dispute

Similarly disturbing connections have been found between dairy—especially milk—and ovarian cancer. In November 2004, research published in the *American Journal of Clinical Nutrition* by Swedish researchers concluded that "our data indicate that high intakes of lactose and dairy products, particularly milk, are associated with an increased risk of serious ovarian cancer, but not of other subtypes of ovarian cancer." And just as the original manuscript for this book was being submitted, researchers at the Harvard School of Public Health examined twelve different previously published studies to try to find some trends. The results, published in *Cancer Epidemiological Biomarkers and Prevention* in February 2006, noted that while no associations were observed for intakes of specific dairy foods or calcium and ovarian cancer risk, "A modest elevation in the risk of ovarian cancer was seen for lactose intake at the level that was equivalent to three or more servings of milk per day." The researchers noted that because three servings is exactly what the dietary guidelines recommend, "the relation between dairy product consumption and ovarian cancer risk at these consumption levels deserves further examination."

I wish we could say for certain what conclusions can be drawn from so many conflicting studies that suggest connections without proving cause. Unfortunately, we can't. All I can do is point them out in the hope that they will at least cause people to reflect on whether the "all milk all the time" mantra of the dairy industry ought to be taken with a grain of salt. Or two. Or three.

It's also worth pointing out that in all these studies, it's unlikely that the majority of the milk drinkers were drinking the raw, organic, unpasteurized, and non-hormone-treated milk I recommend. Does that make a difference? It's anyone's guess. My personal belief is that it probably does. That's why milk—or meat or cheese—from factory-farmed cattle is not food I will ever recommend.

I do, however, recommend yogurt. In a perfect world, we'd make it ourselves, or get it from the same grass-fed animals that provide raw milk and healthy meat. But even commercial yogurt can contain large amounts of healthy bacteria—called probiotics—and for this reason alone, yogurt is worth including. (There are other reasons as well—see below.) And both organic butter and ghee, for all the reasons listed, below, remain among my favorite fats.

 # Butter/Ghee

I love butter. And back when I first wrote this section—in 2006—I knew that my positive take on butter was going to cause apoplexy among the diet dictators, conventional dietitians, doctors, and other members of the diet establishment. And it did. But that was then, and this is now. Two powerful meta-analyses, one published in the *American Journal of Clinical Nutrition* in 2010, the other in the *Annals of Internal Medicine* in 2014, both concluded that there was no clear evidence that saturated fat had anything to do with cardiovascular disease, leading *New York Times* food writer and consumer advocate Mark Bittman to title a column "Butter is Back."

The fact is that butter—from pasture-fed, organically raised cows—is a wonderful, healthy food.

Butter

To understand why real butter is a healthy food, you have to unlearn a great deal of what you've been taught about saturated fat. Now the argument over saturated fat is way too complex to go into here, but I'll give you the CliffsNotes, and if you're interested in reading further, some suggested sources. Number one, yes, butter contains saturated fat. Number two, yes, saturated fat raises cholesterol somewhat, but that is turning out to be less important than previously thought, and newer, more modern cholesterol tests are showing that saturated fat may actually have a good effect on cholesterol overall. Three, whether an increase in cholesterol translates into higher rates of heart disease or greater rates of mortality is a hotly debated topic whose subplots, political intrigue, and warring factions make the arguments over *The Da Vinci Code* look like a household discussion over which television channel to watch. If you're interested in exploring this issue further for yourself, I'd like to throw in a shameless plug for my 2012 book (with cardiologist Stephen Sinatra, M.D.), *The Great Cholesterol Myth*. It's a great place to start.

Some Saturated Fat Is Good for Us

So yup, butter has saturated fat, and nope, let's not debate the whole saturated fat issue here. Sure, we can always use more research, and sure, we don't have the absolute final word on any of this stuff. My opinion is that the fear of saturated fat that gripped the country for about four decades was way out of proportion to any harm it does. Some saturated fat is good for us and necessary in the diet. To remove healthy foods such as butter, avocado, eggs, coconut oil, palm oil, and grass-fed meat from the diet simply because they contain saturated fat, is, in my opinion, extremely unwise, not to mention unjustified by the research data.

Now that that's out of the way, here's the good stuff on butter. Butter is a rich source of vitamin A, which is needed for many functions in the body, not the least of which are optimal functioning of the immune system and maintaining good vision. Butter also contains all the other fat-soluble vitamins—E, K, and D. Vitamin D deficiency is being called a "silent epidemic" by nutritionists these days, many of whom don't believe we get nearly enough of this cancer-fighting, bone-building nutrient.

WORTH KNOWING

I recommend that you get only grass-fed butter. There are some great ones on the market. I personally use and like Kerrygold butter, but my friend Dave Asprey—the inventor of Bulletproof Coffee and a big fan of high-quality butter—recently pointed out that up to 3 percent of Kerrygold cows' diets may be from GMO feed. Kerrygold is also not organic. However, both Asprey and I still recommend Kerrygold because it's so much better than other commercial butters, the amount of GMO is very small, they don't use antibiotics or hormones and their Irish dairy cows graze outdoors on grass all day long for up to 312 days a year! (Thanks, Dave, for making this information available. I should mention that neither Dave Asprey nor myself have any financial relationship with Kerrygold.)

CLA in "Good" Butter Can Keep You Trim

When you eat animal products that come from healthy, grass-fed animals, you are getting the benefits of the animal's diet. Real feed for cows is green grass, not grains. Foods like butter that come from grass-fed cows are rich in the fats proven to be healthful, such as omega-3s, which are virtually absent from their grain-fed counterparts. Food that comes from grass-fed animals also contains CLA (conjugated linoleic acid), a particularly healthy fat that has demonstrated anticancer properties. Research has also shown CLA to have a lot of promise in fighting weight gain, particularly around the abdomen.

The promise of CLA is so great that it has been the subject of an entire research conference (Perspectives on Conjugated Linoleic Research, Current Status and Future Directions), which is posted on the National Institutes of Health's Office of Dietary Supplements website. Butter, milk, and meat from grain-fed animals contain virtually no CLA, while food from grass-fed animals is a rich source of this health-promoting fatty acid.

The fat in butter is rich in health-giving properties. For years, I've bucked the diet dictators and recommended butter as a "good fat," alongside nuts, eggs, fish, coconut, avocados, and certain oils. Butter has been used for centuries. What's more, 30 percent of the fat from butter is from monounsaturated fat (the same kind that's in olive oil). The late Mary Enig, Ph.D.—a respected lipid biochemist—pointed out that the fat in butter inhibits the growth of pathogens, and that butter is a source of several kinds of antimicrobial fats, including lauric acid, which disables many pathogenic viruses. In her writings, she also noted that butter has glycolipids, which have anti-infective properties, as well as the aforementioned CLA (conjugated linoleic acid), which has anticarcinogenic properties. In her textbook on fat she states: "Butter is definitely a fat with health-potentiating properties."

I couldn't agree more.

Ghee

Ghee is clarified butter, which means it's basically butter with the milk solids removed (more on this in a moment). But to treat ghee as just a form of butter doesn't properly acknowledge the fact that this food has been used specifically for its health-giving properties for thousands of years in an honorable and esteemed medical tradition.

Ghee has a long and respected history as a medicinal and healing food in Indian (Ayurvedic) medicine, a tradition that dates back nearly 5,000 years. According to Dharma Singh Khalsa, M.D., author of *Food as Medicine*, ghee is highly regarded in yoga nutritional therapy, where it is valued as both a nutrient and a preservative for food and medicine. In Ayurvedic medicine, ghee is believed to strengthen the ojas, our vital energy cushion at the root of our well-being and immunity.

WORTH KNOWING

According to Dharma Singh Khalsa, M.D., an easy way to make ghee is to simmer unsalted butter over medium-low heat for 10 to 20 minutes until an almost transparent crust forms on top. Then skim off the crust and strain the golden liquid that remains into a container. Make sure you discard the white sediment at the bottom. Or, you can do what I do and buy ready-made ghee in most natural food stores. It doesn't need to be refrigerated, and in fact, according to some traditions, has more healing properties if you leave it out at room temperature.

Happy Cows, Healthy Ghee

Remember that in India, the cow is revered as a sacred being. There are no factory farms for cattle in India—all cows are grass fed. Therefore, all the health benefits of grass-fed butter discussed under Butter (page 196), apply completely to ghee. As Amadea Morningstar explains about the cow in her excellent book, *Ayurvedic Cooking for Westerners*, "her milk and her butter, clarified as ghee, are like mother's milk in Ayurveda, absolutely essential for health and well-being. They must be pure to do this. Many Westerners are concerned that the use of ghee will increase their cholesterol or add unnecessary amounts of fat to their diet. Used within the context of an Ayurvedic lifestyle, this is unlikely to happen." Annemarie Colbin, Ph.D., would agree. In her book, *Food and Healing*, she says that ghee is one of the three best-quality fats to use.

In Ayurvedic medicine, ghee is believed to help stimulate the healthy flow of fluids throughout the body. It is considered an important rejuvenative tonic for the mind, the brain, and the nervous system. And, because it has all the milk solids removed, it can be used for cooking at higher temperatures. Ayurveda describes ghee as one of the finest cooking oils; it increases "digestive fire," thereby improving assimilation and enhancing the nutritional value of foods. It also doesn't go rancid. I keep a container of ghee out on my kitchen counter all the time, unrefrigerated, and dip into it for a spoonful almost every day.

Like butter, ghee contains butyric acid, a fatty acid that has antiviral and anticancer properties and that raises the level of the antiviral chemical interferon in the body.

Cheese

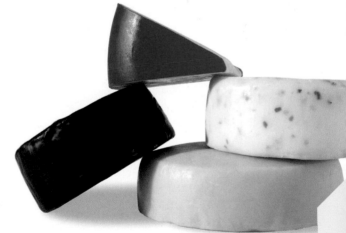

When it comes to cheese, here's a good thing to keep in mind: It's all about the source. Unfortunately, the generic name "cheese" covers a lot of territory. Just as "carbs" include lollipops and cauliflower, the cheese section of the deli is a pretty big umbrella, containing everything from phenomenally wonderful natural cheeses made from the raw and unpasteurized milk of sheep and goats to single-sliced "cheese foods" that bear no resemblance to anything that should ever be put in the human body.

Why Some Cheeses Don't Make the List

There's a great deal of diversity among foods labeled cheese, from raw organic milk cheese to Velveta "cheese products." Sorting out the types and kinds and their origins could fill a book on its own, and if each healthy type were given its own entry, there'd be no room for anything else. So this general introduction to the category will have to suffice.

Cheese falls into four main categories, according to production techniques and maturity: soft, unripened (cottage, ricotta, Neufchâtel); soft, ripened, either mold ripened (blue vein, Brie) or salt cured (feta); firm (Cheddar, Swiss); hard (Parmesan or Pecorino).

Some nutrients that are in all classes of cheese include calcium, magnesium, zinc, selenium, and folate. Natural cheese also has all four fat-soluble vitamins: A, E, K, and D. The mineral content of cheese is influenced by the addition of salt, optional ingredients, the method of coagulation, the treatment of the curd, and the resulting acidity.

French Cheese Has More Cancer-Fighting, Fat-Reducing Fat

French cheeses are especially high in CLA (conjugated linoleic acid), a cancer-fighting, fat-reducing fat that has been widely studied for its health benefits. A 1998 survey found that CLA levels in French cheese range from 5.3 to 15.8 mg/g of fat. American cheese from conventional dairies has half this amount. Why? French dairies are more likely to raise their cows on pasture, which results in naturally high levels of CLA.

The benefits of cheese from healthy animals extends beyond CLA. Unpasteurized Camembert is a natural source of probiotic *lactobacilli*, the very same protective bacteria we find in yogurt and naturally fermented food.

Full-Fat Dairy Doesn't Increase Risk

In 2017, a study published in the *European Journal of Epidemiology* examined the real-life consequences of eating full-fat dairy products, those same ones we've been advised against for decades. It basically found . . . nothing. Study researchers concluded that consuming full-fat versions of cheese, milk, and yogurt didn't increase the risk of heart attack or stroke a whit.

This follows several similar studies, including one in 2010 that reviewed 16 years of data on more than 1,500 adults to investigate the relationship of dairy consumption to mortality. Disappointingly, there was no consistent association between total dairy intake and mortality. But investigators found that those in the study who had the highest intake of full-fat dairy (about 339 g, or 12 ounces, per day) had a 69 percent reduction in their risk for death from cardiovascular disease compared with those who consumed the lowest.

Full-fat dairy contains a fat called palimiteric acid that may have a protective effect against diabetes. Palimiteric acid seems to lower the amount of fat produced from carbohydrates in the liver—a driver of metabolic syndrome and fatty liver disease. Much of the research on full-fat dairy has been done by cardiologist Dariush Mozaffarian, the dean of the Friedman School of Nutrition Science and Policy at Tufts University. In 2016, Mozaffarian and his team published another study of dairy fat in the journal Circulation. "People who had the most dairy fat in their diet had about a 50 percent lower risk of diabetes" than people with the least, he told NPR in an interview.

The take-home point? Once again, consider the source. Sheep and goats are less likely to be factory farmed, so their milk and cheese may contain a lot less drugs and antibiotics. Natural, raw milk cheeses—whether from cow's milk or any other animal—are likely to be richer in healthy fats such as omega-3s and CLA, especially if the animals graze on grass.

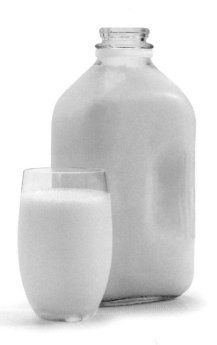

 # Raw Organic Milk

Raw, certified organic milk—unpasteurized and unhomogenized—is one of the true health foods on the planet. It's a wonderful source of protein and calcium, the fat in it is perfectly acceptable, and it tastes absolutely delicious.

Raw milk is loaded with nutrients, including beneficial bacteria such as *Lactobacillus acidophilus*. Because it isn't subjected to the high heat of pasteurization, those good bacteria—along with wonderful beneficial enzymes—aren't destroyed.

Raw milk virtually always comes from grass-fed cows. Milk from grass-fed cows contains higher levels of cancer-fighting CLA (conjugated linoleic acid) and will be richer in the full gamut of vitamins and minerals. Vitally important nutrients like vitamins A and D are greatest in milk from cows eating green grass. And the healthy enzymes contained in raw milk help the body assimilate all those great nutrients, including, by the way, calcium. According to Connecticut naturopath Ron Schmid, N.D., author of *Traditional Foods Are Your Best Medicine* and *The Untold Story of Milk: Green Pastures, Contented Cows and Raw Dairy Products*, enzymes are a critical component in recovering from disease and establishing and maintaining health. "I have become more convinced than ever of the value and importance of raw milk in the diets of people of all ages," says Schmid.

Milk from Grass-Fed Cows Much Higher in Omega-3s

The fat content of the milk from organically raised, grass-fed cows is wholly different than that of their factory-farmed brethren. Studies have shown that the omega-3 fat content of grass-fed, pasture-roaming cows is as high as 50 percent. It's virtually nonexistent in factory-farmed animals. And research at the University of Aberdeen in Scotland and at the Institute of Grassland and Environmental Research (IGER) at Aberystwyth, Wales, showed that organic milk contains between 71 percent and a whopping 240 percent more omega-3s than nonorganic milk, plus it has a much better ratio of omega-3 to omega-6 fats than conventional milk. This is probably because the pasture-fed cows graze on a diet rich in red clover silage as well as their natural diet of grasses.

DAIRY

While it's always possible to become sick from any contaminated food—just read the newspapers—raw milk seems to have been unfairly singled out as a risk. Consider this, from the Weston A. Price Foundation website:

Except for a brief hiatus in 1990, raw milk has always been for sale commercially in California, usually in health food stores, although (there was) a period when it was even sold in grocery stores. Millions of people consumed commercial raw milk during that period and although the health department kept an eagle eye open for any possible evidence of harm, not a single incidence was reported. During the same period, there were many instances of contamination in pasteurized milk, some of which resulted in death.

Raw organic milk is hard to find—see below. But more and more people are turning to small farms and collectives. At this writing, there are nearly forty such farms licensed to sell raw milk in Pennsylvania alone. It's worth looking for.

A Note on Goat's Milk

Goat's milk has more easily digestible fat and protein content than cow's milk. This increased digestibility of the protein is of great importance to infant diets as well as for invalid and convalescent diets. It also has 18 percent more calcium, 41 percent more magnesium, 22 percent more phosphorus, 42 percent more potassium, and almost twice the vitamin A. What it doesn't have is much folic acid or B_{12}, something to consider if you're using it for an infant's diet. And many people who are allergic to cow's milk do fine with goat's milk. Plus, it tastes great.

However, the same caveats exist as with cow's milk. Much of commercial goat's milk is not only pasteurized but ultrapasteurized. That gives it a ridiculously long shelf life, but unfortunately, according to

Ron Schmid, N.D., "turns a great food into something that's basically useless."

Camel Milk

Camel milk is beginning to be available in the United States. I've tried it, and it's delicious. It is the closest thing to human mother's milk, and contains higher levels of calcium, iron, magnesium, copper, zinc, and potassium, vitamin A, B_2, E and C.

It's been used medicinally in some cultures for centuries, and research has shown it to be effective in treating diabetes by reducing blood glucose, insulin resistance, and hemoglobin A1C—a long-term measure of blood sugar used to diagnose diabetes.

It also has potential therapeutic effects on the immune response in hepatitis B patients, autoimmune diseases, food allergies in children, and autism.

Camel milk has exactly none of the two components—beta-lactoglobulin and beta casein—which are the main cause of allergy in cow's milk. In addition, camel milk contains various protective proteins—mainly enzymes that have antibacterial, antiviral, and immunological properties.

Be aware that camel milk is not cheap. (That's an understatement.)

WORTH KNOWING

A great source for locating real, raw, organic, certified milk in your area is www.realmilk.com.

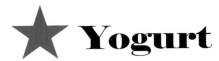

★ Yogurt

(kefir, lassi)

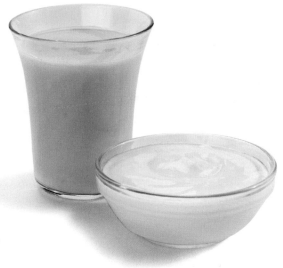

When I was a kid, I remember hearing stories of long-lived robust mountain people in the plains of Bulgaria who regularly consumed this weird white food that was evidentially the secret to their longevity and health. The food, I later found out, was yogurt, and as far as I was concerned, it tasted horrible. Of course, those were my five-year-old taste buds speaking. Now, decades later, yogurt comes in a zillion varieties including, of course frozen yogurt, and it no longer has to fight for shelf space in the American grocery store—it's practically become a staple. Whether this is the same food that the robust, rugged centurians of Bulgaria ate is quite another matter. Read on.

As long ago as the turn of the twentieth century, a Russian scientist named Metchnikoff wrote of yogurt's benefits in his 1908 book *The Prolongation of Life.* He believed that bacteria in the gut produced toxins that would shorten our life span and promote disease and that the good bacteria in yogurt would displace the bad bacteria and improve our health. More than a century later, abundant research has shown that he was on to something.

According to many experts in health and nutrition, all health begins in the gut, which is, after all, the site of digestion and the absorption of nutrients and is a huge part of the body's immune system. As Metchnikoff intuited, the gut is the site of a turf war between bad and good bacteria. You can never completely get rid of the bad bugs, but you can balance them with good bacteria and create a healthy environment that promotes digestion, increases immunity, fights against Candida overgrowth (*Candida albicans,* or yeast, is one of the bad bacteria), and strengthens the immune system.

Probiotics in Yogurt Make for a Healthy Gut

Yogurt—real yogurt, that is (more about that in a moment)—is a wonderful, rich source of those good bacteria. They're called probiotics, which literally means "for life." Because of their critical importance in supporting overall health, and because most people don't get nearly enough in their diet, many nutritionists consider probiotic supplements to be among the most important supplements a person can take on a daily basis. That's probably true—however, you can go a long way toward creating a healthy gut environment by consuming foods that are rich in these amazing, health-promoting microorganisms. Which is where yogurt comes in.

First a bit of history and some definitions. The word yogurt (or yoghurt) probably derives from the Turkish adjective meaning "dense and thick." Yogurt is basically fermented milk. Any milk can be used as a starter—goat's, sheep's, or cow's—but it's the fermentation of milk sugar (lactose) into lactic acid that gives yogurt its texture and tangy taste. Traditionally fermented foods—such as yogurt, sauerkraut, and miso—are among the healthiest foods in the world. They're rich in enzymes and other live microorganisms that have a wide array of health benefits.

The yogurt that the hardy centurians in Bulgaria were eating was very rich in a particular bacteria called *bulgaricus*. *Bulgaricus*—also known as *B. bifidum* or bifidobacteria—is part of that larger class of "good" bacteria known as probiotics (see above). Bifidobacterium primarily work their magic in the large intestine, while another probiotic genus—lactobaccili—are found mainly (though not exclusively) in the small intestine. Examples of *lactobacilli* species are *Lactobacillus acidophilus*, *Lactobacillus casei*, and *Lactobacillus plantarum*. (David Perlmutter, M.D.—the integrative neurologist and author of *Brain Maker*—highly recommends that any probiotic supplement you use include *Lactobacillus plantarum*.)

In any case, it's the presence of these live cultures that are responsible for the main health benefits of yogurt.

Yogurt Ups Your Immunity

And what a list of health benefits it is. Various members of the *Lactobacillus* class have been found to support and improve immunity in a number of studies. One Austrian study published in the *Annals of Nutrition and Metabolism* found that daily yogurt consumption had a stimulating effect on cellular immunity in healthy young women. Another study in the *American Journal of Clinical Nutrition* demonstrated that yogurt containing *Lactobacillus* and *bifidobacteria* can suppress *H. pylori*.

The research on gut health has been exploding since the original publication of this book, and talk of the microbiome is everywhere. (The microbiome is the name scientists give to the whole ecosystem of non-human microbes that reside in your gut and on your skin.) The health of the microbiome has been shown to impact obesity, mood, schizophrenia, and autism—and the list continues to grow. Our knowledge of the specifics of probiotic therapy is still in its infancy. We don't yet know exactly how to use which strains of probiotic bacteria for which purposes. Still, just about everyone in the health space agrees that maintaining healthy gut flora—with food, supplements, or a combination of the two—is of central importance in human health. Eating fermented foods, such as yogurt with real live cultures, is the least controversial and most accepted way to do just that.

Why You Should Look for the LAC Seal

All yogurt taking up shelf space in American supermarkets is not created equal. Far from it. There are food products with the word "yogurt" in them that bear absolutely no relationship to real yogurt except for the fact that the letters on the label are the same. Yogurt-covered pretzels? Yogurt raisins? "Yogurt" with 37 g of sugar and "fruit" on the bottom? People, let's get serious.

For yogurt to have any benefit it has to actually contain real live cultures. The National Yogurt Association (NYA) has developed a "Live and Active Cultures" (LAC) seal for the yogurt label to identify yogurt that contains significant levels of live and active cultures. Be aware that a label stating "made with active cultures" does not mean the same as the LAC label. All yogurt starts with active cultures—the question is whether any remain after the processing. The LAC label means that the yogurt contains at least 100 million cultures per gram of yogurt at the time of manufacture and after pasteurization.

Some yogurt products may indeed have live cultures but not happen to carry the LAC seal. To determine whether the yogurt you buy contains living bacteria, check the labels for "active yogurt cultures," "living yogurt cultures," or "contains active cultures."

Two brands that contain live cultures are Stonybrook Farms and Dannon (plain). Remember, don't be fooled by the words "made with active cultures." All yogurts are made with live cultures, but no live cultures survive heat treatment.

The Fewer Ingredients in Yogurt, the Better It Is for You

The best nutritional deal is plain yogurt, which has only two ingredients: live cultures and milk (whole, low-fat, or skim). The longer the ingredients list, the more calories and the less nutrition. Certain highly sweetened yogurt have more calories in the sweetener than in the yogurt. Read the protein and sugar values on the nutrition panel. The higher the protein and the lower the sugar content, the more actual yogurt you're getting in the container.

WHAT'S THE DEAL WITH GREEK YOGURT?

Both Greek yogurt and "regular" yogurt start out with the same basic ingredients. You heat the milk, you cool it to fermentation temperature (106°F to 114°F, or 41°C to 46°C), you add the bacterial cultures and you leave it to ferment. The difference is that when you make Greek yogurt, you strain it more times, removing some of the whey (and the lactose) and resulting in a thicker, and more concentrated yogurt. That's why Greek yogurt has more protein than regular yogurt. (It also has more fat, which is something that doesn't concern me one bit.)

Greek yogurt also has less sodium, and fewer carbohydrates than regular yogurt, due to the additional straining.

You can pick Greek versus regular based on personal taste. Some people find it too thick and tangy—others like it just fine. Because it's thicker, some people use it instead of sour cream.

I advise avoiding the no-fat and reduced-fat kinds, whether regular or Greek. Almost always, manufacturers add more sugar when they take out the fat, and almost always there was nothing wrong with the fat they took out to begin with. Studies done by Dariush Mozaffarian, M.D., the current dean of Tufts University's Friedman School of Nutrition Science and Policy, have shown that people with the highest levels of dairy fat in their blood had up to 46 percent lower risk of developing diabetes. Of course, it almost goes without saying that the best full-fat yogurt you can eat is from grass-fed cows (for all the reasons I've mentioned when talking about beef and milk). I'm happy to say that grass-fed yogurt is in fact becoming much more available in supermarkets, although you may have some problems finding grass-fed Greek yogurt.

The NYA has been urging the FDA not to allow products that do not contain live and active cultures to be called yogurt. The LAC label ensures consumers that the healthful properties of the organisms are present at the time they eat the yogurt, not just at the time of manufacturing.

Those Who Are Lactose Intolerant Can Still Enjoy Yogurt

Besides live cultures, yogurt is also a good source of protein and a great source of calcium and potassium. Depending on brand and type, it also has some B vitamins and a little of the important cancer-fighting mineral selenium.

Remember, live yogurt culture contains enzymes that break down lactose, so many individuals who are otherwise lactose intolerant find that they can enjoy yogurt with no problems.

One more thing: In case you haven't guessed by now, I'm not a fan of no-fat foods, and that certainly includes yogurt. Many vitamins and minerals—including calcium—are better absorbed with some fat. As I've pointed out many times, if the total number of calories in your diet does not exceed what you need, the percentage of calories from fat is of no real importance, provided it's not damaged fat like that found in fried foods, or horrible fat like trans fats. Yogurt with some fat in it fills you up; it is much more satisfying than the no-fat kind; and, it generally contains a lot

less sugar to boot. If you're still squeamish about the fat, at least go for low fat rather than no fat.

Some of the types of yogurt available include:

- **Bulgarian yogurt.** Known for its specific taste, Bulgarian yogurt contains the important probiotic *Lactobacillus bulgaricus*.

- **Greek yogurt.** Greek yogurt is made the same way regular yogurt is made, but strained an extra time or two, removing some of the whey and leaving a more concentrated, higher-protein yogurt (see box on page 205). The traditional Greek tzatziki sauce is made from yogurt, cucumber, and garlic.

- **Lassi** is a yogurt-based beverage that originated in India and comes in two varieties: salty and sweet. The salty kind is usually flavored with the wonderful spices cumin and chile peppers; the sweet kind often has fruit juice.

- **Kefir** is another traditionally fermented milk drink sometimes billed as "drinkable yogurt."

- **Goat's milk and sheep's milk yogurt** have the properties of the milk they were made from; they're definitely worth trying as well.

WORTH KNOWING

If you like the taste of frozen yogurt, or yogurt-covered peanuts and raisins—all of which may indeed be delicious—by all means eat them. But don't kid yourself that they have any of the health properties of real yogurt. They're sweet treats masquerading as a health food.

THE EXPERTS' TOP TEN LISTS

Stephen T. Sinatra, M.D., F.A.C.C., C.N.S.

Stephen Sinatra is a board-certified cardiologist, a certified bioenergetic psychotherapist, and a certified nutrition and antiaging specialist. Sinatra integrates conventional medicine with complementary, nutritional, and psychological therapies that help heal the heart. In my opinion, his classic *Heart Sense for Women* should be required reading. He and I coauthored *The Great Cholesterol Myth*.

Sinatra couldn't choose among his top twelve, so I let him list all twelve! All foods listed below are organic, natural, wild, or free range. These are the foods that he eats in everyday life.

1. **Asparagus:** These are loaded with folic acid, vitamin C, and are glutathione precursors.

2. **Avocado:** This contains lots of vitamin E, glutathione, and monounsaturated fat that doesn't require an insulin response.

3. **Onions:** Slice raw onions on salad. They contain many important flavonoids, especially quercetin, which supports the immune system, improves prostate health, and it is perhaps the major nutrient responsible for the "French Paradox" (page 294).

4. **Spinach:** Spinach contains lutein, which helps prevent macular degeneration and is instrumental in both lung and heart health. It is also one of the best sources of calcium.

5. **Wild blueberries:** Blueberries contain flavonoids that not only improve the macula and retina of the eye, but also help neurons in the brain communicate with one another.

6. **Pomegranate juice:** Pomegranate is a powerful antioxidant that has been shown to assist in plaque regression in both the carotid arteries and the heart.

7. **Free-range buffalo:** This is an outstanding source of protein with minimal saturated fat. No hormones, antibiotics, or chemicals are added. Grass-fed buffalo also contains precious omega-3s.

8. **Wild Alaskan salmon:** This is an outstanding protein source with the vital carotenoid called *astaxanthin*. This carotenoid prevents lipid peroxidation and assists in mending DNA breakdown products. It is seventeen times more powerful than pycnogenol and fifty times more powerful than vitamin E. It is the carotenoid that gives salmon its orange color.

DAIRY

9. **Broccoli:** This vegetable contains sulfur compounds that assist in detoxifying the body. It is a major source of cancer-preventing compounds, such as sulforaphane and indole-3-carbinol. Steamed with fresh garlic and olive oil, broccoli is a heart saver.

10. **Almonds:** Great monounsaturated fat containing precious gamma-tocopherol, a vital nutrient that neutralizes the perioxynitrite radical, a dangerous free radical that causes destruction to cellular endothelial membranes.

11. **Seaweed:** This contains all fifty-six minerals and especially natural iodine, which are needed for the thyroid gland. Magnesium, chlorophyll, and alginates are also vital for optimum health.

12. **Garlic:** Whole baked garlic cloves not only help blood pressure and cholesterol, but help detoxify the body from heavy metals, especially mercury and cadmium. Garlic was used during World War II as Russian penicillin, as it also neutralizes dozens of bacteria, viruses, and fungi. It is a perfect nutraceutical.

CHAPTER 8

MEAT, POULTRY, AND EGGS

Sorting through the terminology of the local natural food store can be a minefield. Let's see whether we can make sense of the labels.

First there's "natural." You can completely forget about this term, which has no legal meaning or definition. It is used randomly by food manufacturers for marketing purposes, and it means absolutely nothing. There are plenty of things that are natural that I wouldn't want to put in my body—for example, gasoline and poison mushrooms. When you see "natural" or "all-natural" on a food product, just roll your eyes and know it's meaningless.

Organic, on the other hand, has a real, legal definition. The U.S. Department of Agriculture put into place a set of national standards that must be met in order for a food to be labeled "organic." Those standards apply whether the food was grown in the United States or imported from other countries. Organic food is now defined as follows:

Organic food is produced by farmers who emphasize the use of renewable resources and the conservation of soil and water to enhance environmental quality for future generations. Organic meat, poultry, eggs, and dairy products come from animals that are given no antibiotics or growth hormones. Organic food is produced without using most conventional pesticides; fertilizers made with synthetic ingredients or sewage sludge; bioengineering; or ionizing radiation. Before a product can be labeled "organic," a government-approved certifier inspects the farm where the food is grown to make sure the farmer is following all the rules necessary to meet USDA organic standards. Companies that handle or process organic food before it gets to your local supermarket or restaurant must be certified, too.

One of the most significant things to know is what organic food is not—it's not GMO. Any food that is legally labeled "organic" cannot be genetically modified. That's important because the organic label is often the only way you can be sure you're not buying GMO foods. Unless it's labeled organic, it's a good bet that the corn and soy you're buying—and the products made from them—are GMO.

Even the word "organic" has been dumbed down and diluted. After all, you can now get some version of organic crispy choco-nutty cereal, and my local health food store is filled with organic soda. More specifically, when it comes to meat and poultry, what does organic really mean? Clearly, from the definition, it means the animals were given no antibiotics or growth hormones, and that's a great thing! But is it enough? And how does the term "organic" dovetail with other catchphrases such as "free range," "cage-free," and, in the case of meat, "grass fed"? Which of these terms really matters, and which should we be paying attention to?

Glad you asked.

Some Organic Meat Still Comes from Grain-Fed Cows

I'm glad there are standards for organic food. I buy organic food whenever possible, although I'm quite aware that the term is sometimes used in questionable circumstances. (Organic chocolate cereal, I'm talking to you!) I'm glad that organic meat is now available, and I'm glad that when we buy it, we're not getting a nice additional dose of hormones, steroids, and antibiotics with our protein. But is that enough to guarantee a healthy product? I don't think so.

Why? Because the inescapable fact is this: Cows aren't meant to eat grain. It's just not their natural diet. You can make them eat it, just like you can make lions eat Cheerios, but it's not what they normally eat, and they won't do real well on it.

The meat and milk that comes from cows that primarily spend their lives being fattened up on grain at CAFOs (confined animal feeding operations, or factory farms) is simply not the same meat or milk that comes from their pasture-fed, grass-grazing brethren. The fat content is different, the nutrients are different, and except for the protein, it's just not the same food. Though I suppose eating a steak that comes from a cow that was fed organic grain is marginally better than eating a steak that comes from a cow that was fed nonorganic grain, eating a steak that comes from a cow that ate grass beats both of those options by a longshot.

Grass-Fed Meat Always Wins

Organic meat may be free of unwanted chemicals, but it is nutritionally inferior to grass-fed meat. When a ruminant is taken off pasture and fattened on grain, it loses a number of valuable nutrients. For example, compared with grass-fed meat, grain-fed meat has only one-quarter as much vitamin E, one-eighth as much beta-carotene, and one-third as many omega-3 fatty acids. It doesn't matter whether the animal is fed ordinary grain, genetically modified grain, or organic grain. Feeding large amounts of any type of grain to a grazing animal will have this effect simply because grain has fewer of these nutrients than fresh pasture. Grain-fed animals also produce far more of the proinflammatory omega-6s and far less of the anti-inflammatory omega-3s. The balance between these two types of fats is essential to human health. We get far too many omega-6s and far too few omega-3s. The fat in grass-fed animals is much closer to a healthy balance. The fat in grain-fed animals makes the situation worse.

Compared with grass-fed products, organic grain–fed products are also relatively deficient in a cancer-fighting fat called CLA—conjugated linoleic acid. CLA has been widely studied for its anticancer and tumor-fighting ability, as well as for its ability to reduce the accumulation of abdominal fat. (CLA supplements are among the most popular weight control supplements on the market.) When you feed a ruminant grain—even as little as 2 pounds (907 g) a day—its production of CLA plummets. CLA may be one of the most potent cancer-fighting substances in our diet. In animal studies, as little as 0.5 of 1 percent CLA in the diet has reduced tumor burden by more than 50 percent.

Now that we've talked about cows, let's move on to the chickens and the eggs. Free range? Omega-3? Let's take a look.

The Advantages of Organic, Free-Range Chicken and Eggs

I've always bought free-range chickens and the eggs that come from them. The advantages are enormous. Just like the natural diet of humans is that which we can hunt, fish, gather, or pluck, the natural diet of farm animals is what they can graze or forage for (insects, worms, wild plants, and grass). This diet guarantees a healthful ratio of omega-6 to omega-3 fats—which according to much research, is one of the most important dietary metrics. An exclusive diet of grain is no more the natural diet of chickens than it is of cows—or humans, for that matter.

Theoretically, free-range chickens are allowed to run around and forage and eat their natural diet (which means pecking at worms and insects and incorporating all those good omega-3s into their system as a result). Because they get exercise, they're not as fat. Because their quality of life is theoretically better than what it would be if they were confined to tiny, dark cubicles in close quarters for all of their natural life, it's reasonable to assume that they're healthier. Organic, free-range chickens are theoretically less likely to be filled with the growth hormones and antibiotics that the poultry industry routinely uses on factory-farmed animals. And if you're one of those bleeding hearts—like me—who actually cares about the welfare of animals, it's easier to make peace

with eating animals that have had reasonably healthy, happy lives and quick and painless deaths.

The operative term here is "theoretically."

Can We Trust the Term "Free Range"?

In a word, no. Or at least, not always.

There's been quite a controversy as to exactly how free range free-range chickens really are. Birds raised for meat ("broilers") may be considered "free range" if they have USDA-certified access to the outdoors. Note the word "access." According to Michael Pollan's fascinating book *The Omnivore's Dilemma* (which should be required reading for anyone interested in where his or her food comes from), free range is an option few chickens actually choose. "Since the food and water and flock remain inside the shed," he writes, "and since the little doors remain shut until the birds are at least five weeks old and well settled in their habits, the chickens apparently see no reason to venture out into what must seem to them an unfamiliar and terrifying world. Since the birds are slaughtered at seven weeks, free range turns out to be not so much a lifestyle for these chickens as a two-week vacation option."

Today's "free-range" chicken has little in common with the chickens I saw on the small sustainable farms I visited as a kid where chickens ran around pecking at stuff to their hearts' content and produced delicious eggs and meat that were relatively toxin-free. According to *The Washington Post Magazine* in 1995, the term "doesn't really tell you anything about the (animal's) . . . quality of life, nor does it even assure that the animal actually goes outdoors." Richard Lobb, spokesperson for the National Chicken Council, admitted, "Even in a free-range type of style of production, you're basically going to find most of them inside the facility."

No Guarantees with Organic, Just the Possibility of Something Better

So why do I continue to buy and recommend organic meats (hopefully grass fed) and free-range organic chickens? One word: hope. I continue to hope against mounting evidence that companies held to a standard of organic will produce chickens, meats, and eggs that are at least marginally better than the chickens, meats, and eggs that come from companies that maintain unspeakably horrible factory-farm conditions. I realize this may not be true.

Organic" doesn't guarantee much when it comes to animal products—certainly not the quality of life I like to imagine it does. I'm hoping to get something better by buying organic meats and poultries, or eggs that have been "omega-3 enriched," or eggs from chickens that have been fed organic feed whose manufacturers at least made a stab at trying to reproduce the nutrients found in the chicken's natural diet. If I had access to a small sustainable local farm, believe me, I'd just get my stuff there.

Now what if, like most people, you don't have access to organic and free range? What if you can't afford it, or even find it? What if you're on a budget? What if you're a single mom with two kids who's not inclined to go shop at the natural organic supermarket far from your home and pay considerably more for marginally better stuff? Should you never eat chicken or eggs that are conventionally farmed or produced?

Free-Range, Organic Chicken or None at All?

So what do you do when the only choices are to eat factory-farmed or nothing? It's a tough call. Chicken, for example, is still an important source of protein, and eggs are still arguably the most complete and perfect food on the planet (or one of them). So we do the best with what we have. The message here is this: Changing the way our food is produced and delivered to us is going to take a superhuman effort on the part of an awful lot of people over a very long period of time. And it's going to be about more than just slapping the term "organic" or "free range" on something and then watching the food companies do everything they can to comply with the letter—rather than the spirit—of the regulations.

I think the effort is worth it.

Meanwhile, we have to eat.

The Smart Fat Compromise

When Steven Masley, M.D., and I published our book, *Smart Fat: Eat More Fat, Lose More Weight, Get Healthy Now*, we came up with a compromise about meat and fat that's worth mentioning here.

We believe that all factory-farmed meat is a toxic waste dump of chemicals, most of which live in the fat of the meat, and we could never recommend eating fat from factory-farmed meat (or non–free range, nonorganic chickens, eggs, milk, etc.) But when factory-farmed is the only kind of meat available, we recommended one of two things: choose the vegetarian main course, or eat the meat and cut away all the fat. I normally never recommend "lean" anything—I'm a big fan of fat. But I'm certainly not a big fan of toxic fat. If you're eating grass-fed meat or organic/free-range chickens, then I say "bring it on!" (I never order the lean meat when I'm buying grass-fed at my local farmer's market.)

But when it comes to ordinary, factory-farmed meat, that's when it's time to cut the fat away and go as lean as you can go.

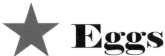 # Eggs

I can't say enough good things about eggs. They're nature's most perfect food. Eggs are plentiful, inexpensive, easy to prepare in a zillion different ways, and loaded with vitamins. They're also one of the best sources of protein on the planet. On three of the four scientific scales for protein quality used in the past few decades—Protein Efficiency Rating, Biological Value, and Net Protein Utilization—eggs consistently score highest in the quality of their protein, soundly beating milk, beef, whey, and soy. (All are tied with a perfect score of 1.00 on the fourth, the Protein Digestibility Corrected Amino Acid Score.)

Why Egg Yolks Are Actually Good for You

So what's so great about eggs? Well, besides the aforementioned fact that they're a perfect source of protein, containing all nine essential amino acids, they're also loaded with vitamins and nutrients that help your eyes, your brain, and your heart. They're one of the best sources of choline, which, though it's not a vitamin, is an essential nutrient that must be consumed in the diet to maintain good health. Choline is essential for cardiovascular and brain function and for the health of your cell membranes. It's an essential part of a phospholipid called phosphatidylcholine; the popular supplement lecithin is about 10 to 20 percent phosphatidylcholine. Without adequate phosphatidylcholine, both fat and cholesterol accumulate in the liver.

Have you picked up on the paradox yet? People avoid egg yolks because they're afraid of the cholesterol, but the choline in the egg yolk actually helps prevent the accumulation of cholesterol and fat in the liver! Egg yolks and beef liver are two of the richest dietary sources of phosphatidylcholine. One large egg provides 300 mcg of choline all in the yolk—and it also contains 315 mg of phosphatidylcholine.

There's more to the choline story. Choline forms a metabolite in the body called betaine, which helps lower homocysteine, a risk factor for heart disease. And phosphatidylcholine is one of the most liver-friendly nutrients on the planet. In Europe, phosphatidylcholine is used to treat liver disease, and many nutritionists recommend it as part of a liver support program. Most liver metabolism occurs on cell membranes, and phosphatidylcholine is the universal building block for cell membranes. Phosphatidylcholine helps protect the liver from a wide range of toxic influences. And choline is also needed for the synthesis of acetylcholine, one of the major neurotransmitters in the body. Acetylcholine is critical for memory and thought. According to the *Physicians' Desk Reference*, adequate acetylcholine levels in the brain are believed to be protective against certain types of dementia, including Alzheimer's disease. So eggs—like fish—are truly brain food!

Eggs for Healthy Eyes

Eggs are also eye food. Eggs contain lutein and zeaxanthin, two of the new superstar nutrients when it comes to eye health. Lutein, present in the macula of the eye's retina, appears to filter harmful, high-energy blue wavelengths of visible light from both natural sunlight and indoor light. Michael Geiger, O.D., a New York optometrist and author of *Eye Care Naturally*, says that lutein and zeaxanthin have been found to be among the most effective supplements for eye health. That's true—but according to research in the *Journal of Nutrition*, lutein bioavailability is even higher from eggs than it is from supplements.

Carotenoids are always better absorbed with some fat, and lutein is a carotenoid—hence, the lutein in egg yolks (which already have some fat) is more bioavailable than the lutein in spinach (which has none, unless you add it). If you're interested in getting the most bang for your buck in terms of eye health, eat eggs and spinach together—you'll get the maximum amount of these nutrients from two potent sources, and the fat from the egg yolks will help you absorb them. Lutein and zeaxanthin are always found together in nature and are generally measured as a unit—one jumbo egg has 215 mcg.

Eggs May Protect Against Breast Cancer

Eating eggs was one of two major dietary patterns found in one study to be protective against breast cancer. A study in *Cancer Epidemiology Biomarkers and Prevention* looked at the difference in breast cancer incidence in Chinese women as they migrate from China to Hong Kong to the United States. Guess what happens? Their incidence of breast cancer more than doubles.

In this study, the researchers looked at changes in diet and discovered two significant patterns: The women eating the most fruits and vegetables were significantly less likely to have breast cancer. No surprise there. But—get this—the women eating the most eggs were also least likely to have breast cancer: Eating six eggs per week vs. two eggs per week lowered their risk of breast cancer by 44 percent.

In addition to the high-quality protein, the lutein and zeaxanthin, the choline and phosphatidylcholine, eggs also contain trace amounts of more than fifteen vitamins and minerals; one jumbo egg contains 18 percent of the Daily Value for riboflavin (vitamin B_2), 14 percent of the Daily Value for vitamin B_{12}, and 29 percent of the Daily Value for the important cancer-fighting trace mineral selenium. Not only that, eggs make you look good! Their high sulfur content promotes healthy hair and nails. Many people report finding their hair growing faster after adding eggs to their diet, especially if they were previous deficient in foods containing sulfur—or vitamin B_{12}.

What about Omega-3 Enriched Eggs?

Recently, there has been an influx in the supermarkets of omega-3 enriched eggs (for more on that, see my introductory essay on meat and poultry, page 209). Chickens that roam free produce eggs that are higher in omega-3 fats, and some companies are offering eggs that have been omega-3 enriched. If you can find these omega-3 eggs, by all means get them.

Full disclosure: I frequently eat my eggs raw. I throw them in a smoothie (à la Rocky!) or I add them whole to vegetable juice and drink them down. Before you gasp, understand that eggs from healthy chickens are rarely contaminated with Salmonella. In fact, according to a study by the USDA, published in the 2002 *Risk Analysis* only .03 percent of the 69 billion eggs produced annually are contaminated at all. According to my friend Joe Mercola, D.O., if you are obtaining high-quality, cage-free, organically fed, omega-3-enhanced chicken eggs, the risk virtually dis-

appears. Salmonella only comes from sick birds, and the risk of sickness decreases when animals aren't kept in dark, crowded, sickening conditions.

You may have noticed that many of the experts who contributed top ten lists to this book mentioned eggs but noted a specific way of cooking them. That's because the less you scramble or expose the yolk to oxygen, the less the cholesterol gets oxidized. For health athletes—those looking for the absolute best, healthiest way to do everything—minimizing oxygen exposure is probably a good idea. Poaching is one way to minimize oxidation; boiling is another; and of course, so is eating them raw (though I imagine I'm not going to win many converts over to that method). Personally, I take a middle ground. I make scrambled eggs all the time, but I eat them as soon as they come out of the pan, minimizing the time they spend sitting around in the air. On the other hand, I rarely eat scrambled eggs from an open hot buffet where they've been sitting out exposed to air for hours—and you shouldn't either. As always, fresh is better.

WORTH KNOWING

One more thing. Do me a favor. Stop with the egg whites already. If I see one more healthy, robust, well-muscled, athletic young person ordering an egg-white omelet for breakfast, I'll scream. Listen carefully: The egg yolk is good for you! It's part of the package. Still worried about cholesterol? According to the *Harvard Medical School Guide to Healthy Eating*, "No research has ever shown that people who eat more eggs have more heart attacks than people who eat few eggs."

Free-Range Poultry

(chicken and turkey)

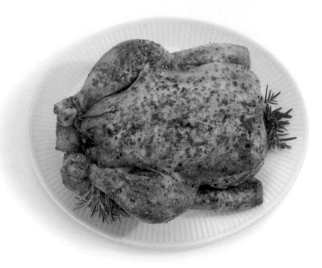

Chicken is a great source of protein, and it has an awful lot of other nutrients in it as well. Plus you can make one of the world's healthiest prepared foods out of it: chicken soup.

Now, obviously, I'm not talking chicken "nuggets" of indeterminate composition. I'm talking the real bird. I prefer free range and organic, but everything I'm about to say about chicken and turkey applies to the plain, old-fashioned, grocery store kind as well.

Four ounces (115 g) of skinless, boneless chicken breast has almost 35 g of high-quality protein as well as small amounts of calcium, magnesium, zinc, and iron. Those 4 ounces also contain 255 mg of phosphorus and 287 mg of heart-healthy potassium. One large (6-ounce [168 g]) chicken breast contains more potassium than there is in a medium banana, plus a whopping 53 g of protein. Skinless dark meat contains somewhat more calories and fat; add the skin and you're talking seriously more fat and calories. Nutritionally, turkey is fairly similar.

Chicken (but not turkey) is also an excellent source of niacin, a B vitamin that's important in energy metabolism and in biochemical functions needed to maintain healthy skin and a properly functioning gastrointestinal tract and nervous system. It's also involved in the metabolism of fats. Four ounces (115 g) of chicken provides three-quarters of the RDI for niacin.

Light vs. Dark Meat

The fat in boneless, skinless chicken is mostly mono-unsaturated. There's about 4 g of fat per 4 ounces (115 g) of boneless, skinless chicken breast, and only 1.1 g of that is saturated fat. The rest is mostly mono-unsaturated, with a smattering of polyunsaturates in the mix. Light-meat turkey has even less fat than chicken breast, but the dark meat has about the same, with a marginally higher percentage of saturated fat.

Then there's selenium. I consider selenium—a trace mineral—one of the single most important nutrients in the human diet. First, selenium is a powerful antioxidant. Second, epidemiological data indicate clearly that low dietary intake of selenium is associated with increased incidence of several cancers, including lung, colorectal, skin, and prostate cancers. And there are in vitro animal and human data showing that supplemental selenium can protect against some cancers. There's a lot of interest now focusing on these findings, given gathering evidence that selenium intakes may be declining in some parts of the world, including some areas of the United States, the United Kingdom, and other European countries.

I believe most people would be a lot healthier if they consumed at least 200 mcg of selenium daily. (The current RDI for selenium is 70 mcg.) Four ounces (115 g) of chicken breast provides 30 mcg, and one large breast contains 47 mcg, making chicken an excellent source of this cancer-fighting mineral. Turkey has even more: 36 mcg for 4 ounces (115 g) of light meat, 45 mcg for 4 ounces of dark meat. (The dark meat of turkey also has more zinc than the light meat.)

Where the Vegans Have It Wrong

Speaking of protein, I'm always amused by the vegan propaganda about how animal protein causes bone loss and osteoporosis. Actually, the opposite is true.

The Framingham Osteoporosis Study investigated protein consumption over a four-year period among 615 elderly men and women with an average age of 75. The amount of protein eaten daily ranged from as low as 14 g a day to as high as 175 g. Those who consumed more protein had less bone loss, and those who consumed less protein had more bone loss, both at the femoral bone and at the spine. The study also found that "higher intake of animal protein does not appear to affect the skeleton adversely."

Calcium is better absorbed on a higher-protein diet, even if there is somewhat more urinary calcium excretion. High-protein diets in two studies resulted in significantly more calcium absorption than the low-protein diets they were compared to. And a study in *Obesity Research* compared a low-protein diet to a high-protein diet to determine whether the protein content of the diet impacted bone mineral density. It did. The folks in the low-protein group had greater bone mineral loss.

Because of the toxins, antibiotics, steroids, pesticides, and growth hormones used in factory farming, I'm reluctant to recommend unlimited amounts of nonorganic meat and poultry. But let's not kid ourselves—protein is a critical part of a healthy diet. Of course, we should try to get it from the healthiest sources we can (which definitely doesn't include fast-food restaurants).

While it's certainly possible to be healthy on a vegetarian diet, it takes more planning than you might imagine. And many people—perhaps not all, but many—just do better with some animal products in their diet. It's been that way since the beginning of the human genus, and until our digestive fuel tanks"undergo significant genetic alteration, I suspect it will remain that way.

WORTH KNOWING

Urban legend department: Everyone thinks that the reason we get tired and fall asleep after Thanksgiving dinner is because of the tryptophan (an amino acid) in turkey. Nope. Four ounces (115 g) of turkey has less than half a gram of tryptophan. We get sleepy after Thanksgiving dinner because we eat too damn much; we zone out while all the blood leaves our head to go down to the digestive tract, where it has a ton of work to do. It has nothing to do with tryptophan.

Grass-fed Beef

Beef is beef and carrots are carrots, right?

Wrong, grasshopper.

Whether your food is animal, vegetable, plant, fish, or fruit, where a food comes from, how it's raised (or grown), what it ate (or was fed), what soil it was grown on (or grazed on), how it is processed, prepared, and cooked (or not cooked) is vitally important to its nutritional content an absolutely central to its effect on your health.

Which brings us to beef.

The natural diet of cattle is grass. It is absolutely not grain. Yet most of the beef that comes to us via traditional routes has been eating nothing but grain. When a ruminant like a cow is taken off its natural diet of pasture and fattened on grain, it loses nutrients. According to one reputable source, grain-fed meat has only one-quarter as much vitamin E, one-eighth as much beta-carotene, and, probably most important, one-third as many omega-3 fatty acids. (This makes sense—grain has far fewer of these nutrients than fresh pasture!)

Grass-fed Beef Ranks Higher in All Nutritional Categories

The fat content of grass-fed beef is different from that of grain-fed beef because the diet of the animals significantly alters their fatty acid composition. Cattle that are primarily fed grass enhance their omega-3 content by 60 percent. A large amount of research indicates that omega-3 fatty acids reduce inflammation and help prevent certain chronic diseases such as heart disease. The ratio of omega-6 fatty acids to omega-3 fatty acids in our diet is of enormous importance to our health. The wrong balance of these fatty acids (a high omega-6 to omega-3 ratio) contributes to the development of disease, while a proper balance helps maintain and even improves health.

Our Paleolithic ancestors consumed a ratio of roughly 1:1 omega-6 to omega-3, which is believed to be optimal. Research by Artemis Simopoulos, M.D., published in the *World Review of Nutrition and Dietetics* (volume 100) suggests that the present

Western diet ranges from 15:1 to an astonishing 20:1 ratio in favor of the proinflammatory omega-6s. No wonder we're experiencing an epidemic of inflammatory-related illnesses! The fat of grass-fed beef has a much more favorable omega-6 to omega-3 ratio than the fat of grain-fed cows.

And the benefits don't stop with higher omega-3s. Ruminants such as cows produce another very important fat called CLA (conjugated linoleic acid), which has long been investigated for its anticancer activity as well as for its ability to reduce fat accumulation, particularly around the abdomen. The antiatherosclerotic activity of CLA was first reported in 1994, and evidence for its health-promoting properties has continued to grow since then. CLA comes mainly from the meat and milk of ruminants (cows). Problem is, grain-fed cattle don't make nearly as much CLA as their grass-fed cousins do. At least four studies have shown that grass-fed ruminant species produce two to three times more CLA than ruminants fed in confinement on grain diets.

Grass-fed Farmers Organic "in Spirit"

A final reason to choose grass-fed meat is that most grass farmers avoid the use of many of the chemicals, hormones, and antibiotics that we'd like to keep out of our food. They might not always be striving to reach the organic certification: they often use nitrogen fertilizers on their fields or may treat their animals with relatively benign medications. Nonetheless, they generally conform to the spirit of organic (see my essay on page 209). And feeding a cow "organic" grain means nothing as far as I'm concerned, except that he was fed a less-contaminated version of a food he shouldn't be eating in the first place. Given a choice between organic and grass fed, I'll go with grass fed every time. Of course if I can get both, I'll take them.

Though the nutrient composition of beef depends somewhat on the cut of the meat, all beef is a great source of protein, a good source of B vitamins—especially vitamin B_{12}—and a good source of heme iron, the most absorbable form of iron you can get from food. About half of the fat in beef is heart-healthy monounsaturated fat. Beef is also high in zinc, with almost any kind of 3-ounce portion providing more than half the Daily Value for this important nutrient.

If you're interested in learning more about grass farming and its benefits to your health, a great place to start is www.eatwild.com. Another good source is the Weston A. Price Foundation (www.westonaprice.org). I also highly recommend the excellent book by Michael Pollan, *The Omnivore's Dilemma.*

WORTH KNOWING

The original energy bar was a food called pemmican, which was developed by the Indians and other indigenous cultures like the Inuit in Greenland. It's a high-energy food that can be transported easily and lasts for many months. Meat from buffalo—or occasionally moose and caribou—was dried, then pounded into a fine texture and mixed with animal fat and sometimes berries. This created a high-calorie, highly nutritious food for traveling. The meat was all wild game and by definition pasture fed, and it was as healthy as the day is long. I eat pemmican as a snack all the time. You can get it from the same place I get it—U.S. Wellness Meats, which only uses grass-fed animals. There's a link to U.S. Wellness Meats on www.jonnybowden.com.

Lamb

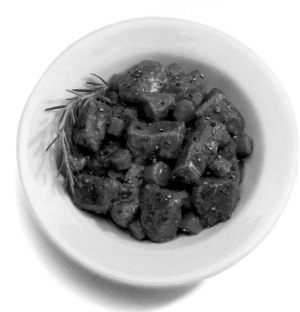

For a meat eater, lamb has a lot to recommend it. For one thing, almost all lamb is grass fed. In parts of the United States, lambs that don't make it to sufficient weight to be marketed may be fattened up on grain; this also happens in other countries when there are adverse conditions such as a drought. But grass is the natural diet of cattle and sheep, and the meat of animals that are grass fed has a higher amount of omega-3 fatty acids, not to mention the absence of hormones, steroids, and antibiotics. Meat from a grass-fed animal, organically and humanely raised on its natural diet, is far superior to its grain-fed, factory-farmed brethren.

For another thing, growth hormones are not used on sheep. (Lambs are sheep that are less than one year old.) And if you purchase organic lamb—highly recommended—you are buying meat from animals that are not dipped, sprayed, or dermally dosed with insecticides, and they are the closest to the kind of animals our Paleolithic ancestors hunted. Problem is, the simple term "organic" doesn't really guarantee all that much. According to The Natural Food Hub (www.naturalhub.com), the closest we can come to ideal is what might be called "certified organic meat," which implies not only avoiding medicines and insecticides, but also extends to a philosophy that prohibits the use of artificial fertilizers on the pasture.

The cut of lamb and the tenderness of the meat are the best indicators of fat content. Lamb has fewer retail cuts than beef. In general, leaner cuts—the foreshank and parts of the leg—are less tender than cuts from areas where the muscles are not used as much, such as the loin and rib. But even leaner cuts of lamb tend to be more tender than similar cuts of beef.

Lamb Is Low in Calories and High in Protein

Lamb is not a high-calorie food, and it's loaded with protein. One 4-ounce (115 g) portion of fresh, lean loin, trimmed to ⅛-inch fat, cooked, is only 217 calories. For that you get about 30 g of high-quality protein, plus some calcium, magnesium, phosphorus, selenium, almost 50 percent of the RDI for niacin, and 90 percent of the amount of potassium in a banana! Less than half of the 9 or so g of fat in that 4-ounce (115 g) portion of meat is saturated fat; most of the rest is heart-healthy monounsaturated fat and the remainder is polyunsaturated.

That 4-ounce (115 g) portion of lamb also

contains 25 percent of the RDI for zinc and more than one-third of the RDI for vitamin B12. Zinc is an essential mineral that is found in almost every cell and stimulates the activity of approximately 100 enzymes, substances that promote biochemical reactions in your body. It's essential for a healthy immune system, which is adversely affected by even moderate degrees of zinc deficiency. (Men take note: Zinc is needed for the production of healthy sperm, which may be one indirect reason why high-zinc oysters got their reputation as an aphrodisiac!) Vitamin B12 is necessary to bring down homocysteine, a nasty metabolic compound that puts you at risk for heart disease and memory impairment. Vitamin B12 is most absorbable from animal foods; vegetarians—despite what they tell you—are most at risk for deficiency.

Although lamb is the principal meat in parts of Europe, North Africa, the Middle East, and India, it is much less popular in the United States. On average, we consume a pound (455 g) of lamb per person annually, a fraction of our beef consumption. By contrast, in New Zealand, the per capita consumption of lamb and goat averages more than 60 pounds (27 kg) a year.

Liver (calf's liver)

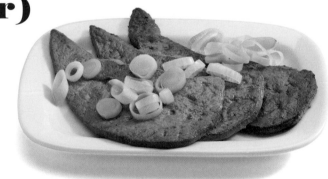

Some cultures place such a high value on liver that human hands are not allowed to touch it; rather, special sticks are used to move it. The Li-Chi, a handbook of rituals published during China's Han era (202 B.C.E. to 220 C.E.) lists liver as one of the Eight Delicacies. I realize that might be a hard concept to sell to your liver-hating teenager. But liver is a great food. Gram for gram, it contains more nutrients than any other food!

Go through any college nutrition text and look up the best food sources for practically every B vitamin and you'll see liver at the top of almost every list. A small 3-ounce (85 g) serving of braised liver provides all the Daily Value for vitamin A (preformed), riboflavin, copper, and vitamin B12. It also contains 93 percent of selenium, a valuable trace mineral that's one of the most powerful cancer-fighting nutrients on the planet. That same 3 ounces (85 g) also has 55 percent of the Daily Value for zinc, 50 percent of niacin, a surprising

50 percent of folate (which is usually associated with vegetables and fortified foods), 40 percent of thiamin and B₆, and about a third of the RDI for iron. For goodness' sake, it even has some vitamin C! And, of course, liver is a superb source of protein.

Remember, though, that the liver of any animal—including humans—is ground zero for detoxification. So, when you're dealing with animals that have been raised on feedlot farms and fed all kinds of things they shouldn't be eating (such as grain) and shot full of all kinds of things they shouldn't be shot full of (hormones, antibiotics), all that stuff is going to wind up in their livers. That's why it's especially important to only eat liver from grass-fed animals.

When it comes to liver, I recommend organic and/or pasture raised to reduce the risk of contaminants. If that's not an option, then I recommend only young animal liver. If supermarket, factory-farmed liver is your only option, choose calf's liver, because U.S. beef cattle spend their first months on pasture.

Now let's talk for a minute about the common advice to avoid liver while pregnant because of its vitamin A content.

Should Pregnant Women Avoid Vitamin A?

There were some very early studies on mice that showed that vitamin A was associated with fetal abnormalities, and based on this, women have been advised for years that large doses of vitamin A could be toxic, especially to their unborn child. And just in case they're right, no one who's pregnant is going to take a chance. I don't blame them. But I think the warnings against vitamin A are vastly overblown.

Re-examining the Study

Why do I believe the dangers of vitamin A have been overstated? Several reasons. One, I went back and read the original mice studies. The amount of vitamin A given to the rodents was so huge that when my assistant and I tried to translate it into IUs (the units in which we commonly measure vitamin A), we simply couldn't do it—the number of zeros was greater than the calculator could work with. Many of these studies used intravenous injections of synthetic vitamin A in massive quantities. No one—repeat, no one—consumes that amount of vitamin A, ever.

Second, the natural vitamin A found in liver does not seem to cause the same toxicity problems that synthetic vitamin A does. In fact, the amount of vitamin A in one slice of liver is a little less than that in two carrots, for goodness' sake. Third, a study carried out in Rome (published in *Teratology*, January 1999) found no congenital malformations among 120 infants exposed to more than 50,000 IUs of vitamin A per day. Fourth, a study from Switzerland published in the *International Journal of Vitamin and Nutrition Research* in 1998 looked at blood levels of vitamin A in pregnant women and found that a daily dose of 30,000 IUs resulted in blood levels that had no association with birth defects. (One slice of liver has about 21,000 IUs; a carrot has 12,000.)

Interestingly, textbooks on nutrition written before World War II recommended that pregnant women eat liver frequently. I personally use high-dose vitamin A (50,000 IUs) every time I feel a cold coming on, and so do a dozen nutritionists I know. Point is that the amount of vitamin A in calf's liver—substantially less than we're talking about here—poses no risk to anyone. But that's just my opinion. If you're pregnant, you should of course check with your health professional about your diet and supplements—but please make sure the reasoning for avoiding liver isn't based on old prejudices.

Wild Game
(buffalo, venison, elk, bison)

Everything said so far regarding grass-fed, pasture-raised beef applies to wild game as well. Humans are genetically adapted to eat what our Paleolithic (Old Stone Age) ancestors, the hunter-gatherers, ate. And that was quite simply this: food you could hunt, fish, gather, or pluck. According to Loren Cordain, professor of health and exercise science at Colorado State University and author of the excellent book *The Paleo Diet*, "Just 500 generations ago—and for 2.5 million years before that—every human on Earth ate this way. It is the diet to which all of us are ideally suited, and the lifetime nutritional plan that will normalize your weight and improve your health."

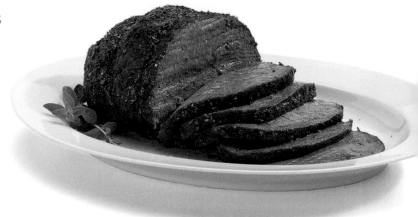

Believe it or not, our Paleolithic ancestors were lean, fit, and free from heart disease, diabetes, and other health issues that are plaguing Western countries. Did they die earlier than we do? Sure. But probably more from the harsh elements and the dangers of wooly mammoths. Is our life span longer? Absolutely. And that's probably due as much to reduced infant mortality, protection from the elements, and the ability of modern medicine to keep us alive longer.

Meanwhile, compare our ancestral diet to our modern diet and then look at the laundry list of degenerative diseases that now plague modern man and modern woman, yet were virtually unknown as recently as a couple of hundred years ago. The point is, if you want a blueprint for what fuel mix the human digestive system was designed to work best on, you need look no further than the basic food source that nourished the human genus for a couple of million years. And that food source was a mix of what we could hunt—wild game—and what we could gather—natural foods such as roots, berries, nuts, wild vegetables, and fruits.

Wild Game Can Help Lower the Risk of Heart Disease

So, what did Paleolithic man actually eat? Wild

animal foods dominated their diets, and these foods provide a higher proportion of good fats compared to other types of commercial meat. That included, by the way, some saturated fat as well! Meat from grass-fed animals has two to four times more omega-3 fatty acids than meat from grain-fed animals.

Wild game is a good source of protein and contains large quantities of B vitamins, including B12, and absorbable heme iron. It also provides potassium (which helps the body's cells work properly) and phosphorus (essential for healthy bones and teeth), zinc, and the valuable, cancer-fighting trace mineral selenium (3 ounces [85 g] of bison or buffalo contains more than 40 percent of the Daily Value for this important mineral). With its healthy ratio of omega-3 to omega-6 fats, game can help decrease the risk of heart disease. Wild game doesn't spend time on facto-ry-style feedlot operations, and therefore is not loaded with antibiotics, steroids, growth hormones, and other toxins that are a by-product of the modern CAFO (confined animal feeding operations, or the modern factory farm).

Remember, we've been eating wild game for as long as we've been on the planet. The modern super-market food we know today—freeze-dried everything, juice concentrates, self-cooking meals, TV dinners, "cheese food," packaged snacks, high amounts of sodium, sugar, trans fats, artificial colorants, and sweeteners—came of age in the late twentieth century. Before 1961, no one ever heard of the Golden Arches. But we've eaten wild game for as long as we've been on the planet.

Do the math: Which way of eating is really more natural?

THE EXPERTS' TOP TEN LISTS

Mary Dan Eades, M.D., and Michael Eades, M.D.

Michael and **Mary Dan Eades** are great friends of mine, and two of the smartest and most committed M.D.s in the country. They are iconic low-carb advocates, and authors of the classics *Protein Power*, *The Protein Power Life Plan*, *Staying Power: Maintaining Your Low-Carb Weight Loss for Good*, and *The Low-Carb CookwoRx Cookbook*. They can be reached at www.proteinpower.com.

1. **Grass-fed beef, pork, lamb:** These are sources of good protein and quality fat, devoid of hormones, antibiotics, and toxins.

2. **Cage-free chicken and eggs:** These are humanely produced, inexpensive, and a source of high-quality protein and cholesterol.

   (Note from JB: This is not a misprint. Cholesterol from the diet helps regulate the production of cholesterol in the body; if you don't get it from the diet, you will make it. And cholesterol is the parent molecule of many important hormones.)

3. **Sardines packed in sardine oil:** Of all fish, these are the lowest in heavy metals and other toxins, while still being rich in essential fats. They are best packed in their own oil, but those packed in olive oil or water are okay, too. Avoid varieties in soybean or vegetable oil.

4. **Coconut oil:** This oil is rich in lauric acid and important for immune health, stable at high temperatures, and great for sautéing, frying, and baking.

5. **Broccoli sprouts:** No food is higher in sulforaphane than these sprouts. They are great on salads or in wraps. If you are short on these tiny powerhouses, eat cruciferous vegetables (broccoli, cauliflower, and cabbage).

6. **Spinach (and other dark-green leafies):** Spinach is packed with nutrients, especially folate, without a slug of carbs.

7. **Tomatoes:** Full of potassium and lycopene, tomatoes are so versatile you can serve them at any meal.

8. **Pomegranate:** This powerful antioxidant is delicious to boot.

9. **Celery root:** This contains all the benefits of potatoes and are used in much the same way, but without the starch load.

10. **Berries:** These are the king of fruits, chock-full of antioxidants, fiber, and flavor.

CHAPTER 9

FISH AND SEAFOOD

Given how confusing and contradictory health advice from the "experts" can frequently be, it's refreshing to find a principle upon which absolutely everyone agrees. One such principle is to eat more vegetables and fruit. Another is that seafood is one of the healthiest foods on the planet.

Fish in general is a high-protein, low-calorie food that provides a range of health benefits, but some fish are real superstars. Fish high in omega-3s that are caught or farmed in an ecologically sound manner and are low in contaminants include wild salmon from Alaska (fresh, frozen, and canned), Atlantic mackerel and herring, sardines, sablefish, anchovies, and farmed oysters.

White-fleshed fish, on the other hand, is loaded with vitamins and minerals, and it is incredibly low in calories. In addition, most fish are naturally low in the proinflammatory omega-6 fats (a possible exception being farmed salmon—see page 240). As of this writing (2017), the FDA recommends avoiding king mackerel, marlin, orange roughy, shark, swordfish, tilefish from the Gulf of Mexico, and bigeye tuna because they are the fish with the highest mercury levels.

Fish for Smarter Babies

Scientific findings presented at a conference sponsored by the governments of the United States, Norway, Canada, and Iceland, and assisted by the United Nations' Food and Agriculture Organization, supported the notion that all people—especially pregnant and nursing women and children—should eat seafood twice a week, despite concerns about pollution contamination (see "What about Mercury?" page 243). Nutrients such as omega-3 fatty acids, iodine, iron, and choline, present in fish such as wild salmon, shrimp, pollock, cod, canned light tuna, and catfish, are important to brain development; researchers have found that they may lessen the effects of dyslexia, autism, hyperactivity, and attention deficit disorder. Some studies have linked those nutrients with increased intelligence in infants and young children.

Aim for Two Servings a Week

The American Heart Association recommends that we eat at least two fish meals a week. This recommendation is also included in the USDA's dietary guidelines. The nutrients found in seafood help reduce risk of death by heart attack and prevent a host of chronic health problems and terminal illnesses. Seafood cuts the risk for heart disease, cancer, Alzheimer's, stroke, diabetes, and inflammatory diseases such as rheumatoid arthritis.

In fact, in 2016 a study in the *Journal of the American Medical Association* found that eating fish—and other seafood—even once a week may help lower the risk of Alzheimer's disease. This is despite higher levels of mercury in the brain from the fish. "This study provides evidence that the increased mercury exposure is not correlated with increased brain pathologics associated with dementia," lead researcher Martha Clare Morris, M.D., told *Life Extension* magazine.

By the way, I hope you know that when I'm waxing on and on about the virtues of fish, I'm not talking about "mystery fish nuggets deep fried in recycled vegetable oil" or some similar Frankenfood from the local fast-food emporium or food court. I'm talking the real deal. Research shows that more nutrients are retained in fish that is baked or broiled, rather than processed and/or fried. But you knew that, didn't you? And to protect against viral and germ contamination, handle uncooked seafood with care and properly cook fish or shellfish, as you would any meat or poultry.

Back in the 1980s, William Castelli, M.D., director of the famous Framingham Heart Study, said this: "I have no qualms about the American public eating three or even four meals of fish a week."

Today, that statement sounds remarkably conservative, but understandably so. We really don't know quite as much about nutrition and health as we think we do, and a lot of the time we're just making our best guesses. Consider what Dariush Mozaffarian, M.D., dean of Tufts University's Friedman School of Nutrition Science and Policy, told the *New York Times* on July 5, 2016, regarding nutrition: "Twenty years ago . . . we knew about 10 percent of what we need to know. And now we know about 40 or 50 percent."

Maybe in twenty years we'll find out that fish is really bad for you. Or maybe we'll find out that the recommendation to eat it twice a week should be doubled. No one knows, but if I were a betting man, I'd bet on the latter.

Crustacea

(crayfish, prawns, shrimp, lobster)

Crustaceans are one of two main classifications of shellfish (the other being mollusks). They're a class of arthropods which characteristically have segmented bodies. And they're very, very tasty. Enjoy.

Crayfish (also called crawfish) are freshwater cousins of the lobster, found in most parts of the world. According to the Natural History Museum of Los Angeles County, more than 70,000 different species of these crustaceans have been identified. The most biologically diverse concentration of crayfish species in the world is found in the southeast United States. You can prepare them in the same style as lobster—steamed, boiled, fried, blackened, or baked. They're a big favorite in Louisiana.

Prawns are basically really large shrimp, though there are regional differences of opinion about the distinctions. (In Europe and some Asian countries, prawns are considered large decapods with long antennae and toothed beaks, some varieties of which have slender bodies, with tails that don't curve under as much as typical shrimp tails; but in the United States they're just big shrimp.) One particularly desirable type is called the Black Tiger, a huge prawn that can grow to over a foot in length. Its name comes from the distinctive coloration of its shell: black with alternating bands of yellow. They're usually sold frozen, with most commercial supplies coming from Asian shrimp farms.

Shrimp are one of about 740,000 known species of crustacea, the only group of arthropods that is primarily marine. They're the most popular shellfish in the world, and they are probably one of the most popular varieties of seafood, period. And no wonder—they're lean, high in protein, rich in nutrients, and delicious; some might say an ideal food.

First things first: Shrimp are a great source of protein, and a low-calorie one at that. One small 3-ounce (85 g) serving has 17 g of protein and only 90 calories. Shrimp have all nine essential amino acids, plus small to moderate amounts of nine important minerals. They're relatively high in the important trace mineral selenium, with one 3-ounce serving providing 46 percent of the Daily Value for this cancer-fighting nutrient.

Then there's astaxanthin. You probably never heard of astaxanthin, but it's the main carotenoid pigment found in aquatic animals and it is responsible for giving salmon their pink color. The thing of it is, salmon get most of their astaxanthin from dining on crustaceans like shrimp—particularly krill. Why should you care? Because this red-orange pigment, closely related to other well-known carotenoids like beta-carotene and lutein, has stronger antioxidant activity than either of them (ten times higher than beta-carotene, in fact). Studies suggest that astaxanthin can be more than 100 times more effective as an antioxidant than vitamin E. And shrimp are loaded with it. In many of the aquatic animals in which it is found, astaxanthin has several essential biological functions, including protection against oxidation of essential polyunsaturated fatty acids, protection against UV light effects, pro–vitamin A activity, immune response, pigmentation, communication, and improved reproduction. In species such as salmon and shrimp, astaxanthin is considered essential to normal growth and survival and has been attributed vitaminlike properties. We're just beginning to understand its potential in human health, but there's every reason to believe it's really good for you.

Lobsters are large crustaceans. They have hard shells and ten legs, two of which have developed into pincers. Although considered a gourmet food today, lobsters were so plentiful in the nineteenth century that they were used as fish bait or even fertilizer. Lobsters have firm, rich meat in their bodies, tails, and legs. You can also eat the lobster's liver (known as green tomalley) or its roe (known as coral).

Fun fact: Lobsters migrate in autumn to calmer waters, and they do it by marching in single file on the ocean floor for a couple of days and nights! Each individual member of the convey touches the tips of its antennae to the animal in front of them.

Ounce for ounce, lobsters are somewhat similar to shrimp in nutritional value, with a few differences. Three ounces (85 g) of lobster meat has about 95 calories and delivers almost 19 g of high-quality protein, with all nine essential amino acids. It's even higher in the cancer-fighting trace mineral selenium than shrimp is (3 ounces provides 56 percent of the Daily

Value for this valuable nutrient), and in addition provides 32 percent of the Daily Value for zinc, plus small amounts of other minerals. Lobster is one of the best nonanimal sources of vitamin B12, with 3 ounces (85 g) providing 50 percent of the Daily Value for that important B vitamin.

WORTH KNOWING

Shrimp and other shellfish used to be given a bad rap for their high cholesterol content, but thankfully, that is starting to change. The last edition of the Federal Guidelines stated that cholesterol "is not a nutrient of concern," and even mainstream medicine is starting to accept the fact that dietary cholesterol—i.e. the cholesterol in shrimp, eggs, etc.—has little to do with the cholesterol in your blood.

One study, published all the way back in 1996 in the *American Journal of Clinical Nutrition*, tested a high-shrimp diet at Rockefeller University. They fed the subjects 300 g of shrimp a day. Blood cholesterol went up a bit, but HDL ("good") cholesterol went up far more than LDL ("bad") cholesterol, resulting in an improved cholesterol ratio. As an added benefit, subjects on the high-shrimp diet saw a significant lowering of their triglycerides (a significant risk factor for heart disease). Bottom line: For the majority of people, the cholesterol in shrimp and related species isn't a problem.

Note: As with mollusks, you need to be aware of the potential for allergic reaction. But it's also worth noting that seafood poisoning frequently masquerades as an allergic reaction. The take-home point: Get all your seafood from reputable sources, eat it fresh, and prepare it correctly.

Mackerel

Mackerel has long been one of the most underappreciated fish. For example, in 2006 the *New York Times* published a story by food columnist Marian Burros, placed prominently on the cover of its "Dining In" section. The headline? "Holy Mackerel And Other Guilt-Free Fish." The story—a paean to the health benefits and environmental friendliness of this terrific fish—began like this: "Like the shy kid at the dance whose charms are not readily apparent, unpopularity has kept some species (of fish) in circulation, waiting to be discovered. Atlantic mackerel wears its reputation like a pocket protector and horn-rimmed glasses, but a little attention reveals its sweet side."

Mackerel live in both the Atlantic and the Pacific. The Atlantic mackerel (also known as Boston mackerel) is preferred, and it is the variety I recommend (more on that in a moment). A relative of the tuna, the Atlantic mackerel is found in the Atlantic's cold waters, where it forms large schools and can live up to an astonishing seventeen years. Before 1870, all mackerel caught in New England waters was salted on board and sold that way in Boston. Fresh mackerel is very perishable, and it must be kept on ice or it develops a really fishy flavor.

Mackerel is a sleek, oily fish with a forked tail. It contains two kinds of meat: the red outer meat and the light inner meat. You can get it canned, whole, as fillets, and as steaks. Atlantic mackerel is often used in sashimi. Pacific jack mackerel (also called horse mackerel) is often canned. Spanish mackerel has only a small percentage of red meat and a milder taste than other kinds of mackerel. King mackerel (also called kingfish or cavalla) has a firm texture and distinct taste. Wahoo (also known as ono) is a very close relative of the king mackerel; it is a subtropical fish with a delicate flavor that is often used in sashimi. Cero mackerel (also called cerro or painted mackerel) is caught in waters along the coast of Florida; it has leaner flesh and a more delicate flavor than most varieties. Pacific mackerel (also called American, blue, or chub) is an oily fish with a strong flavor.

Mackerel Low in Environmental Contaminants

Mackerel is delicious and extremely healthy. One of the reasons why the *New York Times* article was so excited about it is that the Atlantic version was, at the time, on the list of "Best Seafood Choices" on the Oceans Alive website. Oceans Alive was a division of the Environmental Defense Fund. The Oceans Alive website is no more, but Seafood Watch—a website dedicated to healthy, sustainable choices in seafood—has ten "best choice" recommendations for mackerel.

Mackerel is high in omega-3 fatty acids, and it's also low in environmental contaminants. Atlantic mackerel come from marine fisheries, not fish farms, are primarily caught with purse seines and trawls, and have relatively low "by-catch." They can safely be eaten more than once a week. All good news.

Three ounces (85 g) of mackerel has roughly 20 g of protein and plenty of good healthy fat, though there are some slight differences. Three ounces of Pacific mackerel has 6 g of monounsaturated fat and about 1½ g of omega-3, while 3 ounces (85 g) of Atlantic mackerel contains 3 g of monounsaturated and a little more than 1 g of omega-3. But both are very good sources of the cancer-fighting trace mineral selenium, providing more than 50 percent of the Daily Value. And while Pacific mackerel has a respectable amount of vitamin B_{12} (60 percent of the Daily Value), the Atlantic variety is a B_{12} heavyweight, providing more than five times that amount.

WORTH KNOWING

Herring are like mackerel nutritionally, though they taste a lot different and are usually prepared a completely different way. However, they too are loaded with good fat, protein, and vitamin B_{12}.

Mollusks

(clams, mussels, scallops, oysters)

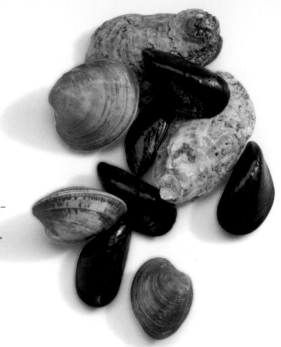

Mollusks include all the shelled creatures of the sea (except for barnacles). They form one of the largest groups in the animal kingdom, with more than 80,000 known species.

Mollusks have always been a readily available food source for humans. Mussel and oyster beds, clam flats, and other abundant shellfish reserves have traditionally provided an easy, accessible source of food, as evidenced by many of the archaeological digs that have uncovered huge middens heavy with shells. Mollusks are almost pure protein, naturally low in fat, and rich in a host of minerals, including zinc and copper.

Clams, Mussels, and Scallops

Clams are one of the richest sources of iron on the planet, containing many times the amount found in beef liver. And 3 ounces (85 g) of clams provides a whopping 700 percent of the Daily Value for vitamin B_{12}, plus 66 percent of the Daily Value for iron. A comparable 3 ounces (85 g) of oysters contains 271 percent of the Daily Value for vitamin B_{12}, and 43 percent of the cancer-fighting trace mineral selenium. And 3 ounces (85 g) of raw blue mussels provides more than 100 percent of the Daily Value for manganese, an important trace mineral that's essential for growth, reproduction, wound healing, peak brain function, and the proper metabolism of sugars, insulin, and cholesterol. Mussels also have a decent amount of selenium, providing more than 50 percent of the Daily Value. Finally, scallops, while not being a superstar in the nutrient department, are more than 80 percent protein, providing a rich 15 g per low-calorie 3-ounce serving, plus trace amounts of at least eighteen vitamins and minerals.

Oysters

Oysters are often referred to as the "milk of the ocean." They're one of nature's most concentrated packages of zinc: A 1-cup (248 g) serving of drained oysters supplies many times more than 100 percent of the Daily Value, much more than the same amount of beef liver. Adequate zinc is crucial for a strong immune system. It's also crucial for fertility and male sexual health, which might be the origin of oysters' reputation as an aphrodisiac. (Another might be the odd fact that oysters are sexually fluid—they

WORTH KNOWING

A running theme in this book has been that the source of your food—where it comes from, what it eats, where it is grown, how it is harvested—is of huge importance in determining its quality. Nowhere is this more true than in the area of fish, especially shellfish. Bacteria multiply at a phenomenal rate in dead shellfish, making them dangerous to consume. So, for example, if you're buying live oysters, make sure that they are indeed alive as advertised! Also, if they're harvested improperly or come from contaminated waters, watch out … *Vibrio vulnificus* is a bacterium that lives in warm seawater and was responsible for more than 300 infections between 1988 and 1995 in the Gulf Coast states alone, where most of the cases occurred, and it can be found in oysters and shellfish in warm coastal waters during the summer months. It's especially dangerous to immunocompromised people.

The point is not to be afraid of shellfish, but to buy it from only extremely reliable sources—restaurants and suppliers you trust—and prepare and consume it properly. Fresh shellfish from clean waters prepared and served properly is a delight and a nutritional bonanza. But be smart: As in the case with consuming other raw animal protein products, there is a risk associated with consuming raw oysters, clams, and mussels. If you suffer from chronic illness of the liver, stomach, or blood, or have immune disorders, don't eat them raw.

change sex one or more times during their life span. They always start life as males, and usually end up as females. Go figure.)

And oysters really are a brain food, helping to boost your mental energy and acting as a mood elevator. The protein in oysters is rich in the amino acid tyrosine, which your brain converts to the feel-good, energizing neurotransmitter dopamine.

Some oysters produce nacre (a combination of calcium and protein), with which they coat any irritating sand or grit that gets trapped within their shell. This substance hardens into a smooth ball . . . we know it as a pearl.

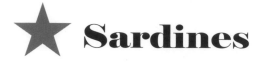 # Sardines

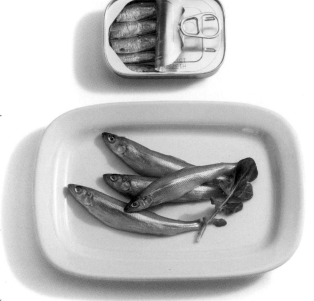

Sardines are a health food in a can.

I first discovered this way of thinking about sardines in Florida. My friend, the great New York celebrity nutritionist and author Oz Garcia, Ph.D., and I were jointly leading a seminar on nutrition for personal trainers in Miami Beach. We were driving around near the hotel looking for something remotely healthy to eat and couldn't find anything promising. Garcia, who is a Miami native, stopped the car at a local bodega and came out with two cans of sardines and a couple of plastic forks. They were delicious and filling and ever since have been on my top ten list of the healthiest and most convenient foods on the planet.

Sardines Are Full of Healthy Omega-3 Fats

Sardines are loaded with omega-3 fats. The benefits of omega-3s are legion (see a lengthier discussion in the section on salmon, page 240). Epidemiologic studies in the United States report that a mere ½ g a day of these fats can significantly decrease cardiovascular risk. (The average American gets much less.)

Omega-3s help with mood, thinking, circulation, and glucose and insulin metabolism; they lower blood pressure; and they protect against heart disease. They've been referred to by more than one health writer (including myself!) as "wellness molecules." Books have been written on their health benefits. By some estimates, sardines are as high in omega-3 fats as salmon; by other estimates, they are a close second. Either way, you can get all you need of this amazing fat from one little can of sardines.

And that's not all you'll get from one can of these innocuous fish. They are absolutely loaded with calcium—depending on the type of sardines, one can gives you 25 to 38 percent of the Daily Value. They also contain iron, magnesium, phosphorus, potassium, zinc, copper, and manganese, not to mention a full complement of B vitamins. And they are notable for being a superb nonmeat source of vitamin B_{12}: One little can provides a whopping 150 percent of the Daily Value!

Sardines are also a good source of selenium. Higher levels of this important cancer-fighting trace mineral have been found to be associated with lower rates of cancer in numerous studies. A can of sardines provides 58 to 75 percent of the Daily Value of this critical mineral.

Randy Hartnell, a descendent of three generations of Alaskan fishermen and president of Vital Choice, Inc., points out that sardines are highly sustainable "They grow without the need for arable land, fresh water, fertilizers, pesticides, veterinary drugs, artificial colors, flavors, [or] preservatives," he says. "They're among the last truly wild naturally organic foods available to us."

As far as mercury is concerned, you have a lot less to worry about with sardines than with bigger fish. Sardines are small, relatively short-lived, and feed at the bottom of the marine food web, so they don't bioaccumulate hazardous levels of contaminants such as the mercury and PCBs that are found in larger, longer-lived predatory fish.

There are three things to be aware of when buying and consuming sardines:

1. Sardine quality varies widely depending on when it was harvested, whether it was packed from fresh or previously frozen fish, and on the quality of the oil added. Few companies pack in certified extra-virgin olive oil, but some do—look for them. "You get what you pay for" generally applies.

2. Many people think they don't like sardines because they've experienced cheap, lower quality versions that taste bad and misrepresent what a delicious, incredibly healthy food they can be.

3. To minimize cost, some manufacturers will freeze sardines and ship them to low-wage countries for canning (Vietnam, Thailand, etc.), lowering the quality and increasing the "food miles" factor.

WORTH KNOWING

Get sardines packed in their own oil. They're harder to find, but worth it. Do not be afraid of the fat—it's good stuff! If you can't find them in sardine oil, olive oil is a perfectly fine substitute. Do not—repeat, do not—buy the kind that's packed in vegetable oil, which simply soaks them in proinflammatory omega-6 fats from a heavily processed oil that does nothing good for you. If you're really trying to reduce the fat for some reason, go with sardines packed in tomato sauce. Or mustard sauce. Anything but vegetable oil is fine.

One of the best places I know to buy sardines is from Vital Choice. It is also the best place I know to buy salmon and other wild fish. There was a link to Vital Choice on my website, www.jonnybowden.com, back when this book first came out, and it's still there ten years later. I've never found a better source.

Tuna

Canned tuna is the second most popular seafood product in the United States after shrimp. If other healthy foods were that popular, we'd be in good shape.

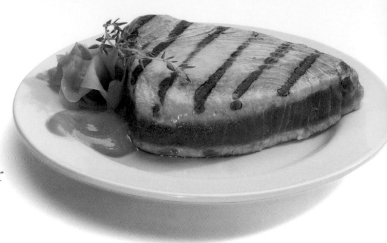

All of the good stuff about seafood applies, of course, to tuna. Although it doesn't have as many omega-3 fats as salmon or sardines do, it's still considered a fatty fish, and a serving of tuna does provide some healthy omega-3s. Here again, the source of the food is everything. The big companies with the household names cook their fish twice, first baking them on a rack, which results in a loss of a lot of the beneficial oils. Then they debone it, can it, stick in flavorings and additives, and cook it again.

Canned tuna from big commercial companies typically has fewer than ½ g of omega-3s. It's better than nothing, but you wouldn't write home about it.

Water Packed or Oil Packed: Which Is Better?

Small specialty companies, on the other hand, usually pack their fish in the can raw and cook them only once, so you're more likely to be getting the natural fats and juices. Small specialty companies are often family owned and catch their tuna in the Pacific by hook. As soon as it's hooked, it's brought aboard the boat and fresh-frozen. Big commercial companies typically fish for tuna in the Atlantic using long lines, which are harvested only once a day.

Then there's the issue of water packed versus oil packed. Many people avoid the oil packed because of a fear of fat, but the oil-packed version is more likely

to retain its omega-3s. That is, unless you drain it, which is what most people do. Then the omega-3s are likely to leak out with the oil and go down the drain. That's less likely to happen with water packed, but on the other hand there might be less omega-3s there to begin with. So, either buy the kind in oil and don't drain it, or buy the kind in water. Better yet, in my opinion, seek out the small specialty companies that produce a better-quality product (such as gourmet or premium canned Pacific tuna) in the first place.

Forty-Two Grams of Protein in Just One Can of Light Tuna

The nutrient content of tuna differs depending on the company that canned it, the type of tuna (Atlantic, Pacific, white, light), and how it's packed (water or oil). Nonetheless, all tuna is a terrific source of protein, containing large amounts of all the essential amino acids and then some. A single can of light tuna canned in water and drained provides an astonishing 42 g of high-quality protein, for less than 200 calories. That same can has more than 100 percent of the Daily Value for niacin, 29 percent of the Daily Value for vitamin B_6, and 82 percent of the Daily Value for vitamin B_{12}.

And tuna is a superb source of the vitally important cancer-protective trace mineral selenium. That water-packed can of light tuna provides almost 200 percent of the Daily Value. Even if you use one can for two portions, you're still getting almost 100 percent of the Daily Value for this vital nutrient.

Tuna steak is likely to be higher in omega-3s but may be higher in mercury as well. (For a fuller discussion of the mercury issue, see page 243.) A 3-ounce (85 g) portion of yellowfin or bluefin tuna is still a nutritional bargain at less than 150 calories and around 25 g of high-quality protein. There are slight differences, though: The yellowfin has almost no B12, while the bluefin contains more than 150 percent of the Daily Value.

All that said, whatever kind is used, tuna is still my favorite fish at a sushi restaurant.

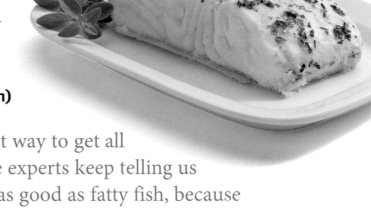

White-fleshed Fish

(cod, flounder, halibut, orange roughy, pollack, rockfish)

White-fleshed fish are a perfect way to get all the benefits of seafood that the experts keep telling us about. They may not be quite as good as fatty fish, because they're not a source of those powerful omega-3 fatty acids found in salmon, sardines, and the like, but they have plenty of other good things to recommend them. And although fatty fish have more omega-3s than lean fish, even lean fish contain some—and these healthful fatty acids are found in very few other foods.

Even white-fleshed fish are extremely rich in high-quality protein while being low in calories. One 3-ounce (85 g) portion of cod, for example, provides about 20 g of extremely high-quality protein, all for less than 100 calories. (A whole fillet is still a nutritional bargain, delivering a whopping 41 g of protein for under 200 calories.) Cod is also rich in B vitamins and minerals, especially the all-important, cancer-fighting trace mineral selenium. One 3-ounce portion of cod provides about half of the Daily Value of this vital nutrient.

Orange roughy is similar to cod in protein and calories, but delivers more selenium—one 3-ounce (85 g) portion has more than 100 percent of the Daily Value for this nutrient, which has been linked to lower rates of cancer. Note that, as of 2017, orange roughy is one of twelve fish that the nonprofit Food and Water Watch website recommends you avoid. (See the sidebar on page 239 for the complete list).

Flounder and sole fall somewhere between the cod and orange roughy in the selenium sweepstakes, but are otherwise competitive on vitamins, minerals, protein, and calories. All are great foods.

Lean fish typically have a mild flavor, making them adaptable to every sort of cuisine. And most of them are similar enough in taste and texture that you can easily substitute one variety for another—cod for sole, grouper for flounder, and so on.

COD

Among the five most popular fish eaten in the United States, Atlantic cod is one of the mainstays of New England fisheries. The flesh is firm, white, and mild. Small cod (less than 3 pounds [1.4 kg]) are sometimes marketed as scrod; they are sweeter and more tender than full-grown cod. Note that, as of this writing, Atlantic cod is one of twelve fish that the nonprofit Food and Water Watch website recommends you avoid.

FLOUNDER

This widely available flatfish, found on nearly every American coastline, has a mild flavor and light texture that have made it a longstanding favorite. The flounder family includes the true sole (caught only in European waters), European turbot, and fluke. Winter flounder from New England is sometimes called lemon sole, and other flounders are offered as gray sole, petrale sole, or rex sole. If you see Dover sole on a restaurant menu, it may be imported from England (and priced accordingly), or it may be a type of Pacific flounder that is sometimes called sole in the United States.

HALIBUT

A flatfish, like flounder, halibut is found in both the North Atlantic and the northern Pacific waters.

ORANGE ROUGHY

This small saltwater fish is imported from New Zealand and sold in the form of frozen fillets. It has become quite popular, probably because its firm, slightly sweet flesh possesses an adaptable neutral flavor like flounder.

POLLACK (ALASKA AND ATLANTIC)

Tons of mild white Alaskan pollack from the Pacific go into fish sticks and surimi (mock crabmeat), making it one of the top fish in the American diet.

ROCKFISH (OCEAN PERCH)

Fish of this large family go by many names: on the East Coast of the United States, Atlantic ocean perch, rosefish, or redfish; on the West Coast, rock cod, Pacific ocean perch, or Pacific red snapper (although they are different from cod, freshwater perch, and true red snapper).

WORTH KNOWING

I highly recommend checking around for the latest warnings on fish. Several consumer groups are constantly monitoring the situation, and some rate fish both for their contamination and for how harvesting them affects ecology and the environment. For more information, start by checking out the nonprofit Food and Water Watch www.foodandwaterwatch.org).

FISH TO AVOID: THE DIRTY DOZEN

Food and Water Watch is a nonprofit organization that evaluated both the health and environmental effects of eating more than one hundred types of fish and shellfish. As of 2017, the group has listed twelve species that failed to meet two or more of its criteria for safer and more sustainable seafood. Here's the list.

1. **Imported catfish**. Ninety percent of the catfish imported to the United States is from Vietnam, which freely uses antibiotics that aren't even allowed here.

2. **Caviar**. Both beluga and wild-caught sturgeon are susceptible to overfishing. Try eggs from American lake sturgeon or hackleback/shovelnose sturgeon caviar from the Mississippi River.

3. **Atlantic cod**. Though vital to the economy of New England fisherman, the stock has been so mismanaged that it's now listed as one step above endangered on the International Union for Conservation of Nature's Red List of Threatened Species.

4. **American eel**. This tends to be highly contaminated with PCBs and mercury.

5. **Imported shrimp**. The dirtiest of the dirty dozen, imported farmed shrimp comes with a "whole bevy of contaminants"—from antibiotics to chemical residues to rodent hair.

6. **Atlantic flatfish**. This includes flounder, sole, and halibut caught off the Atlantic coast that are overfished and tend to have heavy contamination. Go for Pacific halibut instead.

7. **Atlantic salmon**. It's illegal to capture wild Atlantic salmon because of the extremely low stock of fish, which is partly due to the explosion in salmon farming. Farmed fish are to wild fish what factory-farmed meat is to grass-fed. Thousands of fish are crammed into pens, fed grain, and dosed with antibiotics. The pens pollute the ocean, leading to the growth of diseases and parasites. This is why I recommend wild Alaskan salmon. The company I buy mine from—Vital Choice—offers three varieties: wild Alaskan sockeye salmon, wild Alaskan silver salmon, and wild Pacific king salmon. They're all better for you than Atlantic salmon.

8. **Imported king crab**. When it comes to king crab, go domestic. Most imported king crab comes from Russia where there aren't strongly enforced limits on fish harvests. In addition, it's often misnamed Alaskan king crab. Alaskan king crab is much more responsibly harvested than the imported stuff.

9. **Shark**. Sharks are high in mercury, which is reason enough to avoid eating them. In addition, eating sharks seriously damages the ocean's ecosystem. With fewer sharks around, the species they normally eat—such as rays—increases. Rays deplete scallops and other fish that we eat and wreak havoc on coastal communities that depend on those fisheries.

10. **Orange Roughy**. This is high in mercury and wildly overfished—so much so that some restaurant chains refuse to serve it.

11. **Atlantic Bluefin tuna**. A *New York Times* analysis found that Atlantic Bluefin tuna had the highest mercury levels of any variety of tuna. Bluefin tuna are considered critically endangered.

12. **Chilean sea bass**. Greenpeace estimates that unless we stop eating this fish, the entire species could be commercially extinct within five years. On top of that, these fish are high in mercury.

★ Wild Alaskan Salmon

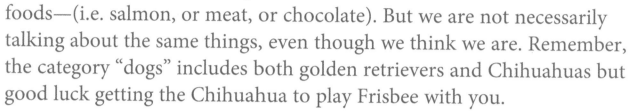

Before we get to salmon, I want to take a minute and talk about definitions. One of the biggest problems we have when we talk about food is that we all use the same basic descriptive words for foods—(i.e. salmon, or meat, or chocolate). But we are not necessarily talking about the same things, even though we think we are. Remember, the category "dogs" includes both golden retrievers and Chihuahuas but good luck getting the Chihuahua to play Frisbee with you.

If you and I discuss the health benefits of salmon, and I'm thinking wild salmon and you're thinking farmed salmon, we may think we're talking about the same food, but we're not. Wild and farmed salmon are two very different animals.

Confused? Read on.

When this book was first published, many people weren't aware of the difference between wild and farmed salmon. People were beginning to realize that salmon was a healthy food, demand for it was increasing, and no one gave a lot of thought to where it came from. At that time, I made a strong case for choosing wild salmon over farmed whenever possible. But the debate continues to this day. (Search "farmed vs wild salmon: which is better?" and you'll see what I mean.)

Demand for salmon has increased exponentially, and to keep up with it, so has salmon farming. In 2015, the *Wall Street Journal* reported that the privately owned agriculture giant Cargill plunked down $1.5 billion for the Norwegian salmon feed producer,

EWOS AS. According to the *Journal*, farmed fish production has already surpassed global beef output and leading the pack is . . . you guessed it, salmon. As of 2017, more than half the salmon sold worldwide comes from fish farms. Meanwhile, global stocks of wild salmon are half what they were just a few decades ago.

It's easy to understand why everybody wants salmon. It's one of the healthiest foods you can eat, because it's chock-full of a particular kind of fat that has more health benefits than almost any other single food on the planet. The type of fat in salmon belongs to a family called the omega-3s, which is the general, family name for a group of three fatty acids. (It's just a coincidence that there happen to be three of them.) Books have been written detailing the benefits of omega-3 fats to human health. (For a more detailed discussion of omega-3s and what they can do for you, see page 330). Omega-3s are helpful for heart health and brain health as well as for inflammation, circulation, memory, thought, and blood sugar control. And we know that salmon is one of the best sources of these omega-3s on the planet.

Not only that, salmon's also a great source of high-quality protein. One 3-ounce (85 g) serving of wild salmon gives you more than 18 g of first-rate protein, not to mention 360 mg of potassium and almost half of the Daily Value of the important cancer-fighting trace mineral selenium. It also contains more than half of the Daily Value for vitamin B12 and 30 percent of the Daily Value for niacin.

Farmed vs Wild: What's the Difference?

The farmed fish proponents loudly proclaim that farmed salmon has just as much omega-3 as wild salmon. That may be true in some cases, but it's not the whole story. If omega-3 content is all you're looking at, it could easily appear as if it doesn't matter whether the salmon on your plate comes from the sea (wild Alaskan salmon) or from a salmon pen (Atlantic salmon, which is almost always farmed).

But it does.

Farm-Raised Salmon Has More Inflammatory Fats

Salmon is an excellent example of a once-great food that has become so popular it is now a commodity. At salmon farms, thousands of salmon are crowded into small, roped-off areas called "net pens" with serious health repercussions for both the fish and the surrounding waters. The fish are packed in like sardines. Disease can spread rapidly in these conditions, so farmed fish receive tons of antibiotics, both in their feed and through injections. Salmon are carnivores—they eat mackerel, sardines, krill, and other fish. But to raise them in pens, salmon farmers do the same thing that factory farmers do with cattle—they feed them grain. Grain is not the natural diet of salmon any more than it is for cows and chickens. The result

is that the fat in farm salmon is completely different from the fat in wild salmon. The fat of farm-raised, grain-fed salmon contains a much higher proportion of inflammatory omega-6s, a fat that we already consume far too much of.

It gets worse.

Wild salmon get their gorgeous pink color from eating krill and shrimp, which are high in a natural pigment called *astaxanthin*. Astaxanthin is a member of the carotenoid family and it has ten times the antioxidant activity of beta-carotene. (Stephen Sinatra, M.D., mentioned astaxanthin as one of his reasons for including wild salmon on his top ten list. See page 207.) But farmed salmon don't get to eat krill and shrimp. They get their color a completely different way. Farmers can pick out the color of their salmon from a color wheel that looks exactly like the ones you see in the paint section of Home Depot. I'm not making this up—I've seen it. It's called the SalmoFan, and it's an actual farmed salmon color wheel where you can choose the shade of red or pink you'd like your "product" to be.

To reduce costs and contaminant levels, farmed salmon are being fed less rendered fish meal and more grain-derived feed than ever before. Unlike their wild cousins, farmed salmon have almost no vitamin D3, and continue to be fed synthetic astaxanthin to color their flesh, pesticides to keep sea lice at bay, and large amounts of antibiotics to combat their extreme vulnerability to disease . . . too often unsuccessfully.

PCBs: Another Reason to Choose Wild Salmon

Then there's the issue of PCBs. According to independent laboratory tests by the Environmental Working Group, seven of ten farmed salmon purchased at grocery stores were contaminated with polychlorinated biphenyls (PCBs) at levels that raise health concerns. These first-ever tests of farmed salmon grocery stores show that farmed salmon are likely the most PCB-contaminated protein source in the U.S. food supply. On average, farmed salmon have sixteen times the dioxinlike PCBs found in wild salmon, four times the levels in beef, and 3.4 times the levels in other seafood. American consumers are exposed to elevated PCB levels by eating farmed salmon.

A 2004 study published in *Science* entitled, "Global Assessment of Organic Contaminants in Farmed Salmon," looked at 700 salmon samples from around the globe. It found that on average, PCB concentrations were eight times higher in farmed salmon than in wild salmon. David Carpenter, M.D., a researcher on the study and the director of the Institute for Health and the Environment at the University of Albany, told *Prevention* magazine that the farmed stuff is "higher in contaminants and even flame retardants." (For more information, go to www.prevention.com/content/which-healthier-wild-salmon-vs-farmed-salmon.)

And if you're concerned about the global impact of farmed salmon, consider this. In British Colombia, hundreds of farmed salmon pens continue to obstruct the migration routes of five different wild salmon species, exposing them to potentially lethal parasites, predation, and diseases that have wiped out wild salmon runs in Norway, Scotland, Iceland, and other areas previously inhabited by healthy wild salmon runs. And it's only likely to get worse—not better.

At the end of the day, both wild salmon and farmed salmon contain plenty of protein, and both have omega-3s. But there the similarity ends. Wild salmon has less calories than farmed, and a lot less proinflammatory omega-6s. Wild salmon eat their natural diet of krill; farmed salmon eat grain and fish pellets, and are a major source of PCBs. Still, there's a serious argument to be made for the fact that salmon is such a great food that even less-than-perfect salmon (i.e., farmed fish) is better than no salmon at all, and that in today's world, not everyone has access to wild salmon, and not everyone can afford it. I'd have to agree with that—if farmed salmon was absolutely the only salmon I could get, I'd probably eat it, and even if you do eat wild most of the time, the occasional farmed salmon fillet certainly won't kill you.

But given a choice between farmed and wild, there's little argument that wild is the clear winner.

WORTH KNOWING

Some people wonder whether the benefits of wild salmon are counteracted by the potential for mercury contamination. That's a tough call, but my answer would have to be no. Here's why: There may be—theoretically—a concern about mercury, particularly for pregnant women. But the health benefits of salmon are so enormous that, in my judgment, they outweigh that concern, especially because salmon is one of the least mercury-contaminated species, and especially because there are companies marketing salmon that routinely screen for every possible contaminant and impurity. One company I'm particularly fond of that harvests toxin-free salmon from pristine Alaskan waters and ships it—and other "clean" fish—direct to your door is Vital Choice. (Find a link to Vital Choice on my website, www.jonnybowden.com.)

WHAT ABOUT MERCURY?

I'm frequently asked what to do about the mercury in fish. Honestly, I don't have a perfect answer. No one is more concerned about mercury than I am. We all know that retooling industrial plants so that they don't spew it everywhere costs a fortune, and we've all watched with dismay as the issue has become a political football, largely because no one wants to pay the enormous price of change. Big business insists that the amount released into the environment is insignificant, politicians continue to curry favor with big business by giving them unacceptably long lead times to clean up their act, and meanwhile our rivers, lakes, and oceans are contaminated with this powerful toxin.

What makes matters worse is that those attempting to avoid responsibility can point to the fact that the stuff travels so effectively via wind and sea that even if they did clean up their act it might not make much difference unless every company on the planet followed suit—mercury and other toxic metals, like cadmium, and industrial pollutants, like PCBs, have been found as far away from their original industrial sources as the waters of the Arctic Ocean. In Greenland, for goodness' sake, 16 percent of the population's blood mercury levels exceed the levels that could have toxic effects on people.

No one—I hope—denies that mercury is a powerful toxin and damaging to the brain. It impairs neurological function. And yes, there's a good chance it's in your fish. The questions are "how much?" and "does it really matter?" In 2004, two federal agencies that have traditionally disagreed about how much contaminated fish is too much were charged with issuing a joint warning advisory. Not surprisingly, the compromise position pleased few people.

Should We Trust the FDA and EPA Guidelines for Mercury?

The U.S. Food and Drug Administration (FDA), which regulates the fish you buy, supposedly has more knowledge of nutrition and tries to weigh the potential harm of eating contaminated fish against the enormous potential benefits. The Environmental Protection Agency (EPA), on the other hand, is concerned with contaminants like mercury and doesn't really concern itself with nutrition—only with toxins and safety. Charged with finding a compromise warning, they issued a joint document in 2004 that set the following limits for women of childbearing age, pregnant women, and nursing mothers:

- No more than two meals (12 ounces [340 g]) a week of most fish, including salmon, catfish, and canned light tuna

- No more than 6 ounces (168 g) a week of albacore (white) tuna

- No swordfish, king mackerel, shark, or tilefish at all

Ten years later, in 2014, they submitted a draft revising their fish consumption advice, but the recommendations were virtually identical. Instead of saying "no more than 2 meals (12 ounces [340 g]) a week of most fish," they now say "Eat 8 to 12 ounces (225 to 340 g) of a variety of fish each week from choices that are lower in mercury."

But as reporter Amanda Schaffer pointed out in her excellent article on Slate (www.slate.com/id/2115878), an average woman could follow these rules to the letter and still exceed the EPA's cutoff for mercury—0.1 mcg of mercury per kilogram of body weight per day—by a sizable margin. "For instance," she writes, "a 140-pound [64 kg] woman who ate just one 6-ounce [170 kg] can of white tuna a week would be

30 percent over the EPA cutoff, defined as a daily exposure level that over time is unlikely to cause appreciable harm."

Mercury Advisories Risk Scaring People Away from All Seafood

None of this would be a problem if fish weren't so damn good for us. It's for just that reason that the Harvard Center for Risk Analysis has recommended that government advisories about mercury in seafood need to walk a fine line and avoid scaring consumers away from seafood altogether. To add to the problem, the warnings have been for specific risk groups (e.g., pregnant women, women of childbearing age) and, it could be argued, do not apply equally to all groups of people. Plus they have a tenfold safety margin built in as a precaution.

According to a 2005 statement by the National Oceanic and Atmospheric Administration, "Women will not put their baby at risk if they avoid eating shark, swordfish, tilefish, king mackerel, tuna steaks and whale meat until after they have delivered and stopped breast feeding." For good measure, women planning to become pregnant should avoid these fish for six months beforehand.

There's one more reason I'm a little less panicked about mercury in seafood than you might think I'd be. And that reason is selenium. That amazing, anticancer trace mineral that I refer to in so many discussions of the foods in this book, is plentiful in seafood. Why does it matter? Because selenium is a powerful chelator of mercury—it helps mitigate the effects. At a 2005 Washington conference sponsored by the governments of the United States, Norway, Canada, and Iceland and assisted by the United Nations' Food and Agriculture Organization, evidence was presented that showed that selenium helps neutralize the effects of mercury acquired from foods

"This very important but little analyzed point helps us to understand how people from the Seychelles islands can eat fish twelve times per week and show no toxic signs," said William E. M. Lands, a retired professor of biochemistry at the Universities of Michigan and Illinois and an expert on the metabolism of fats.

What to Do, What to Do?

The best response to mercury warnings, obviously, is to stay away from the fish that are the most contaminated. Keep your eyes open for the reports of consumer advocate groups who often sound the alarm way in advance of government agencies. (A good place to start is the Food and Water Watch website, www.food andwaterwatch.org). Read the thoughtful books by Marion Nestle, Ph.D., M.P.H., who tends to take a middle ground (*Safe Food*, *Food Politics* and *What to Eat*). Keep your fish consumption to the recommended levels.

And if you're so moved, get involved. Write to your congressperson. Elect people who want to clean up the environment and the food it produces. Join a consumer advocacy group.

But for goodness' sake, do not stop eating fish. The good stuff in it will do you more good than the bad stuff will do you harm, especially if you choose your sources carefully.

THE EXPERTS' TOP TEN LISTS

David Perlmutter, M.D., F.A.C.N., A.B.I.H.M.

David Perlmutter is a board-certified neurologist and the author of several bestselling books, including *Brain Maker* and *The Grain Brain Whole Life Plan*.

In 2002, he was the recipient of the Linus Pauling Award for his innovative approaches to neurological disorders and was awarded the Denham Harmon Award for his pioneering work in the application of free radical science to clinical medicine. He is the recipient of the 2006 National Nutritional Foods Association Clinician of the Year Award and serves as medical advisor for The Dr. Oz Show. He has contributed extensively to the world medical literature with publications appearing in *The Journal of Neurosurgery*, *The Southern Medical Journal*, *Journal of Applied Nutrition*, and *Archives of Neurology*. Here is his top ten list:

1. **Eggs (organic, and pasture-raised).** Egg yolks are a great source of choline, an important nutrient for brain health.

2. **Coconut oil.** Coconut oil is one of the fundamental recommendations of the Grain Brain program. Research shows its consumption is associated with improved cardiovascular parameters and a slimmer belly!

3. **Olive oil.** Olive oil is one of the foods that has the greatest potential to keep us healthy. Consider that it's a staple of both the Grain Brain and highly-praised Mediterranean diet.

4. **Avocado.** The avocado is part of my "anti-Alzheimer's trio," and is an incredible source of healthful fats.

5. **Dandelion greens.** Loaded with antioxidants, including vitamin C and vitamin A (beta-carotene), the health benefits of this plant have been documented as far back as the tenth and eleventh centuries. Most important, they are a rich source of prebiotic fiber.

6. **Blueberries.** These are a healthy, low-sugar fruit, and a way to fight off Alzheimer's.

7. **High-cacao chocolate.** There's nothing wrong with indulging in a few pieces of dark chocolate (greater than 70 percent cacao) every now and then!

8. **Kale.** It's jam-packed with vitamins, antioxidants, carotenoids, good fat, and fiber.

9. **Wild salmon.** This is an excellent source of the omega-3 fatty acid DHA, which turns on the growth of new brain cells while offering protection for existing ones. It's also anti-inflammatory.

10. **Brussels sprouts.** Like kale, Brussels sprouts are in the *Brassica* family and are a relative of cabbage. They're high in fiber, low in calories, and loaded with important antioxidants and plant chemicals such as indoles.

SPECIALTY FOODS

This group of foods is connected only by two facts: One, they are all superbly healthy foods, and two, none of them fits neatly into any of the other categories. Sure, sauerkraut and kimchi are both technically vegetables, but they're also fermented and used as condiments. And olives are a fruit, but no one thinks of them that way. And into what category would bee pollen go?

It seemed simpler to group these misfits into their own category.

So, what we have here is a group of wonderfully nutritious foods that range all over the map, from traditional fermented foods such as sauerkraut and kimchi, to the mineral-rich seaweeds, to juices made from green grasses, to completely modern inventions such as whey protein powder and brewer's yeast. And though this category includes a few foods not found in our Paleolithic diets (our hunter-gatherer ancestors, for example, never came across dark chocolate bars in the wild), a list of the world's healthiest foods would not be complete without any one of them. Eat and enjoy!

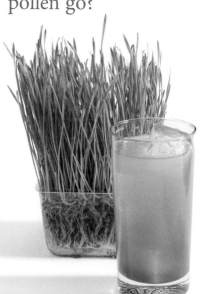

★ Bee Pollen, Propolis, and Royal Jelly

Advocates of bee pollen can be their own worst enemies, claiming that bee pollen can cure everything from cancer to hangnails. But inflated claims aside, a significant body of literature shows that bee products—particularly propolis—do have significant and documented health benefits that help explain why they have been a staple in folk medicine and healing traditions for more than 2,000 years.

Bee pollen is a phenomenally nutritious and well-balanced food that can be consumed by people and domestic animals. It's been called nature's perfect food because it is loaded with vitamins and contains almost all known minerals, trace elements, enzymes, and amino acids. (It actually has more amino acids and vitamins than any other amino acid–containing product like beef, eggs, or cheese.)

This makes sense because bee pollen captures the essence of every plant from which it collects pollen. In addition, bee pollen contains digestive enzymes from the bees. According to Ray Sahelian, M.D., bee pollen contains eighteen amino acids; DNA and RNA; vitamins A, B_1, B_2, B_6, and B_{12}; niacin; pantothenic acid; folic acid; vitamins C, D, E, and K; choline; inositol; rutin and other bioflavonoids; calcium, magnesium, iron, and zinc; ten types of enzymes; coenzymes; and many other nutritional factors. Bee pollen contains flavonoids that have significant antioxidant properties. According to Mark Stengler, N.M.D., bee pollen also contains hard-to-get trace minerals such as silicon, molybdenum, boron, and sulfur. And it's one of the few nonmeat sources of vitamin B_{12}.

Bee Propolis Fights Infection

Propolis possesses a multitude of pharmacological activities. It's created by the bees by mixing a resinous sap from trees with wax back at the hive. Bees use it as a kind of glue or general-purpose sealer—they coat the hive with propolis in much the same way we use paint and caulking on our homes. People began using propolis more than 2,300 years ago for many purposes, the foremost of which was applying it to wounds to fight infection. A review of the biological activity of bee propolis on health and disease published in the January 2006 *Asian Pacific Journal of Cancer Prevention* noted that propolis possesses antimicrobial, antioxidative, antiulcer, and antitumor activities.

Many scientific articles are published every year in different international journals related to the pharmacological properties of this amazing substance. More than 300 compounds have been identified in propolis samples, including polyphenols, and many of these compounds have surprisingly protective effects. One active compound from propolis—caffeic acid phenethyl ester (CAPE) —is known to have anticarcinogenic, anti-inflammatory and immunomodulatory properties. In a study published in the May 2006 *Journal of Nutritional Biochemistry*, CAPE derived from propolis inhibited the cell migration and colony formation of tumor cells, providing direct evidence for the role of CAPE as a potent antimetastatic agent that can markedly inhibit the metastatic and invasive capacity of malignant cells.

Humans Benefit from Bee Susceptibility to Infection

Propolis is well known for its antimicrobial activity. It's been shown to have an antibacterial effect (against *Staphylococcus aureus*) as well as an antifungal effect (against *Candida albicans*, or yeast), and even an antiviral effect (against Avian influenza virus). It's really not so surprising that bee products like propolis would have such powerful antibiotic effects. Any beekeeper will tell you that bees are very susceptible to bacterial and viral infections. From a sheer Darwinian point of view, it makes survival sense that the very material that they "caulk" their hives with would be highly protective against the microbes that could easily destroy them.

One study, in the July 2006 issue of *International Immunopharmacology*, suggested that the anti-inflammatory activities of propolis might make it a novel therapeutic agent for asthma. (One of the flavonoids found in bee pollen is the powerful anti-inflammatory quercetin.) And a paper in the *Journal of Ethnopharmacology* in 2005 found that propolis stimulates antibody production, perhaps accounting for its reputation as an immune system enhancer.

Royal Jelly

Royal jelly is a special creamy substance secreted from the nurse worker bees that stimulates the growth and development of the queen bee; without it, she'd just be a regular old worker bee. When the eggs turn into larvae, they eat this special food for only two or three days and quickly develop into large and healthy bees. But the queen continues to eat this food for the rest of her life, with the result that she grows 40 to 60 percent larger and lives about four to six years, while the worker bees live only about six weeks. These facts may account for the anecdotal reputation of royal jelly as an amazing antiaging substance that can foster health and extend life.

Royal Jelly May Be Overrated

I'm less enthused about royal jelly than I am about propolis and bee pollen, though it is a concentrated source of nutrition. Royal jelly has the appealing property of being a creamy emulsion that is strongly antibacterial, which makes it an ideal component of cosmetics and skin care products. But as some responsible experts point out, internal uses of royal jelly are less promising as the antibacterial activities disappear when the pH is raised to above 6 by the natural buffering systems in the body (which maintain a pH of about 7.4). In fact, no clear evidence exists to support claims of internal usefulness for royal jelly as a therapeutic agent—though one study showed that royal jelly (at approximately 50 to 100 mg per day) reduced total serum cholesterol and serum lipid levels. And neopterin—a substance found in humans that appears to play an important role in the human immune system—has been isolated from royal jelly.

Still, it is a greatly nutritious food—containing all the B-complex vitamins, including a high concentration of B_5—plus minerals, vitamins A, C, D, and E, eighteen amino acids, enzymes, and hormones.

But none of these vitamins or minerals appears to be unique to royal jelly, and there is much less published research on royal jelly than there is on propolis. Its antibacterial activity seems unlikely to be expressed when the food is ingested, yet that same antibacterial activity, along with other properties of the substance, make it a really desirable ingredient in topical preparations and skin creams.

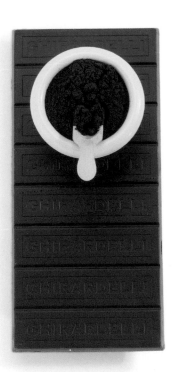

Dark Chocolate

In a fascinating and much-discussed article that appeared in the December 18, 2004, *British Medical Journal*, researchers put forth an idea called the polymeal. They examined all of the research on foods and health to see whether they could put together the ideal meal (the Polymeal) that, if you ate it every day, would significantly reduce your risk for cardiovascular disease. They examined all of the research, did all the calculations, and came up with a theoretical meal that, eaten daily, would not just reduce cardiovascular risk, but reduce it by a staggering 75 percent (there's not a pill in the world that can do that).

The ingredients of this Polymeal? Wine, fish, nuts, garlic, fruits, vegetables, and chocolate.

In fact, they even figured out the risk-reduction contribution of each of the individual foods; the actual percentage of reduction in risk for cardiovascular disease from eating 100 g a day of cocoa-rich chocolate (more about that in a moment) turned out to be a pretty impressive 21 percent.

Flavonoids in Cocoa Prevent Clogged Arteries

Cocoa is loaded with compounds called flavonoids, which are also found in cranberries, apples, strawberries, onions, tea, and red wine, placing chocolate in excellent company. There are more than 4,000 of these flavonoids in the plant kingdom. In plants, flavonoids provide important protection like shielding from environmental toxins, and when we consume plant-based foods that are rich in flavonoids, we also get a lot of the same benefits the plant gets.

The particular class of flavonoids found in cocoa are called flavanols. Cocoa flavanols prevent fatlike substances in the bloodstream from clogging the arteries. When you reduce the blood's ability to clot, you also reduce the risk of heart attack and stroke. (That's why they sometimes tell you to take a baby aspirin—for the same reason.) All these factors make blood platelets less likely to stick together and cause clots. As a bonus, cocoa also contains magnesium, one of the most important minerals for heart health.

Flavanols in cocoa also do something else that's very important. They modulate a compound in the body called nitric oxide. Nitric oxide is critical for healthy blood flow and healthy blood pressure and is a very important compound in the area of cardiovascular health. In one Italian study, dark chocolate was shown to lower blood pressure, and the reason may well be that flavanol-rich cocoa actually supports the body's ability to synthesize nitric oxide. In another study in the *American Journal of Clinical Nutrition*, it was reported that dark chocolate not only decreased

blood pressure but also improved insulin sensitivity in healthy people!

Cocoa flavanols have gotten a lot of attention in the nutrition world since the original edition of this book, and a big part of the reason is the Kuna Indians. The Kuna live off the coast of Panama, and they are unusual in that their blood pressure tends to stay pretty much the same throughout their lives. Unlike Americans and Europeans, the Kuna do not experience the dangerous rise in blood pressure that accompanies aging and increases the risk for heart disease and diabetes. Some researchers—including Norman Hollenberg at Harvard Medical School—think it's because of cocoa. The Kuna Indians drink about 5 cups (1.1 L) of the stuff every day. One study, published in 2011 in the prestigious *British Medical Journal*, found that the highest levels of chocolate consumption were associated with a 37 percent reduction in cardiovascular disease. The researchers concluded that "levels of chocolate consumption seem to be associated with a substantial reduction in the risk of cardiometabolic disorders."

Chocolate and Dementia

A number of studies have found that eating chocolate lowers the risk of dementia, and improves performance on cognitive function tests. Best of all, one of these studies found that it only took about 10 g a day to get the results.

And speaking of cognitive performance, consider this study, one of the most novel and inventive studies on chocolate I've ever seen. Given chocolate's reputation as a cognitive enhancer, Franz H. Messerli, M.D., director of the Hypertension Program at St. Luke's-Roosevelt Hospital in New York, decided to see whether there was any connection between winning the Nobel Prize and chocolate consumption! So he looked at the number of Nobel Prize awards per capita in 23 countries, and compared that with the recipient's country's chocolate consumption. His findings, published in the *New England Journal of Medicine*, showed a strong correlation between chocolate consumption and Nobel Prize winners. Granted, this is a completely whimsical, observational study which certainly doesn't prove cause and effect, but still it's interesting and thought provoking. And a great little factoid to have at your fingertips when you're trying to convince stubborn friends that dark chocolate is a health food.

Eating the Right Kind of Chocolate Is Key

But here's the thing: This endorsement of chocolate comes with a very big qualification. I am not talking about commercial chocolate bars. I'm not talking about those chewy caramel-marshmallow-nut-covered candy bars you see in the grocery store. That's not the stuff that has the health benefits. The health benefits come from the flavanols and antioxidants, and those are found in real cocoa—in fact, that's the stuff that makes cocoa kind of bitter. So if you want the benefits of these flavanols in your diet, you've got to get the real deal chocolate—high-cocoa-content dark chocolate. You'll see the best of these bars with labels that say "60 percent cocoa" (70 percent or higher is even better). Milk chocolate and white chocolate have virtually none of these health benefits. Plus, the commercial candy bars are loaded with extra sugar, fat, waxes, and chemicals that are not what you want to be adding to your diet. And the more chocolate is processed, the more the beneficial flavonoids are lost.

The fat in chocolate is from cocoa butter and actually contains three different kinds of fat. One of them is oleic acid, which is the same monounsaturated fat found in olive oil—a very heart-healthy fat. The second is stearic acid, which has a neutral effect on the body. The third kind, palmitic acid, is probably not the best kind of fat to be eating large amounts of, but it really only accounts for a third of the fat in chocolate, and if you keep your portions small, you won't be taking in a lot.

Remember, though, that cocoa butter is expensive. Cheap brands of chocolate replace the good cocoa butter with milk fats and hydrogenated oils, another reason to seek out the best brands if you're interested in getting the health benefits—and the amazing taste—of real, cocoa-rich chocolate.

Chocolate Is Not for Everyone

Health benefits aside, chocolate is not for everybody. It seems to trigger addictive eating behavior in some people, and if you're one of those, and you know who you are, then remember the old adage "know thyself" and just stay away from this food. But if you can handle it and don't have any medical condition that would prevent you from being able to enjoy it, then having a small—remember, I'm talking small—amount of dark chocolate a few times a week is a great idea. My friend, the well-known cardiologist and nutritionist Stephen Sinatra, M.D., has said that even cardiac patients can enjoy dark chocolate regularly in moderation, if they're not sensitive to caffeine.

I'd recommend you get the darkest, most delicious kind you can find, that is at least 60 percent cocoa, and enjoy an ounce or two (28 to 55 g) a few times a week.

★ Green Foods and Drinks

(cereal grasses: barley grass and wheatgrass; and microalgae: spirulina, chlorella, and wild blue-green algae)

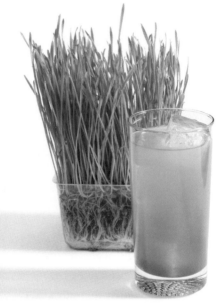

If dogs happen to be a part of your family, you've undoubtedly seen them eat grass. Why? No one really knows. Some people believe that dogs eat cereal grasses because they contain nutrients not found in meat that are essential for the animals' good health. One thing is for sure—grass is a rich source of nutrients, and "green foods" made from cereal grasses and algae are among the healthiest foods I know of for humans.

This unusual category—green foods and drinks—covers a lot of territory, from the perennial health food store favorite wheatgrass juice to the algae such as blue-green algae and spirulina. All have specific nutrient profiles and are used for different (but overlapping) purposes. Let's start with the main thing they all have in common: chlorophyll. Chlorophyll, the substance that makes plants appear green, is a natural blood purifier. What does this mean? Well, consider that everything—from anaerobic bacteria to yeast and fungus—travels through the blood. Our own immune system creates complexes that attack these foreign substances, and chlorophyll assists our bodies in cleaning out the sludge that can cause damage. "Chlorophyll helps manage bacterial growth," Sonja Pettersen, a naturopathic physician in Arizona, explains. "It helps remove unwanted residues and helps activate enzymes. It's a natural anti-inflamma-

tory and it's nutrient dense." Indeed, chlorophyll-containing plants—such as spirulina, chlorella, and wild blue-green algae—are an essential part of the healing armament in traditional Chinese medicine and other Eastern practices.

As far as chlorophyll's reputation as a "blood builder," there may be some scientific basis for this. The molecular structure of red blood cells and chlorophyll is virtually identical except for the center atom—in red blood cells it's iron, in chlorophyll it's magnesium. Chlorophyll is sometimes called "the blood of plant life."

Then there's the issue of acidity and alkalinity. As every gardener knows, the relative acidity and alkalinity of the soil can be determined by measuring its pH. The body also needs a balance of acid and alkaline for optimal health, and pH can be measured in urine, in blood, and in saliva. "I believe the future of preventative medicine is in managing the pH of your body," Pettersen told me. "All kinds of things can cause acidity—stress, rock music, sugar, and many foods. But if you balance your body with alkaline substances—such as spirulina, algae, and chlorella, all 'supergreens' with the benefits of chlorophyll—you can maintain the pH of your body at the right level, which goes a long way toward increasing your resistance to disease. At the proper pH level, enzymes flourish and the body mobilizes all its healing forces."

Cereal Grasses: Barley Grass and Wheatgrass Juice

Barley grass and wheatgrass are both high-chlorophyll foods that are nearly identical, although barley grass may be a bit more digestible. It's worth mentioning that people with wheat allergies are almost never allergic to wheat in its grass stage. Cereal grasses contain many enzymes, as well as the powerful antioxidant enzyme SOD (superoxide dismutase). They also contain large amounts of the mucopolysaccharides (MPs) discussed on page 254.

BARLEY GRASS

Barley grass is a great alternative for those who can't tolerate wheatgrass. It's milder, though bitter compared to the sweetness of wheatgrass. Young barley leaves have a tremendous ability to absorb nutrients from the soil. "Green magma," often found in the green foods/green drinks section of the health food store, is the trade name for one well-known brand of barley grass powder.

WHEATGRASS JUICE

Paul Pitchford and others note that wheatgrass juice is very concentrated, and even one ounce (30 ml) has therapeutic value. He recommends not taking more than 2 ounces (60 ml) at a time—it doesn't increase the effectiveness. Wheatgrass juice is believed to help

IS WHEATGRASS GLUTEN-FREE?

Technically, yes. Gluten is only found in the seed kernel—also known as the endosperm. It's not found in the stem and leaves, which is where wheatgrass comes from. Same thing with barley grass. If the grass doesn't include the seed kernel, you should be fine.

But note that I said wheatgrass and barley grass are technically gluten-free. In their pure form, they absolutely are. But if a farmer lets some of the grasses begin to produce seeds before harvesting them, then bingo—you've got gluten on your hands. And there's always the possibility of gluten cross-contamination, especially when wheatgrass is an ingredient in prepackaged foods.

If you suspect you're gluten intolerant or even gluten sensitive, it's probably a good idea to stay away just as a precaution. Or, at least, make sure that the product is truthfully labeled gluten-free.

And while the grasses are pretty nutrient dense, wheatgrass juice shots are trendy and expensive. You'd probably be better off just eating a bunch of fruit and vegetables. They're nothing in wheatgrass juice you can't get from other plant foods—at, I might add, a fraction of the price.

cleanse the lymph system, restore balance in the body, help remove toxic metals from the cells, and restore vitality. One ounce (30 ml) of the juice is believed to have the vitamin and mineral equivalent of more than 2 pounds (896 g) of vegetables, though I have been unable to substantiate this. It is also thought to contain about thirty different enzymes. It should be consumed immediately after juicing.

Microalgae (spirulina, chlorella, and wild blue-green alga)

These members of the microalgae family contain more chlorophyll than any other foods and were among the first life forms. According to Paul Pitchford in his book *Healing with Whole Foods: Asian Traditions and Modern Nutrition*, microalgae exist on the edge between the plant and animal kingdoms. In addition to chlorophyll they contain protein, beta-carotene, and nucleic acids (RNA and DNA).

SPIRULINA

Rich with chlorophyll, protein, beta-carotene, and the beneficial fatty acid GLA (gamma-linolenic acid), spirulina also contains a pigment called phycocyanin, which has antioxidant and anti-inflammatory properties and which, in one study, was shown to inhibit cancer-colony formation. The cell wall of spirulina is composed of mucopolysaccharides (MPs), which are complex sugars mixed with amino acids, simple sugars, and sometimes protein. MPs contain only completely digestible nutrients, which makes them very different from the indigestible cell wall found in other microalgae and other plants.

CHLORELLA

Chlorella is similar to spirulina but contains just a little less protein, much less beta-carotene, and much more chlorophyll and nucleic acids. It has a tough outer cell wall that is believed to bind with heavy metals, pesticides, and other carcinogens, carrying them safely out of the body. Its chlorophyll content is higher than any food, and it contains higher amounts of fatty acids, about 20 percent of which are omega-3s. Unlike spirulina, chlorella does not contain phycocyanin.

WILD BLUE-GREEN ALGA

This microalga grows wild in Klamath Lake in Oregon. Under certain conditions it can transform into a very toxic plant—it can cause death in animals within five minutes. However, according to experts, wild blue-green alga, has never been found in its toxic state in Klamath Lake, and the products coming out of Klamath Lake are believed to be completely safe, especially because freeze-drying denatures the toxin. (I only mention the toxicity issue in case you have visions of harvesting your own blue-green alga from the wild and you don't know exactly what you're doing.)

WORTH KNOWING

There are many good brands of "green drinks," but the best of them use high-quality grasses, and extracts grown in rich soil, organically. One of my favorite brands is Barlean's Greens, which also comes in a chocolate flavored version that kids actually like! I'm also a big fan of Mighty Maca Plus, a special greens drink that also includes Maca (see page 51) and that's made by my pal Anna Cabeca, D.O. (It's available through a link on my website, www.jonnybowden.com.)

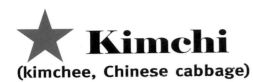 # Kimchi
(kimchee, Chinese cabbage)

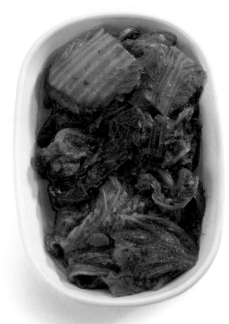

Kimchi is a traditional Korean dish made of fermented chile peppers and vegetables, usually cabbage. It's so popular in Korea that Koreans reportedly say "kimchi" instead of "cheese" when posing for pictures. In Korea, it's served as a popular side dish, but is also used as a cooking ingredient (in pancakes, as a topping on pizza, and in dishes such as kimchi soup and kimchi fried rice). Many Chinese and Japanese eat this dish on a daily basis. Whatever you call it, it's a nutritional powerhouse. *Health* magazine, a magazine I generally like, called it one of the world's five healthiest foods. Want to know why? Read on.

The most common ingredients of kimchi are Chinese cabbage, radish, garlic, red pepper, onion, some kind of seafood (oyster or squid are common), ginger, salt, and maybe sugar. Internationally, it's sometimes just known as Chinese cabbage. The first clue to kimchi's health properties is its ingredients: Cabbage, onions, and garlic are not only all featured in this book as members of the elite group of 150 healthiest foods on the planet, but all three have also earned special mention (stars) for being superstars in their respective categories. All three ingredients in kimchi—cabbage, onions, and garlic—have both significant anticancer properties and significant heart benefits. (Garlic has been shown in research to reduce plaque, lower LDL cholesterol, and inhibit the proliferation of colorectal cancer cells; the indoles in cabbage fight cancer; and onions are one of four foods found to reduce mor-

tality from heart disease by 20 percent!) And other ingredients in kimchi—chile peppers and ginger, for example—have health benefits of their own.

Why Fermented Foods Are Almost Always Good for You

Then there's fermentation. Kimchi is always fermented, which should be our next clue to the fact that this is going to be a healthy food. Virtually all naturally fermented foods are health promoting. The healthy bacteria *lactobacilli* are heavily involved in the fermentation process, and kimchi is a potent source of these healthy probiotics. Various members of the Lactobacillus class of healthy bacteria have been found to support and improve immunity in a number of studies. They help control inflammation, which is an essential feature of so many degenerative diseases, including heart disease. And on top of that, they're essential in maintaining a healthy digestive system.

So kimchi is a superstar in the world of healthy foods. According to a comprehensive review in the *ISHS Acta Horticulturae #482*, it has demonstrated antioxidant, antimutagenic, and anticarcinogenic activities. Pretty darn impressive for a sometimes smelly little cabbage dish! Kimchi also contains high levels of vitamins (vitamin C, the B vitamins), minerals (calcium, potassium, and iron), and dietary fiber.

Licorice

First things first—everyone knows licorice as a candy, which, at least when I was a kid, was very much an acquired taste. But candy confections aside, real licorice root is a serious food and a potent herb and has real health benefits.

Licorice is a perennial herb native to southern Europe, Asia, and the Mediterranean. The herb is extensively cultivated in Russia, Spain, Iran, and India. Licorice is one of the most popular and widely consumed herbs in the world. Ancient cultures on every continent have used licorice, with the first recorded use by the Egyptians in the third century BCE. The Egyptians and the Greeks recognized the licorice herb's benefits in treating coughs and lung disease. It's the second most prescribed herb in China, following ginseng.

Licorice Root Soothes the Throat and Lungs

The most common medical use for licorice is for supporting upper respiratory tract health. It's known for its soothing effect on inflamed mucous membranes. Licorice root, when mixed with water or used in cough drops, soothes mucous membranes like those found in the throat, lung, and bronchial tubes. (When I was a kid, my mom would give me Smith Brothers licorice cough drops at the first sign of a cough.)

According to the *Materia Medica*, licorice root is also used for urinary tract irritation, adrenal fatigue and exhaustion, immune-deficient states, allergies, liver disorders, and detoxification. The Japanese use a licorice preparation to control hepatitis, not surprising given that the *Materia Medica* suggests it is particularly good for conditions in which the patient needs immune system support and has abnormally high liver enzymes (mononucleosis, hepatitis). It is also a wonderful herb for chronic fatigue syndrome.

Licorice Makes Top Six List for Anticancer Activity

The active ingredient in licorice is a member of the saponin family called glycyrrhizin, though according to Louis Vanrenen's excellent book *Power Herbs*, the plant also contains flavonoids (at least twenty-five of them), terpenoids, amino acids, lignans, and plant sterols. (Vanrenen considers licorice one of his "50 power herbs.")

Glycyrrhizin, the most well-known constituent, is both anti-inflammatory and immune stimulating. (It may also raise blood pressure—see "Worth Knowing.") There are dozens of published studies showing the health properties of the flavonoids and other compounds in licorice. One study shows that the flavonoids in licorice help reduce abdominal fat in obese mice. Other studies have shown glycyrrhizin to have antioxidant effects, and a number of constituents in licorice have shown antitumor activity in animal research. In fact, licorice was among six foods and herbs listed as having the highest anticancer activity according to the 1997 report "Phytochemicals: Guardians of Our Health" by the *Journal of the American Dietetic Association* (the others were garlic, soybeans, cabbage, ginger, and the umbelliferous vegetables).

Licorice has also been known to soothe joints and support normal blood sugar. The licorice root extract produces mild estrogenic effects, and it has proven useful in supporting the stress of menopause and menstruation. Licorice also has a beneficial effect on digestive processes.

Note: Don't confuse real licorice root—a medicinal food and herb—with most common licorice candy, much of which is really made with anise and has virtually no real licorice root content. You can find real licorice candy, and it's delicious—but you have to look for it carefully.

WORTH KNOWING

Because the active ingredient in licorice works in ways similar to the hormones of the adrenal glands, it is a double-edged sword. On the one hand it is anti-inflammatory (like the adrenal hormone cortisol), but on the other hand the glycyrrhizin content can easily raise blood pressure (like the adrenal hormone aldosterone). Do not use the herb licorice—or eat real licorice candy on a regular basis—if you have high blood pressure. It's also contraindicated for heart failure, kidney disease, liver cirrhosis, and cholestatic liver disorders.

De-glycyrrhizined licorice is frequently used in supplements for its anti-inflammatory and other beneficial properties. There is 2 to 9 percent glycyrrhizin in licorice root. The de-glycyrrhizined root extract has a maximum of 3 percent glycyrrhizin in it.

Olives

Look up any nutritional textbook and you're sure to find an entry for olive oil, with a massive number of references touting its health properties. Strangely, you don't see as much good press for the lovely little olive from which the oil comes.

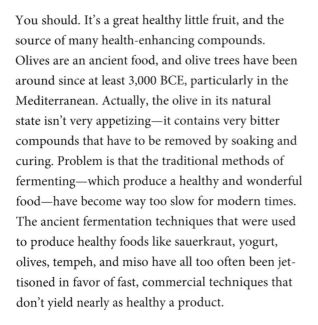

You should. It's a great healthy little fruit, and the source of many health-enhancing compounds. Olives are an ancient food, and olive trees have been around since at least 3,000 BCE, particularly in the Mediterranean. Actually, the olive in its natural state isn't very appetizing—it contains very bitter compounds that have to be removed by soaking and curing. Problem is that the traditional methods of fermenting—which produce a healthy and wonderful food—have become way too slow for modern times. The ancient fermentation techniques that were used to produce healthy foods like sauerkraut, yogurt, olives, tempeh, and miso have all too often been jettisoned in favor of fast, commercial techniques that don't yield nearly as healthy a product.

Choose Your Olives Wisely

Traditional fermentation is a slow process caused by the action of yeast and bacteria, and it produces a food that is brimming with healthy compounds and active cultures that are good for you. But in today's "faster is better" world, olives are much more likely to be treated with lye to remove the bitterness, then packed in salt and canned. Processed olives are those that have been through a lye bath; the more old-fashioned (and way better) method is to cure them in oil, brine, water,

or salt. Those are known as oil-cured, brine-cured, water-cured, or dry-salted olives. If you're willing to look, you can find the good kind in olive bars; they're sitting in dishes, usually in the cheese section of some of the better grocery stores, and they're olives that are still alive with active cultures that your body loves! Those are the ones to go for.

Olives and their oils contain a host of beneficial plant compounds, including tocopherols, flavonoids, anthocyanins, sterols, and polyphenols. Polyphenols are probably what give olives their taste; the polyphenols from olives have anti-inflammatory activity, improve immune function, help prevent damage to DNA, and protect the cardiovascular system. Olives and olive oil are a significant staple of the Mediterranean culture and are associated with countless health benefits, including lower incidence of heart disease and certain kinds of cancer.

The fat in olives (and olive oil, see page 339 is largely the monounsaturated fat oleic acid, which has been associated with higher levels of protective HDL ("good") cholesterol and lower levels of inflammation. A number of studies have shown that people who get plenty of monounsaturated fat are less likely to die of heart disease.

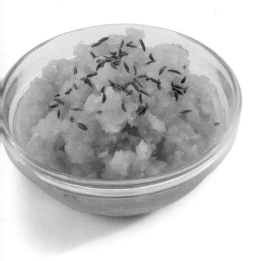

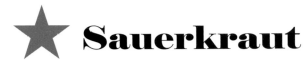 # Sauerkraut

(nonpasteurized)

Sauerkraut combines one of the healthiest foods on the planet (cabbage) with one of most healthy forms of processing on the planet (fermentation). The resultant food is a consistent winner in the health promotion sweepstakes.

Fermentation simply refers to an ancient technique of preparation and preservation in which food is naturally "processed" by microorganisms such as bacteria that break down the carbohydrates and protein in the food and produce the final result—yogurt, sauerkraut, miso, old-fashioned soy sauce, and kimchi being terrific examples. The key to their nutritional value is twofold—the ingredients and the process. Commercial food processors have tried to standardize the fermentation techniques, and many modern mass-produced foods (canned olives, pickles) are not actually fermented but just treated with chemicals, packed in salt, and then canned. Only true fermentation gives you the amazing health benefits of the "live cultures" such as *Lactobacillus*, which are legion for their health benefits.

Live Cultures in Sauerkraut Help Control Inflammation

And what a list of health benefits it is. Bacteria of the *Lactobacillus* genus feed the "good" bacteria in your gut, creating a natural balance of gut flora that improves digestion, immune function, and the absorption and assimilation of nutrients. Various members of the *Lactobacillus* genus have been found to support and improve immunity in a number of

studies. Many of the studies used yogurt as the delivery system for these good bacteria (known as active cultures or probiotics), but any naturally fermented food—like sauerkraut—would be expected to have the same results. These studies have found that active cultures like those found in sauerkraut have a stimulating effect on cellular immunity and can actually suppress *H. pylori*. Sonja Pettersen, N.M.D., a naturopath practicing in Arizona and one of my favorite doctors, explains: "By maintaining good gut flora, you'll prevent all kinds of different diseases, especially chronic degenerative ones. Probiotics (live cultures) help control inflammation, which is a central feature of so many degenerative diseases, including heart disease. Probiotics help increase NK (natural killer) cells, a powerful immune system weapon. They increase antibodies when we have infections. They improve digestion. They have anticancer properties." Probiotics are abundant in naturally fermented sauerkraut.

Cabbage Phytochemicals Ward Off Breast Cancer

Then there's the cabbage from which sauerkraut comes. Cabbage—a superstar vegetable on its own—first came to the attention of researchers after they observed that women living in Eastern European countries surrounding Poland and Russia and eating four or more servings of raw or barely cooked cabbage per week were 74 percent less likely to develop breast cancer than Polish-American immigrants who ate 1.5 or fewer servings of sauerkraut per week. Researchers now believe that the likely reason for the protective effect were phytochemicals found in cabbage called indoles. Years of research have now demonstrated that these indoles in fact alter estrogen metabolism in a favorable way, one that is likely to reduce the risk of cancer.

The anticancer benefits of cabbage don't stop with indoles, though. In a study published in the October 23, 2002, *Journal of Agricultural and Food Chemistry*, Finnish researchers reported that fermenting cabbage produces compounds known as isothiocyanates, shown in laboratory studies (in test tubes and animals) to prevent the growth of cancer. Sulforaphane, a particularly potent member of the isothiocyanate family, increases the production of certain enzymes known as phase-2 enzymes, which can "disarm" damaging free radicals and help fight carcinogens. It's believed that phase-2 enzymes may reduce the risk of prostate cancer. According to research from the Department of Urology at Stanford University published in *Cancer Epidemiology Biomarkers and Prevention*, sulforaphane is the most potent inducer of phase-2 enzymes of any phytochemical known to date.

The Unique Benefits of Red and Purple Cabbage

Though a lot of sauerkraut is made from white cabbage, some is made from the purple kind, which has a whole other set of protective phytochemicals. Red and purple cabbage is a source of anthocyanins, pigment molecules that make blueberries blue and red cabbage red. They're found in many colorful fruits such as grapes and berries. Turns out they do a lot more than make our produce pretty. Anthocyanins (a member of a group of phytochemicals called flavonoids) have considerable bioactive properties, including acting as powerful antioxidants. In one study, anthocyanins were found to have the strongest antioxidizing power of 150 flavonoids studied (more than 4,000 different flavonoids have been identified). And the anthocyanins in red cabbage were found in another study to protect animals against the damages produced by a known toxin. There's every reason to think that they're equally protective for us.

Anthocyanins' ability to act as antioxidants and to fight free radicals makes them powerful weapons against cardiovascular disease. And anthocyanins are also known for their anti-inflammatory effects. Anti-inflammatory anthocyanins can help dampen allergic reactions as well as help protect against the damage to connective tissue and blood vessel walls that inflammation can cause.

Sauerkraut is also a high-fiber food with a ridiculously low number of calories—1 cup (142 g) of undrained sauerkraut provides almost 6 g of fiber for only 45 calories. It also has 150 percent of the Daily Value for the vitally important bone-building nutrient vitamin K, not to mention generous amounts of calcium, vitamin C, potassium, phosphorus, magnesium, and iron.

The downside of sauerkraut—especially the commercial kind—is that it's really high in sodium (salt). And to make matters worse, most of today's commercially available sauerkraut is pasteurized, making it a "dead" food lacking in the very beneficial bacterial that helped earn it a place of honor on this list. Instead of the good stuff, all you get is a lot of salt. (According to Andrew Weil, M.D., if you rinse and soak sauerkraut in cold water before eating, you can lower the sodium content considerably.) But to get all the health benefits this great traditional food is capable of delivering, look for fresh or raw sauerkraut in the refrigerated sections of natural food stores and in barrels in delicatessens that still make their own. Better yet, make your own!

★ Sea Vegetables

(seaweed)

I once heard a traditional healer say that sea plants are "gifts from the sea." She had a point. There is practically no group of plants on the planet richer in nutrients, minerals, and trace minerals. Coastal peoples all over the world have prized seaweed as a source of valuable nutrients— primarily minerals—for millennia. Sea vegetables have long been acknowledged for their ability to impart beauty and health and to prolong life.

As Paul Pitchford points out in *Healing with Whole Foods: Asian Traditions and Modern Nutrition*, the human body is nourished and cleansed by blood that has almost the same composition as seawater. According to ancient Chinese texts, "there is no swelling that is not relieved by seaweed."

Seaweeds have a number of properties in common, and yet each has a distinct nutrient profile. Let's first talk about them as a group. Seaweeds in general contain dozens and dozens of minerals and trace elements integrated into living plant tissue. They contain vitamins and amino acids and are particularly good sources of iodine, calcium, and iron.

Sea Vegetables Protect against Radiation and Environmental Pollutants

As a group, they are known for their ability to detoxify the body. (It's no coincidence that one of the most popular spa treatments is a seaweed wrap.) Some health professionals feel they can help prevent assimilation of heavy metals such as cadmium as well as other environmental toxins. There's good reason to believe that might be true. Canadian researchers at McGill University in Montreal studied a compound called sodium alginate that is present in strong quantities in brown algae. (Sea vegetables classified as brown algae include arame, hijiki, kombu, and wakame.) In their studies, it was found that sodium alginate (prepared from the sea vegetables kelp, kombu, and other seaweeds) reduced the uptake of radioactive particles into the bone. Sea vegetables appear to be very protective against radiation and environmental pollutants.

Seaweed Eaters Seem to Enjoy Lower Risk of Cancer

Seaweeds have also been studied for their possible anticancer effects. One paper published in *Cancer Chemotherapy and Pharmacology* in 2005 investigated the antitumoral properties of a polysaccharide isolated from a brown marine algae *Sargassum stenophyllum*. And kombu and wakame are particularly rich in a substance called fucoidan, a polysaccharide believed to have anticancer activity. (To get the fucoidan in its effective form, the kombu or wakame needs to be eaten raw or dried, without heating. It's worth noting that in Okinawa, Japan, which has one of the lowest cancer mortality rates in Japan, people eat their kombu mostly uncooked.) Breast cancer rates are lower in Japan than in Western countries, and this just might have something to do with seaweed consumption.

Seaweed is also a great source of fluorine (not fluoride), a compound that boosts the body's defenses and strengthens teeth and bones. However, to get the fluorine you have to consume the seaweed raw— even minimal cooking causes the fluorine to be lost. Seaweed is also a good source of the cancer-fighting mineral selenium.

Separately, each brings its own particular nutrient composition and health benefits to the table.

ARAME

A Japanese sea vegetable with a mild flavor, arame is dried and cut into thin strands and can be added to soups or served sautéed as a vegetable side dish. It contains between 100 and 500 times the iodine in shellfish, plus iron, vitamin A, and more than ten times the calcium of milk.

HIJIKI

This contains the most calcium of any of the sea vegetables and is also a rich source of iron and vitamin A. It's very tough in its natural state; you usually get it dried, but when cooked it rehydrates and expands to about five times its dry volume. Like arame and wakame, hijiki contains more than ten times the calcium of milk. It also contains eight times the iron in beef.

KELP

The kelp family includes kombu, wakame, and arame. It's a rich source of iodine, a component of the two main thyroid hormones T3 (triiodothyronine) and T4 (thyroxine). Kelp can contain between 100 and 500 times the iodine in shellfish, and has about four times the iron in beef.

KOMBU

Kombu can be used for soup stock or added to a pot of beans. It helps the beans cook faster and renders them more digestible. It contains potassium, calcium, vitamins A and C, and between 100 and 500 times the iodine in shellfish. According to natural-foods expert Rebecca Wood, kombu should not be eaten excessively during pregnancy.

NORI

Best known to sushi lovers, nori is the seaweed that wraps around hand rolls. It contains protein, calcium, iron, potassium, and more vitamin A than carrots.

WAKAME

This is good source of protein, iron, calcium, sodium, and other minerals and vitamins. After hijiki, wakame is the seaweed highest in calcium, containing more than ten times the calcium in milk. Like kelp, it also has four times the iron in beef.

WORTH KNOWING

Though tests indicate that seaweeds are abundant in vitamin B_{12}, don't believe it. The B_{12} in plant foods is actually a B_{12} analogue—something that looks like B_{12}, but that is not an effective form of the vitamin. Despite all the other wonderful things they provide, seaweeds—or any other plant foods for that matter—are not a viable source of B_{12}.

 # Sprouts

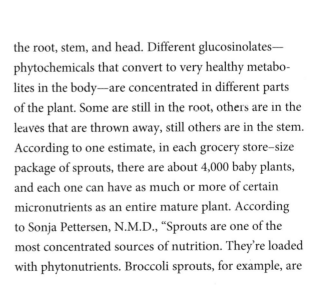

Sprouts are the iconic symbol of what used to be known as "health food." For many people, sprouts conjure up images of granola-eating folks in granny glasses and Birkenstocks wandering around Woodstock and growing organic food. Sprouts. Rabbit food.

Okay, so people make fun of sprouts. But all kidding aside, sprouts are one of the most complete and nutritional foods on the planet. They're rich with enzymes and vitamins and amino acids. And perhaps most important of all, sprouts like alfalfa, broccoli, clover, mung bean, and the like contain concentrated amounts of phytochemicals that can have strong protective effects against disease.

Sprouts Are Baby Plants

When you eat a sprout, you're actually eating a very, very young version of the whole plant. You're eating the root, stem, and head. Different glucosinolates—phytochemicals that convert to very healthy metabolites in the body—are concentrated in different parts of the plant. Some are still in the root, others are in the leaves that are thrown away, still others are in the stem. According to one estimate, in each grocery store–size package of sprouts, there are about 4,000 baby plants, and each one can have as much or more of certain micronutrients as an entire mature plant. According to Sonja Pettersen, N.M.D., "Sprouts are one of the most concentrated sources of nutrition. They're loaded with phytonutrients. Broccoli sprouts, for example, are densely packed with trace minerals, amino acids, and cancer-fighting compounds called indoles (see below). They pack an amazing nutritional wallop."

Researchers at Johns Hopkins University discovered that broccoli sprouts contain anywhere from thirty to fifty times the concentration of protective chemicals found in the mature broccoli plants, including, indole-3-carbinole, one of the cancer-fighting compounds Pettersen was talking about. According to a great deal of research—including a review paper published in *Integrative Cancer Therapies*—indole-3-carbinole arrests human breast cancer cells as well as prostate cancer cells and may lower the risk of hormone-dependent cancers by altering estrogen metabolism. Both broccoli and broccoli sprouts are a significant source of these cancer-fighting indoles.

Broccoli Sprouts Help Our Bodies Fight Carcinogens

In addition, broccoli sprouts are a significant source of sulforaphane. (Two of the experts contributing top ten lists to this book mentioned sulforaphane as one of the important reasons for including broccoli on their lists.) Sulforaphane, a particularly potent member of the isothiocyanate family, increases the production of certain enzymes known as phase-2 enzymes, which can disarm damaging free radicals and help fight carcinogens. It's believed that phase-2 enzymes may reduce the risk of prostate cancer. According to research from the Department of Urology at Stanford University published in *Cancer Epidemiology Biomarkers and Prevention*, sulforaphane is the most potent inducer of phase-2 enzymes of any

WORTH KNOWING

Back in the 1990s, there was a big brouhaha over contamination of sprouts and some outbreaks of foodborne illness in the United States caused by Salmonella or E. coli, which was traceable in some cases to the consumption of raw sprouts. In 2002 the Centers for Disease Control and Prevention (CDC) issued a health advisory warning consumers of the "risks" of eating raw sprouts even though the outbreak was traced to alfalfa sprouts from a single producer, which later issued a voluntary recall and ceased production pending an internal review. Andrew Weil, M.D., a highly respected expert in integrative medicine, weighed in on the side of the CDC, and sprouts fell out of favor for a while. Should you be worried? I think not.

"Sprouts are no different from any other food in the sense that they can harbor bacteria," Sonja Pettersen, N.M.D., told me. "But the 'warnings' on sprouts are based far more on fear than on logic. A potato salad left outside at a picnic probably harbors way more bacteria than the average serving of sprouts." Because of the scare, nonorganic sprout suppliers frequently try to "sanitize" their product by bleaching the seeds from which sprouts grow with chlorine. "It's overkill," said Pettersen. "Chlorine is a very damaging molecule to the human body and much more of a concern than a theoretical exposure to a small amount of bacteria."

Pettersen advocates eating organic sprouts to avoid the chlorine issue altogether. I agree, though I'd probably add that people who are immunocompromised might want to avoid any food that has even a possibility of a little bacteria. For everyone else, sprouts are great. Pettersen summed it up perfectly: "They're as close to a superfood as we have."

phytochemical known to date. In one study, sulfora-phane arrested human colon cancer cells. And feeding sulforaphane-rich broccoli-sprout extracts to lab rats that had been exposed to a carcinogen dramatically reduced the frequency, size, and number of the rats' tumors.

Alfalfa sprouts are a source of another important class of phytochemical, saponins. Saponins are a kind of natural detergent found in a wide variety of plant life, especially beans. Saponins bind with cholesterol, preventing it from being reabsorbed into the system. Studies at the University of Toronto department of nutritional science indicate that dietary sources of saponins such as alfalfa and alfalfa sprouts can be part of a chemopreventive strategy and may lower the risk of human cancers. Interestingly, cancer cells have more cholesterol-type compounds in their mem-branes than normal cells; since saponins can bind cholesterol, they can interfere with cell growth and division. In plants, saponins have a strong effect on the immune system, where they function as a kind of natural antibiotic, and it's more than likely that they have a similar antimicrobial effect in the human body.

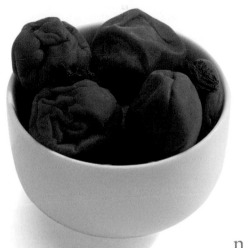

Umeboshi Plums
(umeboshi plum paste)

I first learned about umeboshi plum paste from Annemarie Colbin, Ph.D., the founder of Natural Gourmet Institute for Healing and Culinary Arts and an inter-nationally respected expert in natural foods and healing. One summer we were both speaking at the renowned Boulderfest conference for nutritional medicine, and I attended her fascinating presentation on healing foods, during which she explained that foods have expansive and contractive properties and that certain expansive conditions—such as sugar addiction and crav-ings—could be treated with contractive foods. The contractive food she mentioned most frequently was this umeboshi plum paste, which I could barely pronounce and had never heard of. She later told me she never travels without it and offered to give me some.

Sure enough, it was not only delicious but also had a remarkable dampening effect on my desire to go out and buy a pint of Ben & Jerry's. The word "umeboshi" means dried plum, but it's actually a species of apricot. It's been used as a food and medicine in China, Korea, and Japan.

Umeboshi plums are basically pickled plums. The freshly picked plums are first washed and then dried by the sun on rice mats. The plums are also left out during the night. At that time, dew forms and softens the plums. The next day the sun again dries them, and the process is repeated for several days. As a result, the plums become smaller, and many wrinkles appear.

At that time, the plums are packed in barrels together with white crude sea salt and sometimes the herb perilla, which is high in iron, acts as a natural preservative, and imparts the pinkish color to the plums. The plums are covered by weights and are left to ferment. Though in modern times they may only ferment for a few days and nights, in the traditional methods they could be left to ferment for a full year. During fermentation—through the action of salt and the pressure of the weights—the plums begin to shrink even more, and whatever juice is left is drained out. The result is the umeboshi plum.

Umeboshi Plums Are Aspirin and Apple to Those in the Far East

Umeboshi plums are an ancient Japanese food used to balance and strengthen. They're highly valued for their antibacterial properties and as a digestive aid. Japanese food authority Robbie Swinnerton writes, "Japanese pickled plums have remarkable medicinal qualities. Their powerful acidity has a paradoxical alkalinizing effect on the body, neutralizing fatigue, stimulating the digestion, and promoting the elimination of toxins. This is the Far Eastern equivalent to both aspirin and apple; not only is it a potent hangover remedy for mornings after, (but) an umeboshi a day is regarded as the best preventive medicine available."

And by the way—next time you have a serious sugar craving, try dipping a chopstick or a pinky into a jar of the paste and licking it off. Remarkable stuff!

Wheat Germ

I'll tell you right now, I'm not a huge fan of wheat. As you may have noticed, it didn't make the list of the 150 healthiest foods in the world. (It wasn't even on the list of contenders.) Wheat germ is the nutrient-rich core of a whole wheat kernel. And while it does have some things to recommend it—see below—it still contains gluten and needs to be completely avoided by those with celiac, and probably by those with any kind of gluten intolerance as well.

First, some definitions. Any whole grain consists of four main components. The husk, or chaff, is the inedible outer layer of a grain kernel. That generally gets thrown away. The bran is the main source of fiber in whole grains and can also contain nutrients. (Much of the bran gets removed during the processing of refined carbohydrate cereals, including those that sound healthy.) The endosperm is the main content of a whole grain; it contains protein and starch and is basically the only portion used in refined and processed grain products. And finally, there's the germ: the smallest portion of the grain, rich in vitamins, minerals, and fiber.

So wheat germ is pretty much the best part of a whole wheat kernel. Though it makes up only about 3 percent of the whole wheat berry, nutritionally it's the motherlode. It's rich in vitamin E, zinc, iron, fiber, magnesium, phosphorus, potassium, thiamin, folate, vitamin B$_6$, manganese, and selenium. A ¼ cup (28 g) of wheat germ contain 104 calories, more than 6 g of protein, a little more than 2 g of healthy fat, and almost 4 g of fiber.

The oil in wheat germ is also a source of a compound called octacosanol, which used to be a hot performance supplement back in the 1990s but has pretty much faded from view because it doesn't work. While there are a couple of animal studies suggesting that octacosanol might help with exercise performance, there aren't any human studies, and I think octacosanol as a supplement is overhyped. Octacosanol aside, wheat germ is still a nutritional powerhouse. But because it's high in oil (good oil, but still oil), it can easily go rancid if it's not stored properly. A jar of vacuum-packed wheat germ is fine for up to a year,

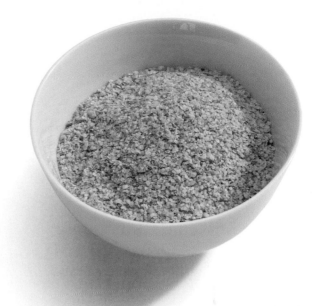

unopened, but opened jars should be refrigerated and used within a few months. If you're someone who uses flour in recipes, consider replacing ½ to a whole cup (64 to 125 g) of it with wheat germ to increase both fiber and nutrients.

Wheat germ has a nice nutty flavor and a crunchy texture and is great in shakes or sprinkled on all kinds for things, from cereal to yogurt. The main reason I don't recommend it more often, or talk about it more glowingly, is because of the gluten. And although I recognize that the majority of people are not technically gluten intolerant, I still think gluten offers zero benefits to anyone—the absolute best thing you could possibly say about it is that it's neutral for some people. For many others—including a large number of people who are unaware that gluten's to blame for many of their symptoms—gluten is bad news. It's pro-inflammatory, offers absolutely zero health benefits, and should be avoided.

★ Whey Protein Powder

Whey protein is hands down my favorite form of protein powder. Not only does it provide extremely high-quality protein, but it has a host of health benefits besides. It can help you lose weight and gain muscle, plus it provides powerful support for your immune system.

I'll assume you already know how important protein is to the body in general, but a quick review: Protein provides the building blocks for hormones and neurotransmitters and antibodies, not to mention being necessary for strong muscles and bones. It is essential for metabolism. Without protein, you would die. (The same is not true of dietary carbohydrate, but that's a whole different story.)

Whey Protein Stimulates the Immune System and Helps Generate a Valuable Antioxidant

On one level, whey protein is just another way to get high-quality protein into the diet and can take its place on the menu along with grass-fed beef and game, fish and eggs, and other protein sources. But whey protein powder has other properties—besides convenience—that make it valuable. It is highly stimulating to the immune system. Whey protein seems to be the best method for obtaining the building blocks of glutathione, arguably the most valuable antioxidant in the body. Glutathione is a master antioxidant—it destroys free radicals and is intimately involved in the detoxification of carcinogens. The white blood cells and the liver use glutathione to detoxify poisons in the body.

Unfortunately, it's been difficult if not impossible to absorb glutathione from the diet or from supplements*. The glutathione in your cells needs to be made by the body, and the best way to do this is to provide the body with the amino acids that glutathione is made from. Whey protein powder has been found to be one of the richest sources of these glutathione building blocks.

Whey protein contains a number of other proteins that positively affect immune function. It contains protein fractions such as beta-lactoglobulin, alpha-lactalbumin, and immunoglobulins, all of which have important disease-fighting effects. In one study done at the department of food science and technology at Ohio State University, it was shown that dietary whey protein protected against oxidant-induced cell death in human prostate cells. Several other animal studies have suggested that whey protein may protect against certain kinds of tumors. A study in the *American Journal of Clinical Nutrition* suggested that whey protein rich in alpha-lactalbumin improved cognitive performance in "stress-vulnerable" subjects (a description that would probably include everyone I know). And in a double-blind, randomized, placebo-controlled trial, doctors from the University of Minnesota Medical School gave otherwise healthy individuals with mild to moderate hypertension 20 g daily of whey protein and observed a significant reduction in their blood pressure levels by the end of the first week. That effect was maintained throughout the study.

Whey and the High-Protein Diet

And then there's weight loss. Quite a few studies suggest that whey may have an impact on food intake through its effect on hormones that influence a feeling of fullness. We already know from quite a lot of research that generally speaking, higher-protein diets help people feel full and satisfied and are very useful as weight loss regimens. But all protein may not be created equal. In one study, researchers consumed a liquid meal containing equal amounts of either whey or casein. Ninety minutes later, allowed to eat freely at a buffet, the whey group consumed significantly fewer calories. Whey protein powder may well be a great tool in the battle to control appetite naturally.

Recently, researchers set up another study to see if whey protein had any special advantage over other sources of protein. They took 48 overweight diabetics and put them into one of three groups. One group had a high-protein breakfast using whey protein, one had a high-protein breakfast using other sources of protein (such as eggs, fish, or soy) and a third group had a high-carb breakfast. Calories were kept the same for all three groups.

The researchers were most interested in what's known as glycolated hemoglobin, or hemoglobin A1C. The A1C test is a kind of long-term measurement of blood sugar, and it is usually used to diagnose diabetes. An A1C level of 5.7 or lower is considered normal; 6.5 or higher gets you a diagnosis of diabetes, while 5.7–6.4 is generally considered prediabetes. In this study, the whey protein group saw the most significant reduction in their A1C levels over the course of almost two years of follow-up. The whey protein group also had the greatest reduction in blood sugar spikes.

"The whey protein diet significantly suppresses the hunger hormone ghrelin," lead study author Daniela Jakubowicz, M.D., told *Science Daily*, in an article published April 2, 2016. "A whey protein drink is easily prepared and provides the advantages of a high-protein breakfast on weight loss, reduction of hunger, glucose spikes and A1C." (The study was presented at the 2016 annual meeting of the Endocrine Society in Boston.)

The benefits of whey have been known for centuries. Thanks to journalist and health reporter Will Brink, I found this wonderful aphorism dating from about 1777 that says the following: "If everyone were raised on whey, doctors would be bankrupt" (Allevato con la scotta il dottore e in bancarott). And that wasn't the first time the health properties of whey were appreciated. According to an expression from Florence, Italy, around 1650, "Chi vuol viver sano e lesto beve scotta e cena presto," which in beautiful Italian means simply this: "If you want to live a healthy and active life, drink whey and dine early."

Collagen Protein Powder

Collagen is the most abundant protein in our bodies. It's found in skin, hair, muscles, tendons, bones—you name it. Lately, collagen supplements have become, as they say, a thing.

So what's the deal? And what's the difference between collagen supplements for the skin or joints, and actual collagen protein powder?

There are at least sixteen different types of collagen, but 80 to 90 percent of the collagen in the body consists of types l, 2, and 3 (Lodish, et al, *Molecular Cell Biology*, 4th edition, 2002). Collagen 1 and 3—which are almost always found together—are mainly in skin. Collagen 2 is mainly in joints, although recent evidence shows it helps the skin as well. That's not a surprise for many reasons, one of which is that the main manufacturer of collagen 2 mixes in about 10 percent hyaluronic acid in their formula, a compound well-known to improve both skin hydration and elasticity. All the collagens and the structures they form all serve the same purpose: to help tissues withstand stretching.

Years ago, we were taught that collagen supplements weren't well absorbed when taken orally, but we now know that's not true—at least not when you're using high-quality collagen supplements. One ingredient manufacturer—Verisol—makes a Collagen 1 and 3 that has been tested in studies. In one study, 114 women aged 45 to 65 were randomized to receive either placebo or 2.5 grams of Verisol once daily for eight weeks. The Verisol group had a statistically significant (20 percent) reduction of eye wrinkle volume compared to the placebo group. A second study, by the same researchers, tested collagen and found it showed a statistically significant improvement in skin elasticity.

Then there's collagen 2. The most respected ingredient manufacturer of collagen 2 is a company called BioCell. A 2015 study at the Center for Applied Health Sciences in Ohio, tested the effects of 3 grams a day of BioCell collagen in a study aimed to evaluate indices of recovery from intense exercise. The researchers looked at three blood markers of muscle tissue damage and found that the people taking BioCell collagen had "a more robust muscular recovery and adaptive response." For collagen supplements, my recommendation is Reserveage Collagen Replenish for skin—which is all Verisol type 1 and 3 collagen— or Reserveage Collagen Booster for joints, which is all type 2 BioCell collagen with hyaluronic acid and chondroitin. I use both every day.

Which brings us to collagen protein powder.

While collagen supplements are a great way to get support for skin and bones, there's recently been a trend toward high-quality collagen protein powders, which offer a much greater dose of the collagen peptides found in the above-mentioned supplements. They're rich in amino acids that are important in building joint cartilage. Clinical studies suggest that 10 grams a day of pharmaceutical-grade collagen reduces pain in patients with osteoarthritis of the knee or hip. One published review concluded that "Collagen hydrolysate is of interest as a therapeutic agent of potential utility in the treatment of osteoarthritis and osteoporosis," adding that "its high level of safety makes it attractive as an agent for long-term use in these chronic disorders." A 24-week long study in 2008, showed improvement of joint pain in athletes who were treated with the dietary supplement collagen hydrolysate.

I think collagen protein is a very promising protein powder that could work well as a high-quality protein source. Several companies make high-quality collagen protein powders. There's not nearly as much research on collagen protein powder as there is on whey, so for the time being, whey protein powder remains my go-to protein powder.

But I consider collagen protein an excellent choice and often use it instead of whey just for variety. It might be a particularly good choice for those who are extremely sensitive to dairy.

Specialty Food Runner-Up

Brewer's Yeast

In the old days when the only people who ate yogurt or organic foods were known as health nuts, before gyms became known as fitness facilities, and before every supermarket had a natural food department with a dizzying array of energy bars, there were only a few supplements and powders that fitness enthusiasts used regularly. One of them was brewer's yeast.

Well, times have changed, fitness has become mainstream, and the menu of supplements, powders, bars, and things to throw into your protein shake has expanded exponentially, but brewer's yeast still occupies a warm spot in the heart of many of those early health nuts.

Brewer's yeast consists of the dried, pulverized cells of *Saccharomyces cerevisiae*, a type of fungus. It's inactive yeast, meaning the yeasts have been killed and have no leavening powder (nor can they create or promote yeast infections, because they're essentially dead). But before the yeast were inactivated, they sucked up a lot of B-vitamins and minerals (such as chromium and selenium) and they continue to have those vitamins and minerals in their deactivated form. That's the main selling point of Brewer's yeast.

Brewer's yeast also contains beta-glucans, which are sugars that line the cell walls of certain fungi and bacteria and certain plants like oats. These beta-glucans are strong modulators of the immune system and may even help stave off the common cold.

Because Brewer's yeast is a good source of B vitamins, people often think it's a good vegetarian source of B_{12}. It's not. Brewer's yeast does not naturally contain any B_{12}, despite what you read to the contrary. (Some manufacturers fortify their yeast with B_{12} to make up for this absence, but most do not.)

According to the Physicians' Desk Reference for Supplements, high-selenium brewer's yeast may have anticarcinogenic activity and high-chromium brewer's yeast has putative antidiabetic activity. The PDR also notes that "beta-glucans in yeast also support the immune system."

WORTH KNOWING

Brewer's yeast fell out of favor largely because better ways of obtaining higher-dose chromium became available (supplements) and because so many people have chronic yeast problems and were afraid of it, even though the yeast is inactive and not related to the *Candida albicans* fungus can cause yeast infection. Brewer's yeast can cause lots of gas in some people. Nonetheless, if you do not have yeast problems (candida) and would like an easily digestible way to get extra B vitamins, amino acids, and minerals, brewer's yeast is a fine food. Look for varieties that contain chromium and selenium.

THE EXPERTS' TOP TEN LISTS

Josh Axe, D.N.M., D.C., C.N.S.

Josh Axe is one of the most trusted and beloved natural medicine gurus I know. His website, draxe.com, is the second most visited natural health website in the world and has more than 10 million monthly visitors. He's a certified doctor of natural medicine (DNM), a chiropractic physician, and a board certified clinical nutritionist. He's also the author of the *New York Times* bestseller *Eat Dirt*.

1. **Bone broth:** I have found bone broth to be the number 1 food you can consume to treat leaky gut syndrome, overcome food intolerances and allergies, and improve joint health and boost immunity.

2. **Dandelion greens:** Dandelion greens are high in fiber, vitamins C and B_6, thiamin, riboflavin, calcium iron, potassium, and manganese. You can also use the root, stem, and flowers to make a delicious and super-healthy tea, which is great for liver detoxification and for healthy skin.

3. **Chicken liver:** Liver is one of the most nutrient-dense superfoods on the planet. It's high in vitamin B_{12} and a fantastic source of iron, vitamin A, phosphorus, and magnesium.

4. **Broccoli:** Broccoli consumption has been shown to help prevent cancer, benefit heart health, improve digestion, and much more.

5. **Salmon:** When it's wild-caught (not farmed), salmon is one of the most nutritious foods we can consume. Not only does it contain a high amount of omega-3 fatty acids, but it's also packed with many other vitamins and minerals.

6. **Blueberries:** Blueberries combat aging, contain substances that are neuro-protective, promote heart health, and benefit the skin. They're also loaded with gallic acid, a powerful antifungal/antiviral agent that's also an antioxidant.

7. **Sauerkraut:** Sauerkraut combines one of the healthiest foods (cabbage) with one of the most beneficial and time-honored food preparation methods ever used (fermentation).

8. **Coconut:** Coconut oil might just be the most versatile health food on the planet. It is my favorite cooking oil, and it can be used as a form of natural medicine, for natural beauty treatments, and more.

9. **Cilantro:** Cilantro has many known healing properties. The vitamin K and calcium content of cilantro helps to build strong bones, teeth, and hair.

10. **Chia seeds:** The chia seed is nutrient dense and packs a punch of energy boosting power. Aztec warriors ate chia seeds to give them high energy and endurance.

SPECIALTY FOODS

CHAPTER 11

BEVERAGES

The best beverage in the world, bar none, is water.

You can't live very long without it, and it's necessary for almost every metabolic process. But that doesn't mean there aren't other beverages that are amazing for your health. There are. And nine of them (ten if you include water) are portrayed in depth in this section of this book.

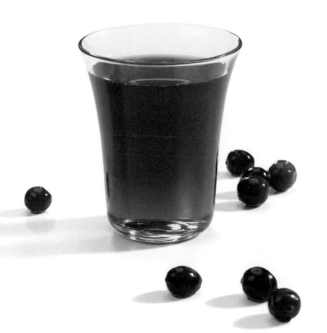

Given that beverages don't grow on trees or come out of the ground, every beverage, by definition, is made from something else (like a plant or a fruit). If I may be frank, one of the difficulties in picking foods and beverages for this book had to do with the following dilemma: When does the source of a beverage (for example, apples) get its own entry, when does the juice made from the source (e.g., apple juice) get its own entry, and when do both get their own entries. (Similar dilemmas existed for oils—e.g., olives vs. olive oil—and nuts—e.g., peanuts vs. peanut butter.) Here's how I tried to solve the problem.

Why Some Fruit and Vegetable Juices Aren't Included

If a fruit—or a vegetable or a plant—was extremely healthy in one form but not so great in another, processed form, I included the one that had the most health benefits and left the other out. Apples are a great example. The fruit itself is a nutritional power-house. The commonly available processed juice sold in supermarkets is a disaster, typically containing about 24 g of sugar in a 1 cup (235 ml) serving. On the other hand, cranberries are a great fruit and are on the list, but so is real, unsweetened cranberry juice, which retains many of the nutritional benefits of the berries (other than the fiber). Therefore, both cran-berries and cranberry juice are listed.

Then there were the exotic berries—noni, acai, and goji. Here the results were inconsistent. Noni berries are impossible to find outside Brazil and taste terrible—but the juice is a nutritional powerhouse. Solution? Noni juice is on the list; the berries are not.

Similarly with acai berries. Goji berries, on the other hand, are easy to find in health food stores and are loaded with nutrients. The juice is perfectly good as well, but way overhyped (and overpriced); hence goji berries yes, goji juice, regrettably, no.

Beverages That Deserve Their Own Entry

The rest of the beverages presented no such dual per-sonality problems. The only way to consume tea is to drink it; same with coffee. Wine, though it comes from grapes (which got their own entry), has proper-ties of its own and in any case has a whole different personality than the fruit it comes from. It deserved its very own entry.

So there you have it—the beverage "system." It's imperfect, and certainly inelegant, but it's the one I came up with and seemed the best solution to a dif-ficult problem.

Drink up and enjoy!

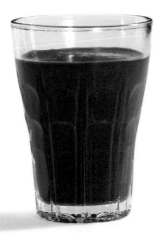

Acai Berry Juice

Acai berries grow on an Amazon palm tree and have been prized by Brazilian natives for hun-dreds of years for their ability to provide a sense of strength and energy and a high nutritional content. The juice tastes like an interesting blend of berries and chocolate.

The acai berry got the best public relations boost any food could possibly hope for when Nicholas Perricone, M.D., picked it as one of his ten top antiag-ing superfoods and it was subsequently featured on *Oprah*, giving this little Brazilian native instant celeb-rity. Does it deserve the hype? The answer is a quali-

fied maybe. I'd never call the acai berry one of the ten top antiaging foods on the planet. But put the acai berry into a search engine and you'll find no short-age of ringing endorsements and glowing testimoni-als about its powerful health benefits. Unfortunately, most of these come from companies that are marketing acai berry juice. That doesn't mean there isn't great stuff in this berry—there is. But it does mean that you should take the hype with a lot more than a grain or two of salt.

Acai Berry Juice Protects Blood Vessels and the Nervous System

There are potential benefits with acai berries. The berry is rich in antioxidants, and also very rich in anthocyanins, a class of flavonoids that have extremely high antioxidant activity and can reduce inflammation and protect blood vessels and the nervous system, including the brain. The berry contains a rich diversity of polyphenols, plant compounds that may reduce the risk of cardiovascular disease and cancer.

When this book was originally published, there were no human trials on acai, although the test tube research was definitely promising. One study in the *Journal of Agricultural and Food Chemistry* showed that extracts from acai berries triggered a self-destruct response in up to 86 percent of leukemia cells in a test tube. But the absence of studies showing that the acai antioxidants were actually absorbed in humans was a problem.

That's no longer the case. Just a year after the original publication of this book, Susanne Talcott and Stephen Talcott, co-researchers at Texas A&M University's nutrition and food science department, published work showing that the healthful compounds in acai juice and pulp are indeed absorbed by the human body.

"Acai is naturally low in sugar, and the flavor is described as a mixture of red wine and chocolate," Susanne Talcott told *Science Daily*, adding "what more would you want from a fruit?"

Aloe Vera Juice

Aloe vera has been recognized for centuries for its remarkable health-enhancing and medicinal properties. It's used in traditional Indian medicine for constipation, colic, skin diseases, worm infestation, and infections; in Chinese medicine for fungal overgrowth; in Trinidad and Tobago for hypertension; and among Mexican Americans for type 2 diabetes. That doesn't mean that it's effective in every one of those situations. But, to my mind, when a substance is believed to have medicinal properties by multiple cultures who have used it for thousands of years, there's probably something to it.

Although known specifically for external application to the skin, aloe juice is also widely used to help a variety of conditions of the digestive tract. And research shows aloe vera to be beneficial for skin conditions, management of burn and wound healing, constipation, diabetes, and gastrointestinal disorders. Aloe is thought to have originated in the Sudan and the Arabian Peninsula. Today, it's cultivated and found in the wild in Africa, the Near East, Asia, and the southern Mediterranean. It's also cultivated in subtropical regions of the United States and Mexico, in the coastal regions of Venezuela, and on the Dutch Antilles.

There are more than 240 species of aloe, and they grow throughout the world. A member of the lily family of plants, aloe has a decided cactuslike appearance. Of the 240 or so species, only four are recognized as having significant nutritional value, with *Aloe barbadensis* miller being the leader. It is used the most in commercial products today that contain aloe. The aloe leaf contains at least seventy-five nutrients and more than 200 active compounds, including twenty minerals, twenty of the twenty-two necessary amino acids, and twelve vitamins.

Aloe Vera Juice Contains Healing Glyconutrients

According to H.R. McDaniel, M.D., who has spent sixteen years exploring the therapeutic nature of aloe, its active ingredients are eight sugars that form the eight essential saccharides: glucose, galactose, mannose, fructose, xylose, N-acetylglucosamine, N-acetylgalactosamine, and N-acetylneuraminic acid. The mannose molecules join together to form a kind of starch (polysaccharide) known by a variety of names: acemannan, acetylated polymannans, polymannose, or APM. The natural sugars of aloe should never be confused with sucrose—common table sugar. The sugars in glyconutrients are not sweet to the taste nor do they elicit a blood glucose or insulin rush. In fact, entire books have been written about the healing and medicinal properties of glyconutrients (see, for example, *Sugars That Heal* by Emil Mondoa, M.D.).

Another compound in aloe, aloeride, contains the essential sugars glucose, galactose, and mannose, as well as another sugar called arabinose.

The gel has the active medicinal sugars and other nutrients listed above. Most of the research on aloe vera has been done on the gel, but there's good reason to suspect that the juice—if it is unrefined or unfiltered—contains a lot of good properties as well. After all, the medicinal part of the plant is the dried juice of the leaves.

Aloe Reduces Inflammation and Speeds Healing

The gel has been shown to reduce inflammation and also shows antibacterial effects. Inside the leaf is this clear, thin, jellylike substance that works great as a skin salve. Applied to the skin, it's a mild anesthetic and relieves itching, swelling, and pain. An animal-based study in the *Journal of the American Podiatric Medical Association* found that both oral and topical aloe preparations speed wound healing. Animals were given either aloe (100 mg/kg body weight) in their drinking water for two months or 25 percent aloe vera cream applied directly to wounds for six days. Aloe had positive effects in both cases. The size of wounds decreased 62 percent in the animals taking oral aloe compared to a 51 percent decrease in the control group. Topical aloe produced a 51 percent decrease in wound size compared to a 33 percent decrease in the control group.

Aloe decreases surgical recovery time, according to a report in the *Journal of Dermatologic Surgery and Oncology*. Eighteen acne patients underwent facial dermabrasion surgery, in which lesions are scraped away. Dressings were applied to their faces, with half of each person's face receiving the standard dressing coated with surgical gel, and the other half with aloe added to this dressing. The half of the face treated with aloe healed approximately seventy-two hours faster than the other side. Dermatologist James Fulton, M.D., of Newport Beach, California, principal author of the report, uses topical aloe in his practice to speed wound healing. "Any wound we treat, whether it's suturing a cut or removing a skin cancer, heals better with aloe vera on it," he states.

Aloe Vera Juice Eases Internal Inflammation

The juice is also believed to have anti-inflammatory action in the digestive system and is often used for heartburn and to ease constipation. Aloe vera juice can be effective for treating inflammatory bowel disease, according to a study in the *Journal of Alternative Medicine*. Ten patients were given 2 ounces (60 ml) of aloe juice, three times daily, for seven days. After one week, all patients were cured of diarrhea, four had improved bowel regularity, and three reported increased energy.

Researchers concluded that aloe was able to rebalance the intestines by "regulating gastrointestinal pH while improving gastrointestinal motility, increasing stool specific gravity, and reducing populations of certain fecal microorganisms, including yeast." Other studies have shown that aloe vera juice helps detoxify the bowel, neutralize stomach acidity, and relieve constipation and gastric ulcers.

According to juice authority Steve Meyerowitz, aloe vera juice contains a wealth of vitamins, miner-als, and nutrients including B_1, B_2, B_3, B_6, C, choline, calcium, copper, manganese, potassium, silicon, and others. But, also according to Meyerowitz, the real uniqueness of the juice lies in its wealth of phytochemicals such as the organic acids chrysophanic, salicylic, succinic, and uric; polysaccharides such as acemannen; enzymes such as glutathione peroxidase; and various resins.

Here are four steps that should help you when you shop for a good-quality aloe vera juice:

Avoid products that put aloe vera through unnecessary and damaging processes such as heating, boiling, freeze-drying, etc.

Look for the International Aloe Science Council seal of approval. Check its website at www.iasc.org to make sure the product is not carrying the seal fraudulently—sad to say, many companies do just that. Make sure the label says the product is a juice or a gel—together with the seal this tells you the product is 95 percent or more aloe vera.

Check the ingredients to make sure aloe vera is the first ingredient, not water or a sugary filler.

Look at the color. It should be similar to fresh-squeezed grapefruit juice.

Coffee

Coffee is one of the entries in the first edition of this book that I decided to re-evaluate this edition. It wasn't so much the substantial amount of research that's been done on coffee in the last ten years, though that was certainly a part of it. It was because coffee is such a good example of how small, incremental changes in our knowledge can slowly increase and deepen our understanding and change the conventional wisdom on a given food.

Back in 2007, coffee was still lumped with alcohol, sugar, and saturated fat as one of the things in our diet we would all be better off without. To this day, you still hear people talking about "detoxing" from caffeine and alcohol. And back in 2007, there weren't many of us defending America's most popular drug. *New Scientist* magazine reported that 90 percent of North Americans consume caffeine on a daily basis, making coffee officially the most widely used legal, psychoactive substance in the world.

So here's how I started the entry on coffee for the original edition of *The 150 Healthiest Foods on Earth*:

If you're surprised to find coffee on the list of the world's healthiest foods, you're not alone. To tell you the truth, so was I.

I went on to say that while I had always suspected that coffee wasn't all that bad for you, I was happy to see that it was actually on the top ten lists of a few of my very forward-thinking experts. And that the research on coffee was promising.

I pointed out that there were things about coffee that I found troubling—like the well-known ability of caffeine to cause nervousness and jitters and interfere with sleep. There was even a study or two showing an association with higher blood pressure.

But that was then.

Now consider this, the opening paragraph of an article about coffee in the June 15, 2016, *New York Times*, almost ten years to the day from when I first submitted the original manuscript:

An influential panel of experts convened by the World Health Organization concluded on Wednesday that regularly drinking coffee could protect against at least two types of cancer, a decision that followed decades of research pointing to the beverage's many health benefits.

Coffee is one of those iconic foods—like butter, or eggs—that nutritionists always seem to be changing their minds about. How often do you read articles that bemoan the fickleness of my profession with statements like, "First they said coffee (or eggs, or butter) was good, then they said it was bad, then they said it was good again—why can't they make up their minds?"

Why indeed. Let's take a look at what's happened with coffee over the past decade or so.

"I'm detoxing from caffeine, alcohol, and sugar . . . "

Although many people lump caffeine in with all the bad stuff they have to detox from, the emerging and extensive research on coffee suggests that our favorite morning drink may have gotten a bad rap. One study shows that those drinking six or more cups a day are significantly less likely to have diabetes. Studies show that folks who drink the most coffee have significantly lower risk of getting the disease, with risk reduction ranging from 23 percent to a whopping 67 percent.

A study—in the 2006 *Journal of Cardiac Failure*—showed that caffeine increases exercise tolerance in patients with heart failure. Other studies have shown it increases alertness and improves mental and physical performance in the short run. According to the Nurses' Health Study, two or three cups a day may lower the incidence of Parkinson's and decrease gallstone formation in men. A study in the *Archives of Internal Medicine* showed that coffee may protect against alcoholic liver disease—for every cup (235 ml) of java (up to four a day) the study charted about a 20 percent reduction in risk of alcoholic cirrhosis.

And if all that weren't enough, there are studies showing that coffee drinkers have a lower risk for Alzheimer's than non-coffee drinkers. Plus, of course, the aforementioned findings of the World Health Organization that regular coffee drinking protects against at least two types of cancer, a finding that echoed the World Cancer Research Fund International finding that coffee protects against multiple types of cancer.

Coffee, the Brain, and Fat Loss

The caffeine in coffee is the reason you feel more energy after drinking it, but do you know why that happens? Well, there's a chemical in your brain called *adenosine* that basically tells you to relax and calm down. Technically, adenosine is called an inhibitory neurotransmitter. It's a neurotransmitter because it sends (transmits) a message in your brain (neuro), and it's inhibitory because that message is to inhibit excitement. Adenosine has little "parking spaces" in the brain (called receptors), but caffeine jumps into those parking spaces like a bad-mannered driver on a New York City street. Once caffeine occupies the adenosine receptors, adenosine can't get in to transmit its message "hey dude, you're tired, relax and take a load off!" Hence, you keep going and (sometimes) you aren't even aware of how tired you really are!

When you use caffeine to mask your exhaustion, that's not a good thing. Not everyone does that—at least not to the point where it would cause problems. A lot of studies show that coffee helps memory, mood, reaction time, and even athletic performance.

And for those who still remain skeptical, consider this: coffee helps you burn fat. At least two studies show that caffeine can boost your metabolic rate by between 3 to 11 percent, and other studies show that caffeine increases fat burning by up to 10 percent in obese folks and an even more impressive 29 percent in lean people. The caffeine actually makes your fat cells break down fat, releasing fatty acids into the bloodstream to be used for energy. Of course, if you're just sitting around all day, those fatty acids won't do you much good, but if you're exercising, the availability of that fat for fuel is a good thing.

Coffee Has More Antioxidant Activity Than Cocoa or Tea

Coffee increases antioxidants in the blood, what scientists call *plasma antioxidant capacity*. In one study, researchers in Italy gave a standard amount (200 ml) of brewed coffee to ten healthy, nonsmoking, moderate coffee drinkers and found that it produced a 5.5 percent increase in plasma antioxidant capacity that was mostly maintained after two hours. Even more impressive, a study in the *Journal of Agriculture and Food Chemistry* in 2001 found that coffee has significantly more total antioxidant activity than either cocoa, green tea, black tea, or herbal tea. Another study in the *Journal of Nutrition* in 2004 looked at the dietary records of 2,672 Norwegian adults and concluded—much to the surprise of the researchers themselves—that coffee was the single greatest contributor to their total antioxidant intake.

Meanwhile, a study published in 2006 consisting of a cohort of 41,836 postmenopausal women concluded that "consumption of coffee, a major source of dietary antioxidants, may inhibit inflammation and therefore reduce the risk of cardiovascular disease and other inflammatory diseases in postmenopausal women." Of course, that study was on a specific subgroup of the population—postmenopausal women—and caution would dictate that we shouldn't necessarily extrapolate the results to the general population. Still, taken as a whole, the evidence for the antioxidant capacity of coffee is compelling at the very least.

Two of the antioxidants responsible for coffee's health benefits are chlorogenic acid and caffeic acid. Both are strong antioxidants, and coffee beans are one of the richest dietary sources of chlorogenic acid in the world. It's been estimated that coffee drinkers might ingest as much as 1 g of chlorogenic acid and 500 mg of caffeic acid on a daily basis. For many people, coffee supplies as much as 70 percent of the total amount of their dietary intake of these important antioxidants.

The Big Reveal: Coffee and Genetics

In the past, we puzzled over the fact that some people were able to drink a double espresso before bed and sleep like a baby while others would get nervous and jittery after a single cup in the morning. But this puzzle may soon be less puzzling: Scientists have identified a number of genes that influence your reaction to caffeine. One gene, for example, encodes for a liver enzyme that is essential for metabolizing caffeine. Another is consistently linked to higher coffee intakes. Apparently some people are fast metabolizers of caffeine and able to consume more of it with no ill effects, while others—like the guy who is jittery all day from one cup of morning java—metabolize caffeine slowly, meaning it stays in their systems longer. Lesson learned: everybody's different.

So if you're someone who can't sleep soundly through the night because you're too wired, you should probably cut back on coffee, or stop drinking it in the early afternoon. But if you're someone who does just fine with caffeine, there's no reason whatsoever to cut it out. Not only does it give you a nice little legal buzz of alertness, but it has multiple health benefits.

WORTH KNOWING

On the negative side—and this is why research is so confusing to so many—one study showed that high doses of chlorogenic acid (about twice what a coffee drinker might ingest) given on a daily basis raises blood levels of homocysteine by 12 percent. Homocysteine is a nasty inflammatory molecule that is believed to be a risk factor for cardiovascular disease. (Just for the record, in the same study, the equivalent of two liters a day of black tea also increased homocysteine by virtually the same amount.) But both coffee and black tea are loaded with antioxidants, and virtually every scientific reference on the subject suggests that chlorogenic acid might actually contribute to the prevention of cardiovascular disease. At this time, it appears to me that moderate coffee consumption has more in its favor than against it.

Cranberry Juice

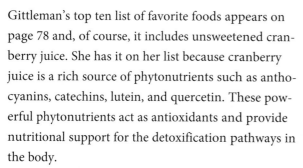

Ann Louise Gittleman, Ph.D., C.N.S., is one of our best-known nutritionists and the author of more than a dozen books. In fact, she's fondly known in America as "the first lady of nutrition." Anyone who's read her work knows that she's a huge fan of unsweetened cranberry juice. Her famous Fat Flush plan relies on copious amounts of cran-water, which is a mix of the unsweetened juice diluted with fresh water in a 1:8 ratio. Fat Flushers drink this stuff all day long.

Gittleman's top ten list of favorite foods appears on page 78 and, of course, it includes unsweetened cranberry juice. She has it on her list because cranberry juice is a rich source of phytonutrients such as anthocyanins, catechins, lutein, and quercetin. These powerful phytonutrients act as antioxidants and provide nutritional support for the detoxification pathways in the body.

Gittleman is certainly right about the rich phytonutrient content of both cranberries and cranberry juice. In one study, biochemist Yuegang Zuo, Ph.D., from the University of Massachusetts–Dartmouth, showed cranberry juice cocktail had the highest total phenol content of the twenty fruit juices tested. Phenolic compounds are natural antioxidants that help neutralize harmful free radicals in the body that are thought to be linked to most chronic diseases, including cancer, heart disease, and diabetes. The researchers state that "cranberry has the highest radical-scavenging capacity among these different fruits studied." In a second study, Catherine Neto, Ph.D.,

assistant professor at the University of Massachusetts–Dartmouth, isolated several bioactive compounds from whole cranberries and found that the flavonoids showed strong antioxidant activity, and newly discovered compounds in the berries were toxic to a variety of cancer tumor cells. "The tumor cell lines that these compounds inhibited most in our assays included lung, cervical, prostate, breast, and leukemia," according to Neto.

Cranberry Juice Prevents UTI Bacteria from Adhering to Bladder Cells

For ages, folk wisdom has held that cranberry juice helps relieve urinary tract infections (UTIs), and there is a great deal of research to support this. Cranberries contain compounds called *proanthocyanidins* that may be responsible for the fruit's and the fruit juice's positive effects on urinary tract infections.

According to a study by Amy Howell, Ph.D., research scientist at the Marucci Center for Blueberry & Cranberry Research at Rutgers University, and Jess

Reed, Ph.D., professor of nutrition at the University of Wisconsin–Madison, an 8-ounce (235 ml) serving of cranberry juice cocktail—but not the equivalent single servings of grape juice, apple juice, green tea, or chocolate—prevented E. coli (the bacteria responsible for the majority of UTIs) from adhering to bladder cells in the urine of six volunteers. (UTIs occur when bacteria in the urine bind to cells of the urinary tract wall.)

In addition, the researchers analyzed the chemical composition of the proanthocyanidins in these foods. According to Howell, "the cranberry's proanthocyanidins are structurally different than the proanthocyanidins found in the other plant foods tested, which may explain why cranberry has unique bacterial antiadhesion activity and helps to maintain urinary tract health."

WORTH KNOWING

Though the health benefits of cranberries are mostly available in the juice, it's important not to confuse real cranberry juice with the highly sweetened cranberry cocktails that are so popular. Anything made with cranberries—even the cocktails—has some benefits, many of the cocktails have less than 20 percent (if that) cranberry juice, and many also contain a lot of sugar. There may be some helpful compounds in there, but their nutritional wallop pales when compared to the real deal: pure, unsweetened cranberry juice that is 100 percent juice and nothing more. Several companies market it: Knudsen's Just Cranberries is one great one, so are Trader Joe's and Mountain Sun.

But be aware of two things. One, real unsweetened cranberry juice is bitter. Two, it's expensive. However both problems are solved by using it in a diluted mix with fresh clean water. A little goes a very long way—a quart (946 ml) of the expensive real stuff can easily be stretched to four quarts (3.7 L) of a nice diluted, healthful mix. And if you really can't stand the tartness, sweeten it with xylitol, stevia, or erythritol.

BEVERAGES

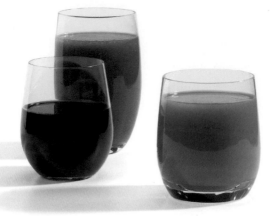

★ Fresh Vegetable (and Fruit) Juice

Consider how many times you've felt frustrated by conflicting advice about food, health, weight loss, supplements, and exercise. One day margarine is good, the next day it's terrible. One day eggs are bad, the next day they're good (actually, they've always been good, but that's another story). Medical and nutritional information seems to change as often as the celebrities on the cover of *People* magazine. So if there was one thing that virtually every expert agreed on, and continued to agree on year in and year out, decade in and decade out, that would be a big deal, right? And worth listening to, correct?

Well, there is. One thing everyone agrees on, that is. And it's this: Eat more vegetables. And while you're at it, eat some fruit. Sorry, but this is the biggest no-brainer in the history of nutrition, for all the dozens of reasons discussed in this book. Let's review: Vegetables and fruits provide fiber. Antioxidants. Phytochemicals. They help control weight, diabetes, and blood sugar. They help fight or prevent cancer. They contain multiple compounds that act as anti-inflammatories. They're associated with significantly lower rates of cardiovascular disease and stroke. They lower blood pressure. They contain compounds such as carotenoids that support the eyes and protect against macular degeneration. Other compounds in vegetables and fruits may help prevent brain aging, dementia, and Alzheimer's.

There is compelling evidence that a diet rich in fruits and vegetables can lower the risk of heart disease and stroke. The largest and longest study to date, done as part of the Harvard-based Nurses' Health Study and Health Professionals Follow-up Study, included almost 110,000 men and women whose health and dietary habits were followed for fourteen years. The higher the average daily intake of fruits and vegetables, the lower the chances of developing cardiovascular disease. Compared with those in the lowest category of fruit and vegetable intake (less than 1.5 servings a day), those who averaged eight or more servings a day were 30 percent less likely to have had a heart attack or stroke. Increasing fruit and vegetable intake by as little as one serving per day can have a real impact on heart disease risk. In the two Harvard studies, for every extra serving of fruits and vegetables that participants added to their diets, their risk of heart disease dropped by 4 percent.

Juicing Adds Healthy Enzymes to the Mix

Are you sold yet? I hope so. So now let's talk about a fabulous way to get most of the benefits of fruits and vegetables, plus the benefits of live enzymes contained in raw food. A terrific way to get a superpotency multiple vitamin and mineral supplement every single day without taking a single pill. A superb solution to the "I don't have time to cook" problem or the "I hate vegetables" complaint.

It's called juicing.

I juice almost every single day—or as often as I can manage it. I honestly believe it's one of the best, most life-enriching health habits I've ever developed. And my decision to include freshly made juices on this list was largely influenced by how strongly I believe in the health benefits of juicing and how much I'd like to see as many people as possible adapt the same habit I've learned to love.

And it doesn't take much work to learn to love it. Juices are absolutely delicious. The best thing about them is that you can disguise almost anything in a juice and still make it taste great. For example, I know a lot of people who just don't like broccoli, but give me a juicer and a few ingredients, and I can mix broccoli's cancer-fighting indoles into a sweet apple-flavored drink faster than you can say, "What's in this thing, anyway?" Listen, if I can fool the teenager in our house into drinking it without grimacing, I can fool anyone.

Hundreds of Healthy Nutrients in a Quick and Easy Package

So here's the deal: There's a slight trade-off when you juice. You lose most of the fiber. (See sidebar on juicing for more details.) That's important—fiber is associated with weight control and reduced diabetes, and may play a protective role in some cancers. You want fiber. But what you gain when you juice is the ability to absorb hundreds of nutrients, phytochemicals, phenols, antioxidants, and enzymes in a quick and easy package that goes down easy and literally fortifies your body with as big a nutritional wallop as any food I can think of or that I've written about in this book.

So, you might be asking, what about sugar? I've warned about the high-sugar fruit juices that I consider to be a scourge on society so many times in the past—how can I be recommending juices made of fruit?

Well, it's like this: Commercial fruit juices are largely flavored sugar water. Homemade, freshly squeezed juices are vitamin powerhouses. Yes, they contain some natural sugar, but you can also modify that by intelligent mixing of low-sugar vegetables (which should constitute the bulk of the ingredients) and some carefully chosen fruits for flavor and additional nutrients. And for all but the most sugar sensitive—or diabetics—the results should be fine.

Add Fish Oil to Your Fruit Juice

And just in case you're still worried, I have another tip for you, one that not only makes the nutrition in fresh juice more complete and makes the nutrients more absorbable, but also lowers the glycemic load—the impact the juice has on your blood sugar. Here's the tip: I add 2 tablespoons (30 ml) of omega-3–rich fish oil to my freshly made juice. (If this sounds disgusting, it's really not. I'll regularly use Omega Swirls formulas by Barlean's. Swirls deliver flaxseed oil or fish oil in a tasty, fruit-flavored base that tastes like dessert and is highly absorbable. Another way to add healthy fat is in the form of coconut oil, MCT oil or omega-7 oil, all of which taste just fine when mixed with juice but also come in Swirls formulations as well.) Any of these terrific fats make the carotenoids in the vegetables and fruits more bioavailable—more usable—to the body. And fat lowers the glycemic load of any food or beverage. Plus you get the independent health benefits of these fats in addition to the benefits of the many compounds found in fruits and veggies. Sometimes,

I'll even throw in a whole egg. The fat in the egg also makes fat-soluble nutrients such as carotenoids easier to absorb—plus I get some protein to boot.

One year, I gave my three best friends juicers for Christmas. They all asked me how to use them. I told them what I'm about to tell you: Use them any way you want! Have fun! Throw absolutely anything from the produce section into them in any combination!

Combinations That Work

Here are a few of my favorite combinations, but remember that any combination works well, and you'll discover all sorts of terrific ways of putting these babies together. There's no right or wrong way—they all work, and though some might be more delicious than others, every one of them is nutritional dynamite.

Any of the following are terrific ingredients for a juice. Experiment and have fun!

Bell peppers (red, yellow, green, orange)

Parsley

Kale

Broccoli

Spinach

Celery

Carrots

Cabbage

Beets and beet greens

Pineapple

Cantaloupe and honeydew

Watermelon

Tomatoes

Apples

Strawberries, blueberries, blackberries, raspberries

Pears

Peaches

Oranges

Lemons (Include a bit of peel. Lots of nutrients in there!)

Limes

Rhubarb

Ginger

JONNY'S FAVORITES (All make two to four servings, depending on how thirsty you are.)

- Green Giant: 6 ribs celery/1 pear/ginger

- Green Giant Deluxe: 2 cups spinach/ 4 ribs celery/2 stalks broccoli/2 apples/ginger

- Spinach Sweetness: 2 cups spinach/1 apple/ 2 to 3 carrots/ginger (variation: add 1 beet with greens)

- Mixed Sensations: ½ of a large red bell pepper/ 2 to 3 stalks broccoli/3 ribs celery/1 apple/ 1 pear/ginger

- Roots of Health: 3 parsnips/2 stalks broccoli/ 3 ribs celery/2 large carrots/1 pear/1 apple/ginger

- Red Juice Deluxe: 2 sticks rhubarb/½ of a red bell pepper/1 pear/1 apple/3 carrots/ginger

- Red Delight: 1 large beet with greens/½ of a large red bell pepper/1 apple/2 to 3 carrots/ginger

JUICING VS. BLENDING

If you're looking for one, single, easy-to-do action item that will give you the most bang for your nutritional buck—and make the biggest difference to your health for the least amount of effort and money—here it is:

Buy a juicer!

By juicer I'm referring to the whole range of household appliances that can turn solid food, like fruits and vegetables, into drinkable beverages. But there are vast differences in how they accomplish this (and vast differences in price). We'll get into all that in a minute.

Nutritionists and health experts may disagree on dozens of details from high-protein diets to the dangers of fat, but there are two things that all of them—from Dr. Atkins to Dr. Ornish—agree on. One, fruits and vegetables are the healthiest substances on Earth. And two, the more the better. If you accept these two facts—and no one I know doesn't—you can easily see why juicing is becoming so popular. It's one of the easiest and most delicious ways to get more fruits and vegetables into your diet.

It's probably not necessary to explain why fruits and vegetables are so important. Data from the Nurses Health Study and the Health Professionals Follow-Up Study clearly show that people who consume more fruits and vegetables have lower risk of coronary artery disease, lower risk of stroke, and lower risk of cancer.

Fresh-made juice—the foundation of any detox diet, by the way—contains a veritable cornucopia of the elements that make fruits and vegetables so doggone good for you: plenty of vitamins and minerals, less known compounds such as flavonoids (of which there are 4,000 in the plant kingdom), carotenoids, anthocyanins, sulforaphane, indoles, isothiocyanates, and probably hundreds more plant chemicals that haven't been discovered yet. Science continues to isolate these compounds and continues to find striking health benefits for most of them.

But you don't have to wait for science to discover what every natural health practitioner from virtually every tradition has known for eons: fresh-made juice is a health bonanza. It can help fight off disease, stimulate immunity, keep cravings at bay, help manage blood sugar, and even make your skin glow.

What kind of juice? And what kind of juicer?

For the purposes of this sidebar, I'm not going to discuss store-bought juices. Though there are exceptions to the rule, most commercial juices are way too high in added sugar, plus they are usually pasteurized—which destroys many beneficial compounds like enzymes. They are also processed in such a way that they require added flavors and fragrances—which are provided by the same companies that formulate perfumes for companies such as Calvin Klein. So let's leave commercial juice out of the discussion and talk about homemade juice, both the conventional kind and the cold-pressed kind.

Blending and Juicing: What's the difference?

There's a world of difference between blending and juicing.

Blending is when you use the whole fruit or vegetable: Nothing is thrown out. There's no separation of juice from pulp, and everything that goes in the container gets liquefied. The most famous machine in this category is the Vitamix, which pretty much dominates what *Business Insider* calls the luxury blender market. In recent years, several other companies—Ninja and NutriBullet, for example—have started aggressively marketing competitive high-end, high-horsepower machines. The best of them can even liquefy an avocado pit! But Vitamix is still the reigning champ.

I have a Vitamix and have owned it for more than a decade. The upside is that you keep all the fiber, most of which gets lost in regular juicing (see below). The downside is, well, you keep the fiber. And that can make blending very tricky. You need just the right amount of water to thin the very thick mixture that results when you liquefy fruits and vegetables. And if you don't get the recipe just right, the result can be bitter and thick. Juicing is much more forgiving.

But, if you've got the patience and follow the excellent recipes available for it, Vitamix (and other high-speed blenders) can provide you with an incredibly nutritious beverage that has all the nutrients and fiber you'd get by eating the actual fruits and vegetables. It just takes some getting used to as it may produce a drink that is thick and pulpy.

Juicing: Cold-Pressed Juice vs. Conventional Juice

Juicing is different from blending in that the fiber is separated from the liquid, and thrown out after you make the juice. This is true for both conventional juicers and cold-pressed juicers, and if there's any negative to juicing, it's that—no fiber.

No one appreciates the importance of fiber more than I do. My book *Smart Fat* recommends 10 servings a day (3 grams each) minimum, and elsewhere in this book (See sidebar on fiber, see 96) I discuss at length why it's so important for our health. But let's get real. The juice from freshly made juice is absolutely loaded with vitamins and minerals, phytochemicals, flavonoids, flavanols, catechins, and polyphenols that have multiple and systemic benefits. That's nothing to sneeze at. I suggest you juice and eat whole fruits and vegetables. And be sure to eat even better sources of fiber—like beans! Why choose between the juicing and eating when you don't have to?

So now that we've established that juicing is great, let's talk about the last key point—conventional or cold-pressed.

Cold-Press Juicers vs Conventional Juicers

For years I had a conventional juicer, the Breville, and honestly, I thought it was great. You put in the fruits and vegetables, the motor roars, out drips the fresh juice, the fiber and pulp collect in a basket, and boom, you're good to go. No complaints there.

Then, in the last few years, a new trend started—cold-pressed juice—and it suddenly became all the rage. Small companies started making it, often locally and in small batches, and these bottled juices started showing up as part of expensive detox programs and on the shelves of pricier stores such as Whole Foods. They were—and are—expensive (about seven to ten dollars a bottle for a single serving).

Then, to complicate things even further, some high-end companies began making cold-press juice machines for the home market to compete with the expensive, ready-made products that were cropping up everywhere.

Why cold-pressed? Does it offer any advantage over conventional juice?

Actually, yes.

Here's the thing. Oxygen and heat destroy nutrients. Conventional, centrifugal juicers extract juice by rapidly spinning the produce around in a chamber exposing them to razor-sharp teeth. The high-speed blades wind up heating and oxidizing the juice, arguably lowering its nutritional content.

On the other hand, cold-pressed juice is made in a completely different way. Commercially, it's made using a hydraulic press without any additional heat or oxygen. Home machines that use a similar technology are often called slow-juicers, an apt term that conveys the much more gentle process by which the juice is extracted. My Hurom HZ slow juicer, for example, uses an auger to squeeze out the juice instead of shredding the fruits and vegetables with high-speed, high-heat blades. The resultant juice is said to retain much more nutrition and much more taste.

I haven't done a lab analysis to confirm the claim that slow-juicing is more nutritious. But I don't need a lab test to tell you about the taste—it's unbelievable.

Now, I won't lie to you. Making daily, fresh-made juice with the Hurom or any other high-end juicer (cold-pressed or conventional) takes a bit of time and effort. It's not like opening a carton of orange juice. But I've learned to embrace that and make it part of my daily routine. I know that from the time I walk into the kitchen to the time everything is cleaned up takes roughly nine minutes. But I also know that the nine minutes spent will reward me with about a quart (946 ml) of one of the most delicious, nutritious beverages on the planet.

Much has been written on the value of making food at home, preparing it mindfully and lovingly, and then enjoying the rewards of your efforts (both physically and mentally). It's all true. I can tell you that when I put in the small amount of time required make the juice myself, it's almost like my own personal Zen tea ceremony. My nine minutes a day spent with my Hurom reward me many times over, and it's an experience I highly recommend both for its calming effects and for the unbelievably delicious and nutritionally dense beverage that it produces.

On a personal note: I'm not much for juicing recipes, even though I included a few suggestions in the book. Basically, I buy a bunch of good-looking produce and just experiment. I'll throw in a pepper along with some raspberries, or I'll add Swiss chard to a bunch of apples. I basically mix and match, and don't measure or count anything. Sometimes I hit the jackpot and come up with something that blows me away. Once in a while, I come up with a combination that's not quite so tasty. But it's never bad and it's always nutritious.

Note well: If you're struggling with the problem of how to get your kid to eat more vegetables, juicing is the answer. If you use apples and carrots as a base, it'll be sweet enough to disguise almost anything else. You can even add broccoli—no teenager will know the difference.

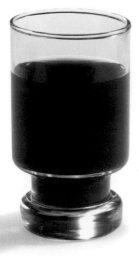

★ Noni Juice

Okay, let me be perfectly honest. I hate multilevel marketing, and I hate "magical" products that claim to cure everything from acne to cancer. The trifecta of my pet peeves is when the they combine, i.e., a multi-level marketing company selling a "magical" product that claims to cure everything. Even when the product isn't bad—which does happen—the multilevel marketers send their salespeople out with such hype and hoopla, quoting "scientific" studies and making claims that are so outrageous and unfounded, that I get turned off before I even try the product.

So I was ready to dislike noni juice. And acai berries, and goji berries, and all the other berries that have been promoted in the last few years—some of them honestly and carefully, some of them outrageously.

But truth be told, marketing gimmicks and practices aside, many of these berries are amazing foods. Especially noni berries.

I ignore the "science" that the companies write about in their brochures because many of the "studies" that they boast about are questionable, biased, unpublished, or, worst-case scenario, made up. I go right to the National Institute of Medicine library, and look for what I can find on my own. And what I found about noni juice was pretty impressive.

Noni Juice Traditionally Used as Medicine

The official scientific name of the noni berry is the Morinda citrifolia fruit. Morinda is actually a genus of about eighty species, mostly of tropical origin. It's known by all kinds of names: hai ba ji in Chinese,

Indian mulberry, noni (in Puerto Rico and Hawaii), nonu (in Samoa), nono (in Tahiti), even—probably because of its potential as an anti-inflammatory—the painkiller tree (in the Caribbean). It's been used for centuries as a food source and has a long tradition of being used for medicinal purposes. And while the fruit itself is pretty vile tasting, the juice products made from it are quite palatable.

You've seen me mention sulforaphane several times in this book. It's a phytochemical that has significant anticancer properties, largely because it increases the production of certain enzymes known as phase-2 enzymes, which can "disarm" damaging free radicals and help fight cancer-causing carcinogens. But a study from the College of Pharmacy at the University of Illinois at Chicago found that a compound in noni fruit was forty times more potent than sulforaphane. If that turns out to be true, that would mean that authentic noni (and noni juice) could have an astonishing amount of cancer-fighting potential.

At least two studies have been published demonstrating that an extract from the Morinda citrifolia fruit (noni) has been found to have an antiproliferative effect on tumor cells. One report in the *Annals of the New York Academy of Science*, titled "Cancer-preventive effect of Morinda citrifolia (noni)," compared the antioxidant activity of noni juice to vitamin C, grape seed powder, and pycnogenol—all very powerful antioxidants. The researchers presented preliminary data showing that Tahitian noni juice mixed in drinking water for one week was able to prevent carcinogen-DNA adduct formation and suggested that the antioxidant activity of noni juice may contribute to its cancer-preventive effect.

Does Noni Juice Prevent Wrinkles?

One study found that constituents of the fruit inhibited the oxidation of LDL ("bad") cholesterol. (Remember that cholesterol only becomes a problem in the human body when it is oxidized.) Another study, in the *Journal of Medicinal Food*, found that a compound in the noni fruit stimulated the synthesis of collagen. The authors stated that this compound—an anthraquinone—was a good candidate as a new antiwrinkle agent. And anti-inflammatory compounds have been isolated from the root of another member of the genus, the Morinda officinalis. If all that weren't enough, researchers at the Beijing Institute of Pharmacology and Toxicology studying Morinda officinalis on a well-known animal model of depression (the forced swimming test) concluded that an extract of the plant possessed antidepressant effects.

As with many fruits, juices, and foods that have been used medicinally for centuries in a variety of cultures, the rigorous scientific study of noni is still emerging. It's likely that the health claims may outpace the evidence for a while. Nonetheless, there's enough solid science—not to mention a long history of folk tradition—to support the inclusion of noni juice on this list. Remember, the taste is off-putting—the best companies making it produce a pure juice that has to be diluted with water or taken in 1-ounce (30 ml) servings.

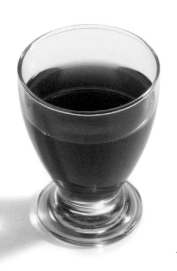

Pomegranate Juice

Only a decade or so ago, pomegranate juice was practically unknown in the US. But in a relatively short time, it's been the subject of a ton of research, and the results have been so impressive that even mainstream medicine is paying attention. It's listed on the Memorial Sloan Kettering Cancer Center website in the integrative medicine section, complete with research references showing that it suppresses inflammation, inhibits tumor growth and breast cancer cell proliferation, and benefits patients with everything from carotid artery stenosis to those with moderate erectile dysfunction.

I'm not kidding about that last benefit. Research published in the Journal of Urology actually examined the effect of long-term intake of pomegranate juice on erectile dysfunction. They established two things: One, that free radicals—rogue molecules that do terrific damage to just about everything in your body from your DNA on down—have a profound effect on erectile dysfunction in an animal model. And two, that pomegranate juice actually helps modulate this effect because it's been found to contain powerful antioxidants that actually fight free radicals and the damage they do. Because of this, pomegranate juice is sometimes called a "natural Viagra."

Controversy exists about whether pomegranate extract in pill form works as well as the juice. The bulk of the research has been on the juice itself, and some wonder if the same benefits apply to the extract in supplement form. No one really knows the answer to that, but it's reasonable to assume that supplements of pomegranate extract are also very beneficial.

THE POMEGRANATE AND ROMANCE

Interestingly, the pomegranate has always been associated with love and erotica. The ancients connected the fruit with procreation and abundance. In Turkey, the bride throws the fruit to the ground, and it's believed that the number of seeds that pop out will predict how many kids she's going to have. Legend has it that the goddess Aphrodite, deity of love, planted the pomegranate on the isle of Cyprus.

The excellent website GreenMedInfo assembled 158 scientific abstracts of studies related to pomegranate, including (but not limited to) studies that investigated the effect of pomegranate on oxidative stress, inflammation, atherosclerosis, prostate cancer, and hypertension. For the most part, the studies are uniformly positive. Pomegranate fruit extract contains polyphenols, which are plant chemicals that have the ability to help protect cells from damage and the ability to lower inflammation.

According to the University of Maryland Medical Center website, pomegranates have been used as medicine for thousands of years. In Asia and in the Middle East, they use the bark, root, fruit and rind of the pomegranate tree as medicine, but in the West, most of the research has been done on the fruit and its juice.

One review article "Potent Health Effects of Pomegranate," published in 2014 in the *Journal of Advanced Biomedical Research*, concluded that pomegranates can help prevent or treat various disease risk factors including high blood pressure, high cholesterol, oxidative stress, hyperglycemia, and inflammation. The researchers noted that the antioxidant potential of pomegranate juice is more than that of red wine and green tea. Pomegranate fruit extract prevents cell growth and induces apoptosis—a kind of programmed death for cells that are no longer needed or are a threat to the organism. It's this ability which may be responsible for pomegranate's anticancer effects.

Pomegranate also seems to protect LDL cholesterol from oxidative damage, which is critical because cholesterol is only a problem when it's oxidized. In one animal study, pomegranate juice slowed the growth of plaque. In other research, it slowed the growth of prostate cancer cells in the lab. Preliminary evidence suggests that the juice may help lower blood pressure, improve cardiovascular risk factors, and enhance immunity. There's even research suggesting that pomegranate's ability to fight inflammation just might stall the progression of Alzheimer's disease, and might have a preventive role in obesity.

How much should you drink? There's no perfect answer to that question. The best advice is to just put pomegranate seeds and pomegranate juice in heavy rotation in your diet. Eat the fruit or drink the juice (or both). Israeli scientists showed blood pressure reduction from drinking as little as two ounces (60 ml) of pomegranate juice daily (Dornfeld, 2001), probably due to decreased activity of angiotensin converting enzyme (ACE). This is worth noting for people who might want a more natural alternative to ACE inhibitors, drugs commonly given for hypertension.

When the first edition of this book came out, pomegranate seeds were not particularly popular, although the juice was getting a fair amount of attention in the nutrition press. Now many supermarkets carry pomegranate seeds in little plastic packages, much like those that contain fresh blueberries or strawberries. They do the tedious work of removing the seeds from the pomegranate for you, so it's now possible to buy the very tasty seeds ready to eat; no muss, no fuss. Just be aware that you'll pay a premium for having the work done for you—a container of pomegranate seeds can be pricey.

Research on pomegranate tends to concentrate on the juice or an extract given in pill form. You don't see too many research reports on pomegranate seeds themselves, though it seems reasonable to assume that many of the same benefits found in the juice would also be available from an equivalent amount of the seeds.

WORTH KNOWING

There is a fair amount of natural sugar in the juice. If you're on a low-carb diet or very sensitive to the effects of sugar, proceed accordingly. For everybody else, pomegranate juice is a superfood. I recommend consuming it regularly.

Red Wine

Plato may have been on to something when he said, "nothing more excellent or valuable than wine was ever granted by the gods to man." Red wine has received a ton of press for its health-promoting abilities and has even been credited for something called the French Paradox. The truth—as always—is more complicated.

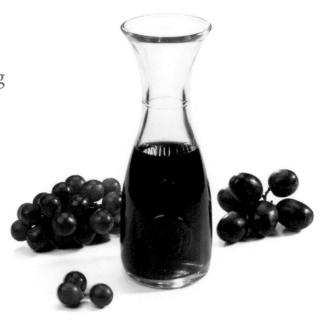

The French Paradox is the term used to describe the well-known fact that the French have less heart disease than Americans, despite the fact that they eat far more high-fat foods, such as cheese.

If you buy into the fact that fat alone is responsible for heart disease (I do not), this indeed looks like a paradox. But, as most nutritionists are now aware, the "fat causes heart disease" paradigm is woefully out of date. Nonetheless, for years it was believed that the reason the French could "get away" with such supposedly unhealthy fare is that they consumed liberal amounts of heart-healthy red wine, which contains numerous compounds that protect the heart and support health. This isn't the place to go into the fallacies of the French Paradox. (There are many.) But it is the place to go into the heart-healthy, life-extending compounds that are in red wine. And the best place to start is with the superstar compound that many consider the number-one antiaging supplement in the world—resveratrol.

Resveratrol: A Powerful Antioxidant That Helps Prevent Heart Disease

Resveratrol is one of the most potent of the polyphenols and is found in red wine and the seeds and skins of grapes (see page 136). It's also found in peanuts, blueberries, and cranberries. Red wine has a high concentration of this powerful antioxidant because the skins and seeds ferment in the grapes' juices during the red wine–making process. This prolonged contact during fermentation produces significant levels of resveratrol in the finished red wine. White wine also contains resveratrol, but the seeds and skins are removed early in the white wine–making process, reducing the amount of resveratrol in the final product.

Antioxidants like resveratrol are beneficial in preventing harmful elements in the body from attacking healthy cells. The antioxidant properties of resveratrol also offer certain health benefits in the prevention of heart disease and the reduction of lung tissue inflammation in chronic obstructive pulmonary disease (COPD). An animal study in Journal of Agricultural and Food Chemistry (volume 54, 2006) suggested that resveratrol can improve blood flow in the brain by 30 percent, thereby reducing the risk of stroke.

Resveratrol also has anticancer activity. Writing in the journal Anticancer Research in 2004, researchers from the University of Texas M.D. Anderson Cancer Center reviewed dozens of studies on resveratrol and concluded that it exhibited anticancer properties against a wide range of tumor cells, including lymphoid and myeloid cancers, multiple myeloma, cancers of the breast, prostate, stomach, colon, pancreas, and thyroid, melanoma, head and neck squamous cell carcinoma, ovarian carcinoma, and cervical carcinoma. The researchers concluded that "resveratrol appears to exhibit therapeutic effects against cancer."

The research on resveratrol has been steadily growing over the past ten years, revealing a picture that is even better than we thought when the first edition of this book was published. In 2010, there was a Resveratrol Conference in Denmark. Almost 3,700 published studies on resveratrol were analyzed and the findings were profound. Experts identified twelve mechanisms of action by which resveratrol may act to combat the diseases of aging and to protect the body against the five leading causes of death among Americans. Among the mechanisms cited:

Resveratrol lowers inflammation.

Resveratrol is a powerful antioxidant.

Resveratrol can prevent damage to DNA.

Resveratrol can stimulate bone formation.

Resveratrol can lower the incidence of hypertension.

Resveratrol is neuroprotective.

Resveratrol has been shown in studies to inhibit the growth of several cancer cell lines and tumors. It's a powerful antioxidant and anti-inflammatory. It ramps up detoxification enzymes in the liver making it easier for your body to get rid of carcinogens, and it protects the heart. It also protects neurons (brain cells). And animal studies show that it slows the accumulation of fat.

Drink Red Wine for a Longer Life

There's a reason why resveratrol may actually work as an antiaging compound. In the past, one of the only things that ever reliably extended lifespan was called calorie restriction (which means exactly what you think it means). Published research has shown that just about every species studied—from fruit flies to yeast cells to monkeys—lives longer when you restrict calories. And the reason is a set of longevity genes known as the SIRT genes.

When calories are scarcer, SIRT genes get turned on.

So if you want to turn on your longevity genes, all you've got to do is eat about one-third less food than you're eating now. How does that sound?

That's what I thought. Not so great. That's why the research of David Sinclair Ph.D., assistant professor of pathology at Harvard University Medical School, generated so much excitement.

Sinclair discovered that there was a molecule found in red wine that actually turned on those same SIRT genes that were turned on by calorie restriction. The molecule was called resveratrol. If there was a way to isolate that molecule and create a drug (or supplement, in this case), one could theoretically get a lot of the benefits of calorie restriction without the angst.

Resveratrol may be one of the best antiaging substances around. And red wine is an excellent way to get resveratrol into your diet.

Besides resveratrol, there are other health-promoting polyphenols in red wine, and many of these are heart protective. Studies investigating the benefits of red wine suggest that a moderate amount of red wine (one drink a day for women and two drinks a day for men) lowers the risk of heart attack for people in middle age by 30 to 50 percent. It is also suggested that alcohol, such as red wine, may prevent additional heart attacks if you have already suffered one.

Other studies have indicated that red wine can raise HDL ("good") cholesterol. Red wine may help prevent blood clots and reduce the blood vessel damage caused by fat deposits. Indeed, studies showed that people from the Mediterranean region who regularly drink red wine have lower risks of heart disease.

Some years back, the *British Medical Journal* published a famous paper on the "polymeal" in which researchers proposed a perfect meal that, if eaten daily, would substantially reduce the risk for heart disease as much as or more than many medications. Wine was a part of it. In fact, the authors calculated that based on the available research, about 5 ounces (150 ml) of wine a day would likely result in a 23 to 41 percent reduction in risk for coronary heart disease.

My follow-up book to this one (*The Healthiest Meals on Earth*, co-written with the Clean Food Coach, Jeannette Bessinger) is based on the polymeal concept—the meals and recipes provide as many of the nutrients found in the seven basic foods (including wine) that made up the original polymeal.

Red Wine and the Risk of Breast Cancer

Okay, before you go out and start guzzling, here's where it gets tricky, especially if you're a woman. The relationship of alcohol consumption to breast cancer risk is murky but troubling. Some studies have found an increased risk of breast cancer in women who drink, even moderately. At least ten studies have looked at the relationship of alcohol and breast cancer and the majority have shown a link between the two.

In general, alcohol does appear to increase the risk of breast cancer in women. The Committee on Carcinogenicity of Chemicals in Food, Consumer Products and the Environment's Non-Technical Summary concludes, "The new research estimates that a woman drinking an average of two units (drinks) of alcohol per day has a lifetime risk of developing breast cancer 8 percent higher than a woman who drinks an average of one unit of alcohol per day. The risk of breast cancer further increases with each additional drink consumed per day."

Both the National Cancer Institute and Walter Willett, M.D., Dr. P.H., professor of epidemiology and nutrition at Harvard's School of Public Health put the increased risk for breast cancer at about 20 to 25 percent for women drinking two drinks a day. This doesn't mean that 20 to 25 percent of women who have two drinks a day will get breast cancer—it means that drinking would increase the risk from about 12 out of 100 women getting breast cancer (the national average) to 14 to 15 per 100. This is a small increase, but no comfort if you're one of those extra two or three people.

How Folic Acid Can Help Reduce Cancer Risk

But there's good news, and it probably explains why there have been some inconsistent results in the breast-cancer-alcohol studies. If you get enough folic acid, the problem with alcohol and breast cancer goes away. According to the Mayo Clinic, folate (folic acid) counteracts the breast cancer risk associated with alcohol consumption. Women who drink alcohol and have a high folate intake are not at increased risk of cancer. Folic acid has multiple protective benefits for everyone, and taking folic acid supplements (or even a multiple vitamin with folic acid) is a great idea—most especially if you're a woman and you drink alcohol. You can get the benefits of red wine and the multiple protective effects of a high folic acid intake.

If you're able to handle it, and if you're consuming it in moderation, red wine can be part of a wonderful healthy lifestyle. The trick is to know when enough is enough.

Or when even a little is too much.

So red wine is antioxidant rich, loaded with healthy polyphenols, and a major dietary source of the anticancer, antiaging compound resveratrol. On the other hand, wine—and alcohol in general—is one of those substances where God truly is in the details, and the dosage makes the poison. Moderate intake of red wine: good. Too much alcohol, especially for those with addictive personalities: unmitigated disaster. Alcohol can raise triglycerides, increase blood pressure, and lead to weight gain. And it's not possible to predict in which people alcohol will lead to alcoholism.

WORTH KNOWING

Under no circumstances should pregnant women drink alcohol. Period. It can harm the baby.

If you're unsure about your relationship to alcohol, stay away. Just about every antioxidant that's in wine can be gotten from fruits and vegetables, and even resveratrol is plentiful in dark grapes, boiled peanuts, and high-quality resveratrol supplements such as those by Life Extension or Reserveage, two companies that make resveratrol supplements that contain a high percentage of trans resveratrol, the active ingredient that you care about.

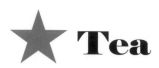

Tea

(green, black, white)

After water, tea is probably the most consumed beverage in the world. Not counting water, it's also probably the healthiest.

The key to the health benefits of tea can be found in a large group of protective plant-based chemicals generally known as phenolic compounds, or polyphenols.

First, some clarifications. All four kinds of nonherbal tea—green, black, white, and oolong (red)—come from the same plant, a warm-weather evergreen known as *Camellia sinensis*. The leaves of this plant contain many chemicals from a general class of compounds called polyphenols.

Polyphenols are powerful antioxidants, many of which have anticancer activity (more about that in a moment). There are more than 4,000 of these compounds, and they fall into many classes and subclasses, including flavonoids, anthrocyanins, and isoflavones. Polyphenols, like other antioxidants, help protect cells from the normal, but damaging, physiological process known as oxidative stress. Although oxygen is vital to life, it's also incorporated into reactive substances called free radicals. These can damage the cells in our body, and they have been implicated in the slow chain reaction of damage leading to heart disease and cancer. Many studies have demonstrated the anticancer properties of polyphenols. They can stop the damage that free radicals do to cells, neutralize enzymes essential for tumor growth, and deactivate cancer promoters.

Tea Color Related to Extent of Processing

What determines whether a tea is green, black, white, or oolong depends entirely on the degree of processing that the leaves of the *Camellia sinensis* undergo after they've been harvested. Here's the short summary: Black tea is fully fermented; oolong tea is partially fermented; green tea is not fermented at all, but panfried and dried; and white tea is barely processed.

White tea is the only one of the four made from immature tea leaves, leaves that are picked right before the buds have fully opened. Silver fuzz still covers the buds, and the silver fuzz turns to white when the tea is dried (hence its name). Depending on the variety of white tea, the exact ratio of buds to leaves can vary—for example, White Peony contains one bud for every two leaves; Silver Needles—which

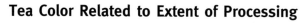

can be expensive—is made entirely from buds picked within a short period in early spring.

Being the least processed of the bunch, white tea in general is highest in polyphenols. Research has found that "certain green and white tea types have comparable levels of catechins with potential health promoting qualities," (according to a study in the *Journal of Food Science*) The take-home point is that there isn't a hierarchy of teas—all teas have benefits.

Green, oolong, and black tea all start with mature leaves that are then "withered" or air-dried. After that, the process differs slightly. To make green tea, the withered leaves are then steamed or panfried, and then dried again. To make oolong (red) tea, the withered leaves are first bruised, then partially fermented, then panfried and dried. And to make black tea, the withered leaves are first rolled, then fully fermented, and then panfried and dried. Black tea represents 78 percent of the total consumed tea in the world, whereas green tea accounts for approximately 20 percent.

Both Green and Black Tea Fight Cancer

The processing changes the chemical composition of the teas, but because the darker teas are more processed, that doesn't mean they're without health benefits. Green tea (and presumably the even less processed white tea) contains a powerful group of polyphenols called catechins. One of these catechins— epigallocatechin gallate (EGCG)—is believed to be responsible for the anticancer effects of green tea. The thing is, the fermentation process that creates black tea oxidizes—or deactivates—this particular catechin. So for a long time, urban legend held that only green tea (and presumably white) possessed anticancer activity, because EGCG wasn't present in black (or oolong) tea due to the fermentation process.

Not so.

We now know that the very fermentation process that deactivates the catechin in green tea creates a whole other set of powerful antioxidants that are present in black tea. Black tea actually contains more complex polyphenols than green tea. The fermentation process needed for the production of black tea produces some unique antioxidants called biflavonols, thearubigens, and especially theaflavins.

Studies show the theaflavins in black tea have just as much antioxidant activity—if not more—than the compounds in green tea. A research report in the *Journal of Nutrition* in 2001 showed that the theaflavins in black tea and the catechins in green tea are equally effective as antioxidants, and a study by the Netherlands National Institute of Public Health and the Environment found a connection between drinking black tea regularly and reducing the risk of stroke. Researchers looked at data from a study examining the health benefits of foods that are high in flavonoids and phytonutrients with antioxidant benefits. Although some of the flavonoids were obtained from fruits and vegetables, 70 percent came from black tea. The study looked at 552 men over a fifteen-year period and found that men who drank more than four cups (940 ml) of black tea per day had a significantly lower risk of stroke than men who drank only two to three cups (470 to 705 ml) per day.

Black Tea Helps Blood Vessels Function, Prevents Stroke and Heart Attack

At Boston University's School of Medicine, Joseph Vita, M.D., conducted a separate study that supported these results. For four months, sixty-six men either drank four cups of black tea or took a placebo daily. Vita concluded that drinking black tea can help reverse an abnormal functioning of blood vessels that can contribute to stroke or heart attack. Furthermore, improvement in the functioning of the blood vessels was visible within two hours of drinking just one cup (235 ml) of black tea.

Finally, a study in *Cancer* found that among 109 Polish women, high black tea consumption was associated with diminished salivary levels of 17 beta-estradiol, the most potent mammalian estrogenic hormone and one that can be carcinogenic in hormone-related cancers. (Lower levels of the hormone were also reported when women consumed high amounts of the catechins found in green tea as well.) In writing about the study, the medical/nutritional newsletter *Clinical Pearls* said the study "suggested that tea consumption may provide a relatively easy dietary intervention for reducing hormone-related cancer risk."

Black Tea Can Help Your Heart

Black tea lowers triglycerides—in fact, it's actually superior to green tea in doing so—and high triglycerides are strongly associated with a high risk of cardiovascular disease. It's also slightly better than green tea at inducing the body's powerful antioxidant superoxide dismutase (SOD). And it appears to help the heart—in a small study published in the *American Journal of Cardiology* in 2004, men who drank black tea experienced improved blood flow in the coronary arteries only a few hours after drinking the tea.

I've spent this much time on black tea only because it's so often overlooked, living in the shadow of its big brother, green tea. But wonderful health benefits of black tea aside, green tea fully deserves its primary place in the sun. It is one of the world's superfoods and has been acknowledged as such by virtually every nutritionist I know. It has anticancer activity. It's helpful in weight loss. It lowers cholesterol. It's associated with significantly lower levels of heart disease. And it has components in it that are helpful with depression and anxiety.

The National Cancer Institute Puts Its Faith in Green Tea

For cancer prevention, evidence for green tea is so overwhelming that the Chemoprevention Branch of the National Cancer Institute has initiated a plan for developing tea compounds as cancer-chemopreventive agents in human trials. For example, in 1994 the

Journal of the National Cancer Institute published the results of an epidemiological study indicating that drinking green tea reduced the risk of esophageal cancer in Chinese men and women by nearly 60 percent. And in 2004, a team from Harvard Medical School reported that EGCG (the catechin in green tea mentioned earlier) inhibits the growth and reproduction of cancer cells associated with Barrett's esophagus. They said that green tea may help lower the prevalence of esophageal adenocarcinoma, one of the fastest-growing cancers in Western countries. Purdue University researchers also concluded that a compound in green tea inhibits the growth of cancer cells.

Of the hundreds and hundreds of green tea experiments that have been conducted, about 10 percent have directly involved humans, and many more have involved observations of populations that drink large amounts of green tea. It's now fairly established that green tea may help prevent the following types of cancers in humans: bladder, colon, esophagus, pancreas, rectum, and stomach.

The studies showing the anticancer and antioxidant effects of catechins in green tea are numerous. Just for example, one particularly exciting study done at the Cancer Chemotherapy Center in Tokyo, Japan, and using leukemia and colon cancer cell cultures, demonstrated that "epigallocatechin gallate (EGCG) strongly and directly inhibits telomerase." Telomerase is the enzyme that "immortalizes" cancer cells by maintaining the end portions of the tumor cell chromosomes. Inhibition of telomerase could be one of the main anticarcinogenic mechanisms of catechins.

The More Green Tea You Drink, the Less Risk of Coronary Artery Disease

The cholesterol-lowering effects of green tea have been confirmed by both animal and human epidemiological studies. Green tea also lowers fibrinogen, which is a substance in the body that can cause clots and strokes. In an article in the *Circulation Journal*

(July 2004) titled "Effects of green tea intake on the development of coronary artery disease," researchers from the department of medicine at Chiba Hokusoh Hospital, Nippon Medical School, Chiba, Japan, concluded that "the more green tea patients consume, the less likely they are to have coronary artery disease."

Green tea may be helpful for anyone who wants to lose weight. In one study, in the American Journal of Clinical Nutrition, men who were given green tea burned more calories than men who were given a similar drink without the green tea, even after allowing for the possible effect of caffeine. The late great nutritionist Shari Lieberman, Ph.D., C.N.S., used to say that green tea stimulates the metabolism way more than caffeine alone. While studies of weight loss using green tea supplements have shown mixed results, in several animal studies, green tea demonstrated the ability to lower blood sugar.

Green Tea Releases Feel-Good Dopamine

A substance in green tea called theanine is helpful in improving mood and increasing a sense of relaxation. In fact, it's used in Japan for just that purpose. Theanine induces the release of a neurotransmitter called GABA, which tends to calm down the brain. Theanine also triggers the release of dopamine, one of the main brain chemicals associated with well-being. Dopamine is the brain's master regulator of reward and pleasure, and the release of dopamine probably contributes to the sense of well-being associated with tea drinking. The calming effect of theanine may be the reason that drinking green tea—even with caffeine—doesn't tend to produce nearly as jittery an experience as drinking coffee.

Since the first edition of this book, there's been even more research on tea, and the evidence is overwhelmingly positive. In 2014, a Chinese group of researchers led by Shoude Zhang published a complete analysis of the multiple bioactivities of green tea, and found that green tea polyphenols affect two hundred

target genes in humans, including those involved in inflammation, diabetes, neurodegenerative diseases, diabetes, and cardiovascular disease. At least two studies have shown that green tea protects against DNA damage while at the same time promoting DNA repair. Large epidemiological studies show that those who are regular green tea drinkers have a significantly reduced risk for heart disease and stroke. And a 2015 study in Molecular Nutrition & Food Research from Penn State University found that green tea kills oral cancer cells.

Finally, numerous studies have cited the connection between inflammation, oxidation, and Alzheimer's disease. Antioxidants have a potent role in the prevention of neurodegenerative diseases. One study, "A review of antioxidants and Alzheimer's disease," in the Annals of Clinical Psychiatry in 2005 reviewed all the research published to date to draw conclusions about the usefulness (or lack thereof) of specific antioxidants in the prevention of Alzheimer's. Researchers scanned more than 300 articles and concluded that there were eight agents that showed promise in helping prevent Alzheimer's. Green tea was one of the eight (the other seven were aged garlic, curcumin, melatonin, resveratrol, Gingko biloba, vitamin C, and vitamin E). And a paper in the Journal of Nutritional Biochemistry (September 2004) examined the neuroprotective mechanisms of green tea polyphenols—especially EGCG—on Alzheimer's and Parkinson's disease.

Matcha: Green Tea on Steroids

Matcha is a kind of super green tea. It's green tea alright—but it's harvested in a special way and consumed differently from other teas. It's also more expensive than standard green tea.

Matcha literally means "powdered tea." It's what's used in the famous Japanese tea ceremony. The tea plants used for matcha are covered with shade cloths for about three weeks, which creates large thin leaves with better texture and flavor. Tea farmers hand select the tea leaves, and steam them lightly (to stop fermentation). Then they're dried and aged in cold storage, which deepens the flavor even more. The "finished" leaves are then ground into a fine, emerald green powder. That's matcha.

Besides the specialness of the leaves used to make it, the main difference between standard teas and matcha is in how they're consumed. With regular tea, you steep the leaves in hot water and then discard them. With matcha, you actually consume the whole tea leaves in the form of the finely ground powder made from them. Nothing is discarded. You're actually drinking the leaves themselves. Not only that, the leaves themselves are the best of the bunch, having been hand-selected and specially processed. The result is a tea that has everything green tea has only in high-

er concentrations. One study indicated that the concentration of EGCG (epigallocatechin gallate)—the catechin in green tea responsible for much of its anti-cancer activity—is 137 times greater than the amount of EGCG available from China Green Tips green tea, and at least three times higher than the largest value studied for other green teas.

To prepare matcha, sift 1 to 2 teaspoons of the matcha powder into a cup or bowl and add about 2 ounces (60 ml) of hot (not boiling) water. Whisk it with a bamboo brush until the mixture froths.

Although purists would probably frown on it, you can make a match latte by preparing the matcha as described above and, once it is well mixed (no clumps), add your desired milk or milk substitute.

DOES PUTTING MILK IN MY TEA DESTROY THE ANTIOXIDANTS?

You can find dozens of articles on the Internet that say that putting milk in tea destroys its antioxidants. But the science on that is not so clear.

It is true that protein can bind with polyphenol/antioxidants, so putting milk (protein) in tea, with its rich polyphenol content, would make some of those polyphenols unavailable. In addition, milk dilutes the tea so the resulting beverage won't be as concentrated in antioxidants because milk isn't as rich in antioxidants as tea is. But milk has antioxidants of its own, so that further complicates the equation. Some studies show that milk reduces antioxidant

value; some studies show it doesn't. One of the most thoughtful analyses of the data on milk, tea, and antioxidants I've read uncovered an element to the tea drinking experience that depletes antioxidants much more than milk does. It's something no one really thinks about—the tea bag. Without question, loose tea has a far higher concentration of health-giving compounds than bagged tea, and even the quality of the bag itself can have an effect.

So if you absolutely love your tea with milk, by all means carry on. Better to drink it with milk than to not drink it at all. The reduction in antioxidants is relatively minor compared to the effect of the teabag, so if at all possible, switch to loose tea.

Everyone Benefits from Tea

I've spent this much time on tea because it is one of the few foods or drinks about which I can say that virtually everyone would benefit from drinking it. It offers powerful antioxidant protection, reduces blood sugar, is anti-inflammatory, lowers cholesterol, protects against heart disease and cancer, and has the ability to stimulate the metabolism.

For an innocuous and common beverage that costs next to nothing, that's a pretty powerful résumé.

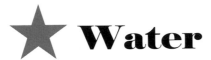 # Water

Okay, consider the following: You're walking in the woods and you come upon a pond. The pond hasn't seen life in ages. There's a brown scummy film floating on it. The water is brown and dirty. It looks stagnant, and there are flies and mosquitos buzzing around it. Now imagine you're on that same walk in the woods and you come upon a mountain glacier. The water is flowing freely down the rocks, with the light of the sun sparkling through, the water looks clean and clear and crisp, and you stand for a moment to admire it as it gushes down the mountain.

Which water would you rather have in your body? Well if you're not drinking enough clean, pure water, the water in your body is more analogous to the pond than the glacier.

Water Runs Your Body

Think about it: Your body is 83 percent water. Your muscles are 75 percent water. Your brain, for goodness' sake, is 74 percent water, and your bones are 22 percent water. You need water for every single metabolic process in the body. Water is necessary to digest and absorb nutrients and vitamins. It carries away metabolic waste. It helps flush fat and toxins through the liver and kidneys.

So doesn't it make sense to constantly replenish that body of yours with the equivalent of the gorgeous clean mountain stream, rather than to let all that water just sit in your body and recycle like the stagnant pond?

Of course it does.

Water can improve energy, increase mental and physical performance, remove toxins and waste from your body, keep your skin healthy and glowing, and may even help you lose weight. If you're dehydrated—and some experts think that most of us are at the very least underhydrated—your blood is thicker and your body has to work that much harder to cause it to circulate. As a result, your brain becomes less active, it's harder to concentrate, and you feel fatigued.

Water is one of the fluids that lubricates and cushions your joints and muscles, protecting them from shock and damage. If the body is dehydrated, it may become more susceptible to ailments. Also, before, during, and after exercise, drinking proper amounts of water can help reduce cramping of the muscles and early onset of fatigue.

Staying Well Hydrated Protects Your Heart

You can live without food for a long time, but try going without water for eight to ten days—you won't make it, and most people would be dead long before that.

And there are health benefits to water beyond the fact that it keeps us alive. Dehydration can elevate at least four independent risk factors for coronary heart disease: whole blood viscosity, plasma viscosity, hematocrit, and fibrinogen. In one landmark study in the May 1, 2002, *American Journal of Epidemiology*, researchers from the School of Public Health at Loma Linda University examined more than 20,000 relatively healthy people over six years. High daily intakes of water (five or more glasses) were associated with significantly lower risk for fatal coronary heart disease events, even after adjusting for smoking, hypertension, and body mass index.

The Eight-Glass-a-Day Rule

In the interest of completeness, I should point out that there are naysayers who argue that the whole dehydration issue has been overhyped. Kidney specialists feel that the "eight glasses" rule is an overestimate and that an average-size adult with healthy kidneys in a temperate climate needs no more than about 34 ounces (1 L) of fluid. And it is true that no one really knows where the "eight glasses a day" rule came from, and that there isn't a lot of science to back up what we nutritionists are saying when we encourage people to drink, drink, drink. These experts also argue that we can get the fluids we need from other sources besides water.

I say phooey. You wouldn't wash your clothes in soda, would you? And though there may not be scientific confirmation on exactly how many glasses a day we need, based on the trillions of cells in the body that need water to function, I'm going to continue to go with the assumption that when it comes to water, more is better. Sure you can go overboard if you drink massive amounts resulting in possible hyponatremia (extreme loss or dilution of sodium) or even water intoxication. But these are rare. Most of us would benefit from more water, not less.

WORTH KNOWING

There's an anecdotal water recommendation for weight loss (and also for general health) that goes like this: Divide your weight in two and drink that number of ounces a day. There's no firm science to back that up, but I've been using it for years, and as a basic guideline, it works quite well.

What about Bottled Water?

Here's the deal. I drink bottled water. I do not, ever, drink tap. This is something I frequently argue with my brother about, and the argument we have is instructive, so I'll repeat it here.

My brother—like many intelligent, well-informed people—argues that the tap water in many parts of America is among the safest in the world and has been deemed perfectly acceptable for drinking purposes. He gently suggests that folks like me who spend all this money on bottled water might be being, well, a bit silly.

Here's my answer.

Politics Can Get in the Way of Safe Water Standards

There are hundreds of chemicals, pollutants, and toxic metals (mercury, arsenic, etc.) that have the potential to wind up in our water; the government determines what an appropriate or acceptable, safe level of these compounds is. If the water has that amount (or less), it is deemed safe for drinking. However, what you have to understand is that there are full-time lobbyists in Washington whose job it is to try to make the "safe" levels of toxins as high as they can reasonably get away with. They fight for much more liberal emissions rules and lobby for much more lenient standards when it comes to environmental pollutants. They spin the research and the science, show that there is no proof that small amounts of certain chemicals cause cancer, and generally try to get regulations made that are as favorable for business and industry as they can. That's their job. Knowing that, I'm not at all sure that I trust the government to decide exactly what level of carcinogenic toxins is "safe" for me to be exposed to, especially when I'm fully aware that their decisions and policies are the result of a marriage of some science and a lot of politics.

Some years ago, fifteen-year-old West Virginia high school student Ashley Mulroy set out to conduct tests for antibiotics in the water supply as a school project; she wound up winning the prestigious Stockholm Junior Water Prize for her essay detailing the extent of antibiotic contamination of American waterways. You think it ends with antibiotics? I don't.

I'm also not confident that all the government standards are particularly up to date, largely because I see how behind the times large agencies and organizations are on other health recommendations. From time to time the government realizes that the amount of a toxin previously considered safe was way too high—whoops! In 2001, for example, the U.S. Environmental Protection Agency lowered the maximum level of arsenic permitted in drinking water from 50 mcg per liter to 10. That means they were previously allowing 400 percent the amount they now know to be "okay." Who knows how many other toxins are currently in our water at levels now considered safe that will later be found to be much too high?

Update: Since this book was written, water safety has become a national issue when lead in the drinking water of Flint, Michigan, caused a mammoth health crisis leading the president of the United States to declare a federal state of emergency. Though I'd like to believe this awful situation was an anomaly, it does not strengthen my faith in the ability of various government agencies to ensure the safety of our water supply.

Cornfield Herbicide Shows Up in American Waterways

Finally, let me offer in evidence the following: Atrazine is a powerful herbicide that, according to Michael Pollan in the *New York Times*, is applied to 70 percent of America's cornfields. At concentrations as low as 0.1 part per billion, the herbicide will chemically emasculate a male frog, causing its gonads to produce eggs. According to Pollan, who is a superb journalist and reporter known for his detail and accuracy, traces of atrazine routinely turn up in American waterways at concentrations much higher than 0.1 part per billion. But American regulators generally won't ban a pesticide till the bodies or cancer cases start to really pile up—that is, until scientists can prove beyond a reasonable doubt that the suspected molecule causes illness in humans or ecological disaster. So atrazine—in the American waterways and food system—is deemed innocent until proven guilty, "a standard of proof," says Pollan, "(that is) extremely difficult to achieve since it awaits the results of chemical testing on humans that we, rightly, don't perform."

So for all these reasons, I'm leaving tap water alone. I'll take my chances with filtered water or bottled water. Are there unscrupulous companies selling stuff that's probably no better or worse than tap? Sure. Is the good stuff expensive? Yup. But compared to a drink at an upscale bar or hotel, or a day's worth of lattes at the local coffee emporium, the best bottle of water in the world is cheap.

Doubly so for the peace of mind it buys me.

THE EXPERTS' TOP TEN LISTS

Fred Pescatore, M.D.

Fred Pescatore's *New York Times*' best-selling books, *The Hamptons Diet* and *The Hamptons Diet Cookbook*, combine the Mediterranean lifestyle with the preferences of Americans, emphasizing a whole-food approach to health and weight management.

1. **Macadamia nut oil:** This is the heart-healthiest fat with a high smoke point and no oxidation or trans-fatty acids.

2. **Avocado:** This is rich in heart-healthy monounsaturated fat.

3. **Alaskan sockeye salmon:** Responsibly caught salmon is high in omega-3 fatty acids. Its mercury and PCB content are either low or nonexistent.

4. **Red/yellow/orange peppers:** These are rich in antioxidants, B vitamins, and flavonoids that are not generally consumed.

5. **Kale:** This green is rich in well-absorbed calcium and vitamin K.

6. **Lean, organic red meat:** Genetically perfect for carnivores and one of the only sources of CLA, this kind of fat that helps people lose weight.

7. **Sea vegetables:** These often-overlooked foods contain iodine and protein and are perfect for vegetarians.

8. **Lentils and beans:** Fiber-rich legumes contain many naturally occurring B vitamins and protein for those who wish to consume less animal protein.

9. **Alcohol:** Every study around the world tells us the same thing: Drinking alcohol in moderation is good for you. Those who drink the least and those who drink the most have the worst health profiles, but those who drink in moderation can lower their risk for heart disease, stroke, and cancer.

10. **Whole foods of any kind:** These are foods that have not been touched by humans or at the very least, minimally processed. They help speed up our metabolism and keep our appetite low, therefore keeping us at our healthiest.

CHAPTER 12

HERBS, SPICES, AND CONDIMENTS

You know the old saying "variety is the spice of life"? Well, it should be the other way around. Spice is the variety of life.

Consider this: There are 25,000 phytochemicals, living plant compounds that continue to amaze with their résumé of significant health benefits. Spices are teeming with these compounds. They're awash with healing properties that are constantly being uncovered. Cinnamon lowers blood sugar; nutmeg relieves nausea; cloves are anti-inflammatory; ginger relieves morning sickness; peppermint inhibits the growth of bacteria; cumin is great for digestion; cayenne pepper increases metabolism; chili powder eases pain; curry powder safeguards your brain; cinnamon stimulates circulation; cardamom soothes indigestion; turmeric is good for practically everything—the list is endless. Spices are truly the variety of life, nature in all its pungent and aromatic glory.

Spices and Herbs Are a Natural Source of Preventive Health Care

Historically, herbs and spices have been used for adding flavors and tastes to foods. They provide unique flavors and enhancing tastes to human diets. But most herbs and spices used in culinary purposes have a long list of potential biological effects on human health. The very spices that make food so delicious and appealing come from plants whose traditional use have included acting as medicinal remedies for preventing or treating human disease for many years. The phytochemicals isolated from plants have been a great resource for discovering a large proportion of commercially available medications for the treatment of a wide range of human diseases, such as pulmonary diseases, cardiovascular diseases, diabetes, obesity, and cancers. Spices and herbs are a natural means of preventive health care; just consider the health effects on human diseases that could be accomplished through daily diets rich in their medicinal phytochemicals. Spices are a great way to get a virtual phytopharmacy into our kitchens.

And these guys seem to work synergistically in ways that are only now beginning to be understood. In an animal study, when curcumin (found in turmeric) was mixed with phenethyl isothiocyanate (a compound found in cruciferous vegetables) the combo had significant protective effects on implanted prostate tumors—though neither compound used alone showed any effect. (Curried cabbage, anyone?) In the *Journal of the American Nutraceutical Association*, researchers tested a spice blend of turmeric, ensian root, hot paprika, and vanillin for its effect on cholesterol, and it was found to have "a beneficial and clinically relevant long-term effect," decreasing non-HDL cholesterol by 16 percent. Which spice was "responsible"? Who knows? Who even cares? Use 'em all!

Plants and spices are literally teeming with health-giving phytochemicals that act and interact in a myriad of mysterious ways, and scientists will probably still be decoding their health secrets decades after everyone reading this book is gone. I think the best take-home point is to use as many of them as possible, use them often, and use them in every combination you can think of.

Cardamom

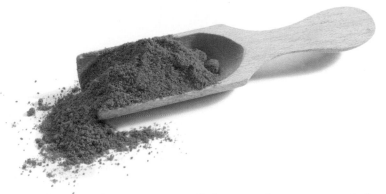

If you've ever eaten at an Indian restaurant, you've probably encountered cardamom. Cardamom is actually the dried, unripened fruit of a perennial member of the ginger family. The pods contain highly aromatic citrus-like, floral-flavored seeds with menthol undertones. Most Indian restaurants have a little dish of these seeds at the entranceway, or at the cash register, much like other restaurants have after-dinner mints. That's because when the seeds are chewed, they're a terrific breath freshener.

As a spice or seasoning, cardamom seeds can be used whole or ground. Cardamom is actually one of the world's most ancient spices. It's mentioned all over the place in The Arabian Nights. It became very popular early in the twentieth century, when about 250,000 pounds were shipped each year to Britain alone. Today, cardamom is used in cooking, as a health remedy, as a coffee flavoring in Egypt, and as an aromatic agent in perfume—especially in France and the United States. And of course, as a parting gift in the above-mentioned Indian restaurants!

But cardamom does a lot more than make your mouth taste good after eating. It stimulates bile flow for liver health and fat metabolism. Health benefits of this delicious spice are legion: It's been used as a digestive aid since ancient times, and is known for easing stomach cramps, stimulating digestion, and cutting mucus. Because it's a carminative—an agent that induces the expulsion of gas from the stomach and intestines—it's a terrific remedy for flatulence.

A wonderful way to consume it is as a tea, which you can easily make by simply pouring boiling water over about 2 teaspoons of the seeds. Let it sit for about 5 minutes, then drain, discard the seeds, and enjoy! (Many ancients believed a cardamom tea to be an aphrodisiac. Feel free to experiment and let me know the results.)

Real cardamom is expensive, second only to saffron in price, and there are lots of inferior substitutes from cardamom-related plants masquerading as the real thing. Only Elettaria cardamomum—its botanical name—is the real deal. Indian cardamom comes in two types—Malabar and Mysore. The Mysore variety contains higher levels of limonene, a valuable phytochemical that boosts the body's synthesis of an enzyme that has antioxidant properties and helps detoxify chemicals. Limonene is also found in citrus fruit peels, cherries, celery, and fennel.

WORTH KNOWING

Health professionals often recommend not using cardamom if you have gallstones, as it could precipitate an attack.

Cinnamon

C. Leigh Broadhurst, Ph.D., is, quite simply, on the short list of the smartest people I know. She's a research scientist at the USDA, and one of my "go-to" sources for the final word on any nutritional controversy. So back when Broadhurst told me about some exciting stuff her team was working on over at the USDA that involved ordinary cinnamon, believe me, my ears pricked up and I started taking notes.

Though cinnamon has a formidable reputation as a health-giving compound (more on that in a moment), the latest buzz about it has to do with its uncanny ability to moderate blood sugar. And in these days, with a growing epidemic of obesity and diabetes, that sort of stuff gets people's attention. According to Broadhurst, plenty of plants and individual phytochemicals can lower blood sugar, but many of them accomplish this by imposing toxic costs on the body. Not this one. Broadhurst and her team identified new phytochemicals in cinnamon called chalcone polymers that increase glucose metabolism in the cells twentyfold or more.

Cinnamon also contains anthocyanins, which improve capillary function. A compound that has a similar molecular composition to the ones found by Broadhurst's team has been shown to inhibit the formation of ulcers and increase blood flow to the stomachs in rats. The chalcone polymers that Broadhurst was so excited about are also powerful antioxidants.

Cinnamon Can Help with Pain and Stiffness in Muscles and Joints

Before I get to the practical use of cinnamon for modifying blood sugar, let me tell you about some other things this wonder spice can do for you. Cinnamon contains the phytochemicals eugenol and geraniol, which, according to registered dietitian and author Laurie Deutsch Mozian, can help combat candida, the overgrowth of yeast in the system that can cause so many problems. This is probably because these compounds have antimicrobial activity that can help stop the growth of bacteria and fungi (including Candida). Cinnamon also contains anti-inflammatory compounds that may ease the pain and stiffness of muscles and joints as well as menstrual discomfort.

Cinnamon is good for digestive function. Both in test-tube and in animal studies, cinnamon functions as what's called a carminative, which means "gas reliever." So if you have abdominal discomfort caused by excess gas, cinnamon would be a great thing to try. In addition, compounds in cinnamon called catechins help relieve nausea. And for whatever reason—we're not really sure why—cinnamon is known for boosting flagging appetite. Maybe it's the delicious smell or the evoked memory of Mom's apple pie. Who knows? What we do know is that it's very "digestive-friendly."

Cinnamon Extract Can Reduce Blood Sugar and "Bad" Cholesterol

Now let's get back to C. Leigh Broadhurst, Ph.D., and the team over at the USDA. They tested the effects on glucose metabolism of forty-nine different herbs, spices, and medicinal plants. As Broadhurst told me, cinnamon was the star of the show. The active ingredient—methylhydroxychalcone polymer, or MHCP—seems to mimic insulin function, increasing glucose uptake by cells and signaling certain kinds of cells to turn glucose into glycogen (the storage form of sugar). The study demonstrating that this active ingredient functioned as an "insulin mimic" was published in the *Journal of the American College of Nutrition* in 2001. Not long after, another study was published in *Diabetic Care* showing that cinnamon reduced not only blood sugar, but also triglycerides, total cholesterol, and LDL ("bad") cholesterol in people with type 2 diabetes. The research hardly escaped the notice of the natural medicine community: The legendary integrative medicine guru Jonathan Wright, M.D., uses cinnamon extract as a component in vitamin supplements he designed for modulating blood sugar.

According to Broadhurst, one of the best parts of the whole cinnamon story is that you can get the best results with the cheapest stuff. In fact, she told me that you're better off getting the really cheap stuff from the supermarket instead of any of the esoteric and expensive oil extracts, which may have some components that could be toxic if taken internally. Cinnamon powder has already had much of the essential oils removed during processing, so it's a nonissue. "Buying cinnamon in bulk is cost-effective and highly recommended," she told me.

Homemade Treatment for Blood Sugar

According to Broadhurst's excellent book on diabetes, the best way to use cinnamon to help lower blood sugar and improve type 2 diabetes is to put 3 rounded tablespoons (about 24 g) of ground cinnamon and ½ to 1 teaspoon of baking soda (less if sodium is a problem for you) in a 32-ounce (946 ml) quart-size canning jar. Fill the jar with boiling water and let it steep at room temperature till it's cool. Strain or decant the liquid, discard the grounds, put a lid on the jar, and stick it in the fridge. Drink one 8 ounce (235 ml) cup of the tea four times per day. After one to three weeks you can drop down to one or two cups a day. Type 1 diabetics can use it too, but should start with only one or two cups per day and increase by one cup per week, monitoring blood sugar closely.

And even if you're not diabetic, this little spice does so many great things that it really deserves the label "superfood."

WORTH KNOWING

Just as the manuscript for the first edition of this book was being submitted, a new animal study was published in the *Journal of the American College of Nutrition* in which dietary cinnamon reduced blood pressure. The researchers suggested that cinnamon may have a role in glucose metabolism and blood pressure regulation; they concluded that adding beneficial substances such as cinnamon to the diet may have a positive influence on blood pressure.

Cloves

If anyone remembers seeing the terrific movie Marathon Man back in the 1970s, you've undoubtedly shuddered at the frightening scene where Dustin Hoffman was subjected to various unpleasantries in a dentist chair at the hands of Laurence Olivier. But you might also recall that the "antidote" that brought immediate pain relief was an oil made from cloves. The medicinal properties of cloves reside in the volatile oil, the same one that brought pain relief to Hoffman's character in the movie. Cloves have long been used as an effective toothache remedy.

A clove is actually the dried, unopened flower bud of a type of tree that originated in the Spice Islands (Indonesia). Cloves look like tiny little nails, which is actually what their name comes from (clavus, which in Latin means "nail"). In Asian medicine, cloves are thought to be among the spices that promote energy circulation and increase the metabolic rate. The Council of Maharishi Ayurveda Physicians recommends one Red Delicious apple pierced with four cloves and boiled as the ultimate energy-enhancing winter dessert (throw away the cloves before eating). They also recommend clove, boiled with milk, to warm you up in winter. Sounds pretty good, actually.

Clove Component Kills Bacteria and Viruses

The highly respected panel German Commission E has approved the use of clove as an antiseptic and as an anesthetic. "The clove herb keeps food fresh because the main active component of cloves is eugenol, which has long been known to help kill bacteria and viruses," says Gary Elmer, Ph.D., associate professor of medicinal chemistry at the University of Washington School of Pharmacy in Seattle. Interestingly, one study investigated the chemoprotective effect of a water solution of cloves on skin cancer and found that the clove solution had an anticarcinogenic effect.

One tablespoon (4 g) of cloves contains the full amount of the recommended dietary intake of manganese for women (and just a smidgen less than the recommended amount for men). Manganese is an important nutrient for bone formation, as well as for protein, fat, and carbohydrate metabolism. A tablespoon (4 g) of cloves also contains 43 mg of calcium, 73 mg of potassium, and 17 mg of phytosterols. And 1 tablespoon (4 g) of cloves contains a little more than 2 g of fiber.

Cumin

There's a lot of confusion about the difference between cumin seeds and caraway seeds; they're actually not the same thing, though they do belong to the same plant family. The seeds look almost identical; in curry recipes, you can pretty much assume that "caraway" means "cumin." You can use cumin interchangeably in the seed or the powdered form.

There are some interesting Trivial Pursuit–type factoids about cumin, some of them having to do with romance: A paste of cumin, black pepper, and honey is considered to be an aphrodisiac in some parts of the Middle East. In Europe during the Middle Ages, cumin was believed to keep lovers from being unfaithful. Soldiers were sent off to war with cumin bread baked by their wives. Cumin was also believed to keep chickens from leaving their yard. And cumin is said to symbolize greed, maybe because its strong flavor can overwhelm a dish.

Almost all the cumin we use in the United States comes from India, but cumin is found in the cuisines of Indonesia, Thailand, and Mexico as well. For the best quality, you should look for it in a specialty market, such as one that specializes in the cuisine of these cultures. Whole cumin blends nicely into dishes like sautéed vegetables, or legumes and beans. Toasting the whole seeds in a skillet really enhances the flavor.

Cumin Decreases Allergy Symptoms

Cumin—also known as black seed or Nigella sativa—is an important medicinal herb. In many Arabian, Asian, and African countries, black seed oil is used as a natural remedy for a whole range of diseases, especially allergies. In four different studies using the oil from black cumin seeds, patients reported significantly fewer allergic symptoms. And one study found that it was effective in inactivating certain kinds of breast cancer cells, at least in a test tube. According to Laura Pensiero, R.D., cumin contains limonene, a phytochemical being studied for its role in blocking certain cancers.

In Indian medicine, cumin is considered to be a cooling herb. And according to Deepak Chopra, M.D., it helps reduce heartburn and improve digestion. You can make a great cup of tea by boiling the seeds and letting them steep—it's frequently used that way to aid digestion. The essential oil of the seeds is antimicrobial. Plus cumin is a good source of iron —1 tablespoon (6 g) has almost 4 mg. It also contains 22 mg of magnesium, 107 mg of potassium, and 56 mg of calcium.

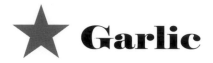

★ Garlic

Garlic is a global remedy. It's one of the oldest medicinal foods on the planet. The world's oldest medical text, the Egyptian Ebers Papyrus, mentions garlic repeatedly. Garlic was fed to slaves and soldiers in the ancient world to keep them healthy. It's been used to fuel the fighting spirit (ancient Greeks); fight leprosy, toothache, and chest pain (Hippocrates); and ward off vampires (almost any Dracula movie you can think of).

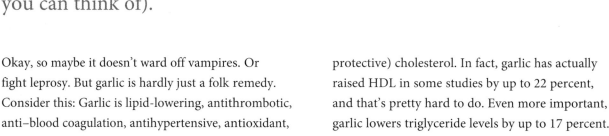

Okay, so maybe it doesn't ward off vampires. Or fight leprosy. But garlic is hardly just a folk remedy. Consider this: Garlic is lipid-lowering, antithrombotic, anti–blood coagulation, antihypertensive, antioxidant, antimicrobial, antiviral, and antiparasitic. Impressive enough for you? All of these benefits have been documented in hundreds of peer-reviewed studies.

Garlic Lowers Cholesterol and Prevents Blood Clots

Garlic is accepted even by conventional, traditional medicine as an agent for lowering cholesterol. For the record, I no longer believe that lowering cholesterol matters all that much, as Stephen Sinatra, M.D., and I argued in our 2012 book, *The Great Cholesterol Myth*.

For those who might be interested, a meta-analysis published in the *Journal of the Royal College of Physicians* showed that garlic supplements lowered total serum cholesterol levels by 12 percent after only four weeks of treatment. Not only that, they lowered LDL (the so-called "bad" cholesterol) by 4 to 15 percent without lowering HDL ("good,"

protective) cholesterol. In fact, garlic has actually raised HDL in some studies by up to 22 percent, and that's pretty hard to do. Even more important, garlic lowers triglyceride levels by up to 17 percent.

Garlic can also reduce plaque, making it a powerful agent for cardiovascular health. In one study, subjects receiving 900 mg of garlic powder for four years in a randomized, double-blinded, placebo-controlled study had a regression in their plaque volume of 2.6 percent; a matched group of subjects given a placebo (an inert substance) saw their plaque increase over the same period of time by 15.6 percent.

One of the active ingredients from garlic—allicin—also has significant antiplatelet activity. That means that it helps prevent platelets in the blood from sticking together. To understand how important that is, consider that many heart attacks and strokes are believed to be caused by spontaneous clots in the blood vessels. The anticoagulant effect of garlic is an important health benefit.

The Anticancer Properties of Fresh Garlic Extracts, Aged Garlic, and Garlic Oil

Then there's cancer. Compounds in garlic have been shown in many laboratory studies to be chemoprotective. Epidemiological evidence shows a decreased risk of stomach and colon cancer in areas where the consumption of garlic and other vegetables in the allium family is high. An article in the *Journal of Nutrition* stated that "evidence continues to point to the anticancer properties of fresh garlic extracts, aged garlic, garlic oil and a number of … compounds generated by processing garlic."

One research article demonstrated the ability of aged garlic extract to inhibit the proliferation of colorectal cancer cells. And yet another study demonstrated the ability of another compound from garlic—diallyl disulfide—to inhibit leukemia cells in a test tube.

Garlic can even help fight the common cold. In one study published in *Advances in Natural Therapy*, a group of seventy patients was given a high-quality standardized garlic supplement for twelve weeks while another group of seventy-two patients was given a placebo. The garlic group had only twenty-four colds over the course of the study, compared to sixty-five for the placebo group. What's more, the average duration of symptoms was less than half for those taking the garlic.

Studies have shown that garlic exerts antimicrobial activity against bacteria, viruses, fungi, and parasites. The antibacterial properties of allicin were written about as far back as 1944 in a paper published in the *Journal of the American Chemical Society*.

Garlic also has a positive effect on blood pressure. The effect is not enormous, but it is significant. A number of analyses have concluded that garlic can modestly reduce blood pressure by 2 to 7 percent after four weeks of treatment. An article in the *Journal of Clinical Hypertension* in May 2004 called garlic "an agent with some evidence of benefit" in reducing hypertension (others were coenzyme Q10, vitamin C, fish oil, and arginine). And the protocols of the Hypertension Institute of Nashville at St. Thomas West Hospital include a particularly high-quality, stable form of garlic called Allicidin by Designs for Health as part of their dietary and supplement regimen for both hypertension and high triglycerides.

Add Garlic to Your Weight Control Toolbox

And get this: New research shows that garlic might hold some promise for weight control. In this research, rats were fed a high-fructose diet designed to make them fat and hypertensive. It worked. Fat and hypertensive they were, with high triglycerides to boot. Then, one of the groups was given allicin (the active ingredient in garlic), while the bad diet continued. The allicin group lowered its blood pressure, insulin, and triglycerides. What's more, even though they were consuming the same amount of food, the rats given allicin stopped gaining weight. Even more impressive, a third group, given allicin from the beginning of the study, gained very little weight despite eating the exact same bad diet.

Even though it's a rat study, that's pretty impressive, don't you think? And no, the take-home message from that isn't to add garlic to your fast-food diet! Meanwhile, another study found that diabetic rats fed garlic oil had increased insulin sensitivity. Garlic may well turn out to be a useful addition to the weight control toolbox.

Crushing or Chopping Garlic Releases Its Full Potential

The key to the astonishingly wide range of health benefits in garlic seems to lie in a compound called allicin. The thing of it is, allicin isn't actually in garlic. Garlic cloves contain an amino acid called alliin.

When the garlic is crushed or damaged, the alliin reacts with an enzyme found naturally in garlic called allinase. Nature designed it so that the alliin and the enzyme allinase live in different compartments of the garlic plant, and they're meant to react only when necessary to protect the plant from attack or when it's crushed. The action of the enzyme allinase on the amino acid alliin produces, presto: allicin, probably the most important of the medicinal compounds unique to garlic and responsible for many of its marvelous health benefits.

Why is this important to understand? Because the preparation of garlic is critical for it to release its health-providing benefits. If you were, for example, to swallow a garlic clove whole—not that you'd want to—not much would happen. The garlic clove has to be crushed, or chopped, the more finely the better, for the compounds to interact.

Allicin starts to degrade after it's produced, so the fresher it is when you use it, the better. Microwaving appears to destroy it completely—sorry. Garlic experts advise crushing a little raw garlic and combining it with the cooked food shortly before serving. Eating it raw isn't recommended because it can be irritating to the stomach.

Now here's the deal with garlic supplements: In a laboratory, dried garlic powder gets added to water so that the alliin and allinase can quickly react to make allicin. The amount of allicin produced is the measure of "allicin potential." But when such garlic supplements are swallowed, the enzyme is destroyed by stomach acid. That's why some garlic products are enteric coated—to protect them against stomach acid.

Unfortunately, many supplements still don't work as advertised and don't release their "allicin potential" as promised. It is entirely possible that the variable results sometimes obtained in studies on garlic supplementation happen because of variation in the quality of the garlic supplements and lack of standardization of the allicin content. This is not to say don't use garlic supplements—absolutely do!—just use very high-quality ones that are standardized for allicin content, not allicin potential.

★ Ginger

In Ayurvedic medicine, ginger is known as the "universal remedy." No wonder. This little plant contains a whole pharmacy of ingredients with multiple health benefits.

Ten years ago, when this book first came out, ginger was mainly known for its wonderful ability to soothe an upset stomach and end nausea. But we've since discovered so many more things about ginger that I've elevated its status and given it a star. My colleague, Kris Gunnars of Authority Nutrition, says "Ginger is one of the very few "superfoods'" that is actually worthy of that term."

The active ingredients in ginger are gingerols, shogaols, gingerdiones, and zingerone, all of which are antioxidants. The zingerone and the shogaol in ginger also have anti-inflammatory properties and might be useful in a nutritional program for arthritis and/or fibromyalgia. And at the Frontiers in Cancer Prevention Research conference, research was presented that suggested that gingerols may inhibit the growth of human colorectal cancer cells. In mice, ginger extract lowered cholesterol, inhibited the oxidation of LDL cholesterol (which is even more important), and slowed the development of atherosclerosis. Not exactly a bad résumé.

Many people are already aware of ginger's awesome ability to soothe an upset stomach and end nausea. By stimulating saliva, it may also help digestion. And ginger ale has long been a favorite for upset stomach for a very good reason: It works. In one study, ginger performed better than Dramamine in warding off seasickness. And the previous mentioned active ingredient gingerol—which is the ingredient responsible for the pungent and delicious taste—is listed in the USDA database of phytochemicals as an antiemetic, meaning it has the property of preventing nausea and vomiting.

Ginger Battles Morning Sickness

Studies from Denmark found that almost 75 percent of pregnant women who used ginger experienced relief from their morning nausea without limiting side effects. Because many drugs are avoided during pregnancy because of risks to the fetus, this makes ginger an excellent herb to have around while you're pregnant.

The benefits of ginger aren't limited to morning sickness—or even sea sickness. It may also help with simple indigestion. It's generally believed that indigestion is more likely to happen to people whose stomachs take a long time to empty. In two separate studies, ginger sped up stomach emptying—which might make it helpful for people with chronic indigestion.

But wait! There's more!

Gingerol does a lot more than just settling your stomach. Research shows it's a powerful antioxidant, and has strong anti-inflammatory properties as well. In one study of 247 people with osteoarthritis of the knee, people taking ginger extract required less pain medication and experienced less pain.

Two grams of ginger powder daily will also lower blood sugar. A 2015 study tested the results of 2 g of ginger powder daily with diabetic patients and found that the people taking the powder lowered their fasting blood sugar by 12 percent, as well as improving their hemoglobin A1C levels by 10 percent over the course of three months. (Hemoglobin A1C is a blood test usually used to diagnose diabetes.)

Animal studies show that ginger can protect against age-related decline in brain function, and in one human study—on sixty middle-aged women—ginger extract improved both working memory and reaction time.

It's effective in helping fight infections. Ginger extract can put a damper on the growth of several different types of bacteria, and it works against the same oral bacteria that is associated with inflammatory gum disease (periodontitis, gingivitis.)

Animal studies on ginger also show that it has antitumorigenic effects and helps boost the immune system; it's an effective antimicrobial and antiviral agent. Studies also demonstrate positive effects on the gastrointestinal tract, the cardiovascular system, pain, and fever. No wonder that a nice hot ginger tea with lemon is a home remedy for all sorts of variations of feeling under the weather.

One benefit that has been noted for thousands of years is ginger's ability to improve circulation. At the Deepak Chopra Center, they routinely give ginger as a remedy for people with cold hands and feet, some-thing that Chinese and Indian physicians have done for eons.

Personally, I put ginger in a lot of things I eat and drink. I almost always include it in juices. And lately, I've taken to infusing my regular drinking water with some fresh lemon peel and ginger root; I keep the lemon and ginger in the water overnight, and drink it during the next day. It's an easy way to get some powerful antioxidants and anti-inflammatories along with your daily H$_2$0.

WORTH MENTIONING

Ginger has very few side effects, but there are a couple of precautions to be aware of. It's possible that ginger increases the absorption of other drugs, but we don't know for sure. If you give ginger to an animal at the same time as you give it a barbiturate, it sleeps longer. (No, I never tried this at home, but it's in the literature!) The explanation is that the ginger probably increases absorption of the drug.

Ginger has a nice blood-thinning effect (like an aspirin in a way), but because of that you should be careful taking it with medications that prevent clotting, such as Coumadin, or even aspirin. According to Joe and Teresa Graedon, Ph.D., authors of *The People's Pharmacy*, the combination of an anticlotting medication and ginger could conceivably result in unexpected bleeding. It's also said to increase bile acid secretion, which is why people with gallstones or gallbladder disease are advised to avoid the herb unless supervised by a health professional.

Mustard Seeds

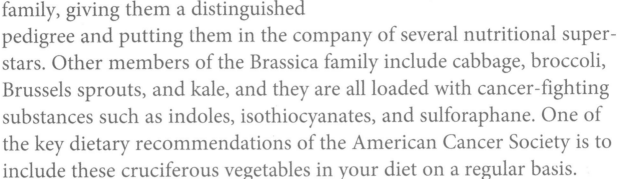

Mustard seeds are, believe it or not, members of the Brassica family, giving them a distinguished pedigree and putting them in the company of several nutritional superstars. Other members of the Brassica family include cabbage, broccoli, Brussels sprouts, and kale, and they are all loaded with cancer-fighting substances such as indoles, isothiocyanates, and sulforaphane. One of the key dietary recommendations of the American Cancer Society is to include these cruciferous vegetables in your diet on a regular basis.

So mustard seeds come from veggie royalty. Other members of the same plant family include horseradish (see page 44) and cress. Mustard seeds, like their relatives, are able to produce isothiocyanates, which are aggressive substances that have the function of a chemical weapon against the plant's predators.

Because these isothiocyanates are dangerous to the plants as well, they are stored in the plant organism as glucosinolates, which are harmless. By an enzymatic reaction that happens whenever the plant tissue gets damaged—like, for example, if it's chewed—the isothiocyanates are quickly formed. Many of these isothiocyanates have been found to have significant roles in human health, as protectors against carcinogens. Mustard seeds are a source of one particular compound, allyl isothiocyanate, which is believed to play a role in the prevention of tumors and the suppression of tumor growth.

Mustard Seed Is Rooted in History

In fact, the use of mustard (and mustard seeds) as a medicinal plant predates all the science on phytochemicals. From its beginnings, mustard was considered a medicinal plant rather than a food; Hippocrates, the father of modern medicine, used mustard in all sorts of medicines and poultices. The ancient Chinese considered mustard an aphrodisiac. And the mustard seed figures prominently as a symbol in the Christian faith, used to signify something small and insignificant that, when nourished, can grow into something of great strength and power.

Mustard itself is only as good as the seeds it was made from. There are many delicious gourmet mustards loaded with phytochemicals. Seek them out! Good mustard can stimulate the appetite and circulation and help neutralize toxins. If you're adventurous, use the seed in cooking. Mustard seeds as a culinary ingredient is popular in Western and Asian cuisines.

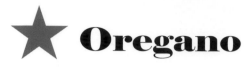

Oregano

Every so often, a doctor or healer gets so excited about one herb, food, nutrient, or ingredient that he or she writes a whole book singing its praises. That's exactly what happened to Cass Ingram, D.O., and the result was a little book called The Cure Is in the Cupboard. The herb that got Ingram so excited that he decided to write a book about it? Oregano.

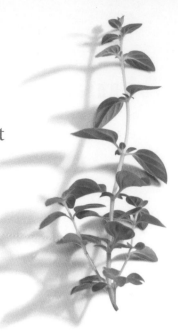

Read the research on this herb and it all becomes clear. Oregano is rich in a host of nutrients, including calcium, magnesium, zinc, iron, potassium, copper, boron, manganese, vitamin C, vitamin A, and niacin. Oregano also seems to be the herb with the highest antioxidant activity. According to a study published in the *Journal of Agricultural and Food Chemistry*, oregano has forty-two times more antioxidant activity than apples, thirty times more than potatoes, twelve times more than oranges, and—maybe most surprising of all—four times more than the amazing blueberries! But that's only the beginning.

Oregano Oil Has Medicinal Benefits

The medicinal parts of this plant are contained in the oil extracted from the leaves or from the herb itself picked during the flowering season and eaten fresh or dried. The essential oil contains thymol (see Thyme on page 324) and carvacrol, compounds that have antifungal, antibacterial, and antiparasitic properties. In one study, 77 percent of patients treated for enteric parasites were parasite free after taking oil of oregano in tablet form for six weeks. As of 2017, it has inhibited the growth of at least ten different microbes, including *Candida albicans* (yeast).

To top it off, oregano—like its relative rosemary—contains the powerful compound rosmarinic acid (see Rosemary, page 322), which has been found to have antimutagenic and anticarcinogenic properties.

Traditionally this herb's oil has been used as a digestive aid and, because of its anti-inflammatory properties, to support joint function. Plenty of health benefits come from using the herb regularly, but for special conditions—such as *Candida* or inflammation—a health professional may suggest oil of oregano supplements.

WORTH KNOWING

In homeopathy, oregano is used to increase sexual excitability. It's also really, really good on pizza.

Parsley

If you've ever chewed on a sprig of parsley after a meal (and before kissing your date), you've experienced its ability to freshen the breath firsthand. What you might not know is that it has the same ability to freshen the whole system.

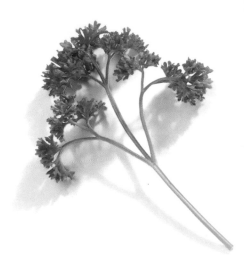

Parsley is known for its detoxification (and deodorizing) properties. It's the world's most popular herb. The Greeks wore parsley crowns at their banquets to stimulate their appetite. Peter Rabbit went looking for some parsley when he overate Mr. McGregor's vegetables. And the Romans believed that nibbling on parsley sprigs would allow them to drink more wine without becoming drunk. From ancient times to the modern dinner table, people have known intuitively of parsley's ability to detoxify. And modern science has begun to confirm what the ancients suspected.

Use Parsley to Purify

Its ability to freshen the breath—and to detoxify the system—comes from the same substance that makes it green: chlorophyll. Dozens of studies have confirmed the ability of chlorophyll to purify and rejuvenate—and it has been shown to stop bacterial growth in wounds, it deodorizes, and it counters toxins, it deactivates many carcinogens, and it builds blood, renews tissues, and counteracts inflammations. In Asian traditions, chlorophyll benefits anemic conditions; it also helps kidney function, probably because it has mild diuretic properties.

Parsley is used by diabetics in Turkey to reduce blood glucose; in one published study, an extract from parsley significantly reduced the blood glucose of rats and reduced their weight! A second study demonstrated parsley's ability to protect the livers of diabetic rats as well. Wouldn't it be interesting if parsley turned out to be another plant weapon in the armamentarium against blood sugar challenges, obesity, and diabetes?

Parsley Part of a Select Group of Cancer Fighters

There's also some suggestion that the volatile oils in parsley—especially one called myristicin—may inhibit tumors. The National Cancer Institute, which has invested millions and millions of dollars researching the anticancer potential of plant foods, found that umbelliferous vegetables (which include parsley) are among a select group of about a dozen foods with the highest anticancer activity.

Ten sprigs of parsley contain 556 mcg of the eye-protective carotenoids lutein and zeaxanthin, as well as 505 mcg of beta-carotene, 164 mcg of bone-building vitamin K, and 842 IUs of vitamin A. Oh, and if you're lucky, while you're shopping you might occasionally come across parsley root, a special variety of parsley grown for its root. It looks like a baby parsnip and usually has the parsley greens attached. I've never tried it, but it's supposed to be delicious in soup as well as having medicinal properties for the stomach.

Rosemary

Rosemary has a poetic and romantic past. It flourishes in the Mediterranean, the south of France, and Portugal. It bears beautiful little blue flowers that are the stuff of legend. Its fragrant properties have been used in aromatherapy since the fourteenth century. And its medicinal properties, known and appreciated by herbalists for hundreds of years, are now being confirmed by research.

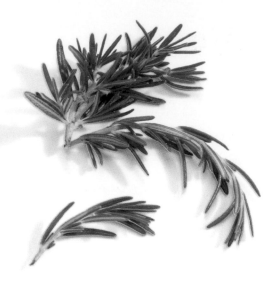

Some of the health-promoting benefits of rosemary come from two of its constituents, caffeic acid and rosmarinic acid, plus plant compounds like diterpenes and monoterpenes, and antioxidants like vitamin E and assorted flavonoids. The acids are anti-inflammatory, and may be helpful in reducing the inflammation that contributes to asthma, liver disease, and heart disease. Exciting research has been done on rosemary's potential for inhibiting cancers such as breast, colon, and skin cancers; animal studies have confirmed that the oil is liver protective, antimutagenic, and tumor inhibiting. The oil is also mildly antibiotic and antiviral, probably because of the diterpenes.

And Shakespeare was on to something when he associated rosemary with memory ("There's rosemary, that for remembrance: pray you, love, remember.") Herbalists have treated rosemary as helpful for the brain as far back as the seventeenth century, when the English physician Nicholas Culpeper wrote that rosemary helps "weak memory, and quickens the senses" as well as "diseases of the head and brain, as the giddiness and swimmings therein . . . ."

Rosemary Works Like an Alzheimer's Drug

As it turns out in the light of modern science, rosemary contains several compounds that prevent the breakdown of acetylcholine, an important neurotransmitter in the brain and one that is needed for memory and healthy brain function. (In fact, one drug used for Alzheimer's—Aricept—works similarly, by interfering with acetylcholine breakdown.)

Besides being used widely as a culinary herb, rosemary frequently lends its distinctive fragrance to soaps and cosmetics. Aromatherapists use rosemary oil in baths and massage lotions, and they consider it to have an enlivening quality that promotes healing and happiness.

WORTH KNOWING

No health hazards or side effects are known with proper use. On rare occasion, a contact allergy has been observed. Though rosemary is perfectly safe in amounts normally consumed in foods, in medicinal dosages it should not be used during pregnancy due to concerns that it might have uterine- and menstrual flow–stimulant effects.

Sage

Sage is a great little herb, which has been valued for more than 2,000 years, both for its medicinal properties and for its ability to spice up foods. In Ayurvedic medicine, sage is considered a purifying herb. Deepak Chopra recommends it for "excessive accumulation of toxic, morbid emotions." On top of that, it also smells great!

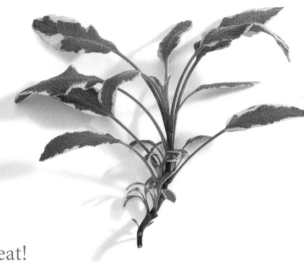

Sage probably got its reputation as a purifying herb because, along with its sisters in the mint family, it has antimicrobial and antiviral activities. Why? Because of its volatile oil. Oil of sage contains a compound called thujone, an effective agent against both *Salmonella* and *Candida*. Sage also contains the phenolic acid rosmarinic acid, which is both an antioxidant and an anti-inflammatory. For this reason, sage has been found to be beneficial for fighting such inflammatory conditions as gingivitis and rheumatoid arthritis.

In animal research, sage has been found to be hypertensive (it lowers blood pressure). In diabetic patients, it's been found to improve glycemic control, lower triglycerides, lower hemoglobin A1C, and raise HDL cholesterol compared to placebo. Something herbalists have known for a long time is that sage works as a memory enhancer. In one study, Alzheimer's patients given sage extract had a significantly better outcome on cognitive function tests than those given a placebo. Sage was also found to enhance memory in healthy young volunteers as well. Sage has been used for combating indigestion, excessive perspiration, and sore throats. And if that weren't enough, it's also been found to be helpful with menopausal night sweats.

WORTH KNOWING

Sage is completely safe, and no health hazards or side effects are known. However, sage may decrease breast milk supply and is considered by some experts to be a uterine stimulant—pregnancy experts advise that sage and sage preparations should not be taken during pregnancy.

Thyme

Although a generation of baby boomers probably first heard the name of this herb through the immortal Simon and Garfunkel song, it's actually been around since the days of the ancient Greeks and Romans, who valued it as an aphrodisiac. In fact, Euell Gibbons, in *Stalking the Healthful Herbs*, said, "According to ancient tradition, if a girl wears a corsage of wild thyme flowers, it means that she is looking for a sweetheart; and according to another tradition, if a bashful boy drinks enough wild thyme tea, it will give him courage to take her up on it!" I don't know about that, but I sure get warm and fuzzy when I hear the Simon and Garfunkel song.

Thyme is one of a naturally occurring class of compounds called biocides, meaning compounds that can destroy harmful microbes. The primary fragrant oil of thyme is thymol, a powerful antiseptic. You've probably felt its medicinal effects if you've ever gargled with Listerine. Research from Canada shows that thymol can reduce bacterial resistance to drugs such as penicillin. And Portuguese researchers have reported that thyme oil—even low amounts of it—act as a kind of natural preservative, fighting against a number of common foodborne bacteria that can cause sickness, while Polish researchers found that thyme oil was very effective against the bacterial strains of *Staphylococcus*, *Enterococcus*, *Escherichia*, and *Psudomas genera*.

Thymol is also a wonderful antioxidant and anti-inflammatory agent. Thyme essential oil fungal cream was found to work on eczema-like lesions in 66.5 percent of those treated with it compared to 28.5 percent of those using placebo. Thyme essential oil also helps kill yeast cells.

It's a terrific aid to digestion: Thyme can help dislodge the mucus coating of the intestinal tract and has a long history in relieving chest and respiratory problems such as coughs and bronchitis—probably why it's used in many over-the-counter vapor rubs or cough drops. Because it is antiseptic, thymol often shows up as an ingredient in natural toothpastes.

The herb itself is typically used for flavoring any kind of slow cooked-dish (soups and stews), and it is a nice addition to a bouquet garni. Rebecca Wood, a noted author and authority on whole food, suggests adding 3 tablespoons (13 g) of dried thyme to boiling water and honey for a homemade cough syrup she swears is more effective than any of the ready-made kinds.

★ Turmeric

If there were ever a contest for a spice that deserved a whole book written about it, turmeric would be the clear winner. It's pretty much my favorite spice, not only for the almost encyclopedic list of health benefits (more about that in a moment) but also for the incredible taste. Turmeric is a staple in India, where 94 percent of the turmeric in the world originates. It's the spice that gives Indian food its distinctive flavor. It's an important part of curry, so every time you're eating anything with a curry sauce, you're eating some turmeric. I use it on just about everything, but my latest discovery is how great it tastes on scrambled eggs and veggie omelets.

Turmeric is a member of the ginger family, and the plant's healing properties reside in its fingerlike stalk. The part of the plant that is actually used is called the rhizome. Turmeric itself contains a bunch of compounds, but the family of compounds thought to be most responsible for turmeric's medicinal effects are the curcuminoids, which are also responsible for giving turmeric its bright yellow color. The most important—and the most studied of the curcuminoids—is curcumin. Some of the studies mentioned below were done on curcumin, but the benefits apply equally to the turmeric plant that contains it.

Turmeric Known for Alleviating Arthritis and Joint Inflammation

Curcumin—the active ingredient in turmeric—is a powerful anti-inflammatory. So powerful that it actually matches the effectiveness of a number of anti-inflammatory drugs. Among its other actions, curcumin blocks a molecule called NF-kappaB, which turns on genes related to inflammation and plays a

role in a host of chronic diseases. It also boosts an important hormone in the brain known as BDNF (Brain-Derived Neurotrophic Factor) which is basically Miracle-Gro for your brain cells. Low levels of BDNF have been linked to both depression and Alzheimer's disease. Trust me—you want a lot of BDNF hanging around in your brain, and curcumin helps that to happen.

Turmeric is part of the healing systems of India, China, and the Polynesian Islands, and occupies a place of distinction in both Ayurvedic and Chinese medicine. One reason is its anti-inflammatory properties, which are believed to be due to the presence of the aforementioned curcuminoids. One of turmeric's many traditional uses has been for the treatment of arthritis, because of its ability to lower inflammation. In one study, curcumin was found to be virtually as effective as the anti-inflammatory medication phenylbutazone. It's used in India to relieve arthritis, and can be useful for muscle pains as well as joint inflammation and even carpal tunnel syndrome. If you're interested in why it works so well, one school of thought is that it exerts its anti-inflammatory effect by lowering histamine levels; other experts are not sure of the exact mechanism. In the long run, who cares? It works as an anti-inflammatory, and does it without any toxic side effects. That's what matters.

And then there's cancer. There are at least thirty published studies indicating that curcumin has an antitumor effect (either reducing the number or size of tumors or the percentage of animals who developed them). Of course these are mostly animal studies, but still, that's pretty promising. And not all the studies are on animals: One study, published in 2006 in the medical journal *Oncogene*, showed that curcumin inhibited the growth of human colon cancer cells. Though no one is claiming that turmeric cures cancer, there is plenty of reason to believe that it is a useful adjunct to the diet of everyone concerned with staying healthy.

Curcumin has powerful antioxidant properties as well as being highly anti-inflammatory. In one rat study, for example, curcumin provided significant protection from cataract development induced by a powerful oxidizing chemical. The group of rats treated with curcumin not only had protection against the damage done by this chemical, but the transparency of the lenses in their little eyes was improved as well. Many other studies have demonstrated curcumin's antioxidant capabilities. In science jargon, curcumin "inhibits lipid peroxidation," which means it fights damage from oxidating substances that age the body and contribute to disease. In other words, it's good stuff.

Why Your Liver Loves Turmeric

This ability to fight inflammation and also to serve as an antioxidant makes curcumin a very liver-friendly food. I like to recommend it for people with various liver ailments, including hepatitis. Though it's not the only thing I would use for serious liver problems, it's definitely part of the arsenal. One study, in the journal *Toxicology*, demonstrated curcumin's significant liver protection in male rats largely through its aforementioned antioxidant properties. Mark Stengler, N.M.D., author of *The Natural Physician's Healing Therapies*, also recommends it for hepatitis and says that it is frequently used to lower elevated liver enzymes.

Turmeric is also one of the easiest spices to use. It has a really pleasing taste and a beautiful color, and it tastes good on almost any food you can think of. Deepak Chopra says that "its traditional purifying effect makes it a useful spice for people participating in a detoxification program." In addition to cooking with it, you can also mix it into a paste with water and apply it directly to irritated skin (including pimples) before bedtime. Chopra also suggests mixing turmeric powder with a little honey and using the mixture to coat your throat at the first sign of a sore throat.

So we already know the strong science behind the pharmacy that lives in the turmeric plant. What does traditional Eastern medicine say about it? According to *The Yoga of Herbs: An Ayurvedic Guide to Herbal Medicine*, coauthored by David Frawley, O.M.D., and the highly respected Indian doctor and herbal authority Vasant Lad, M.A.Sc., "Turmeric gives the energy of the Divine Mother and grants prosperity. It is effective for cleansing the chakras and purifying the channels of the subtle body."

When modern Western science and traditional forms of healing such as Ayurvedic and Chinese medicine both agree on the healthful properties of the same compound, it's time to go to the store.

Vinegar

(apple cider vinegar)

Vinegar was discovered by chance more than 10,000 years ago. It gets its name from the French, vin aigre—meaning "sour wine." Vinegar is made when fresh, naturally sweet cider is fermented into an alcoholic beverage (hard cider). Then it's fermented once again. The result is vinegar. You could say that wine is to grapes what vinegar is to wine.

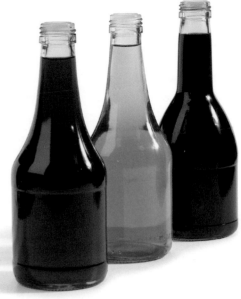

Vinegar can be made from any fruit, or from any material containing sugar that can be fermented to less than 18 percent ethyl alcohol (including such things as honey, maple syrup, beets, potatoes, and coconut). When it's made from apples, it's called apple cider vinegar (more about that in a moment). The U.S. Food and Drug Administration (FDA) requires that any product called "vinegar" contain at least 4 percent acidity. This requirement ensures the minimum strength of the vinegar sold at the retail level. According to whole-food expert and author Rebecca Wood, you shouldn't use aluminum, copper, or cast-iron when cooking with vinegar, because that 4 to 6 percent acidity is corrosive. And if you want to retain the acid flavor of vinegar, stir it in after removing the dish from the heat.

So why is vinegar listed in the world's healthiest foods? Simple. It's a virtual infusion of healthy minerals, vitamins, and amino acids. In fact, unpasteurized vinegar can contain as many as fifty different nutrients, including those that come from the original material the vinegar is made from (such as apples). But note well the term unpasteurized. Remember that pasteurization is basically a process that subjects foods to tremendous amounts of heat. That has the "benefit" of destroying microorganisms, but it's a dubious benefit when it also destroys the heat-sensitive vitamins and enzymes that made it a good food to begin with. To get the health benefits of vinegar, you should look on the label for key terms like unpasteurized, unfiltered, traditionally brewed, traditionally fermented, or aged in wood.

Real Organic Vinegar Beats Common Supermarket Vinegar

Traditionally fermented foods are among the healthiest on the planet, and vinegar is no exception. The clean white vinegar you get at the supermarket is a food chemist's invention made from coal tar and has none of the health properties of real, fermented, organic vinegar. Distilled vinegar is no better. Distilling turns the vinegar into steam and in the process destroys the natural malic and tartaric acids, which are important in fighting body toxins and inhibiting unfriendly bacteria. To get the health benefits of vinegar, get the real thing.

The best known of the vinegars in natural health circles is the kind made from apples. Apple cider vinegar is cheap and easy to use, and it benefits our health in numerous ways. Hippocrates, the father of medicine, thought of it as a powerful elixir and a naturally occurring antibiotic and antiseptic. Ancient Egyptians, Romans, and Greeks used it. And apple cider vinegar is mentioned in the Bible as an antiseptic and healing agent. Even Columbus had barrels of vinegar on his ships for the prevention of scurvy. Indeed, apple cider vinegar has been used for thousands of years, as both a health and a cleansing agent.

Is Apple Cider Vinegar Really a Cure-All?

Books have been written touting apple cider vinegar's benefits for everything from weight loss to osteoporosis to arthritis. Whether it does all the things its proponents claim it does is another matter. I found a humorous "poem" by Patricia Carrol, R.N., M.S., extolling vinegar's many benefits but also offering the following caution: Beware of claims too good to be true—For research backs up but a few.

There's no doubt in my mind that apple cider vinegar is good for you. I'm just suspicious of whether it's a cure-all. That said, there are a lot of terrific things to be said about real, unpasteurized vinegar made from apples. It's nutrient rich, containing minerals such as potassium, phosphorus, natural organic fluorine, silicon, trace minerals, and pectin as well as many other powerful nutrients and enzymes. Over the centuries, oxymel—a combination of apple cider vinegar and honey—has been widely used to dissolve painful calcium deposits in the body, and for other health problems such as hay fever. And while I've had my suspicions about apple cider vinegar's effectiveness as a weight loss product, some people swear by it—and a study in *Diabetes Care* does indicate that it may have some impact on blood sugar and insulin that can only be seen as beneficial.

Studies Examine the Use of Vinegar in Treating Diabetes

In the *Diabetes Care* study, apple cider vinegar significantly improved insulin sensitivity in insulin-resistant subjects. The vinegar also improved insulin sensitivity somewhat in diabetics, but the results didn't quite reach statistical significance. The authors stated that "vinegar may possess physiological effects similar to . . . metformin." (Metformin, the generic name for glucophage, is a drug typically given to diabetics and prediabetics to increase insulin sensitivity.) Insulin resistance is a feature of metabolic syndrome and often precedes diabetes, and anything that makes the cells more sensitive to insulin and helps control blood sugar bears looking into. The authors concluded that "further investigations to examine the efficacy of vinegar as an antidiabetic therapy are warranted."

Carol Johnson, Ph.D., R.D., associate director of the nutrition program at Arizona State University, was interviewed by the *New York Times* (March 29, 2016) on the subject of vinegar and weight loss. She agreed that consuming a small amount of vinegar before a starch-containing meal might blunt a rise in blood sugar by 20 to 40 percent, probably by inhibiting the digestion of starch. (Some skeptics quip that drinking the vinegar makes you so nauseous that you eat less!) Apple cider vinegar is usually recommended because it's more palatable. Johnson recommends diluting it in water: "One tablespoon (15 ml) to eight ounces (235 ml) of water, and ingest it with the first bites of the meal. You want the acid to beat the starch into the intestines."

Nutritionist and researcher Jeff Volek, R.D., Ph.D., whose top ten list of healthy foods is featured on page 362, suggests a salad with vinegar at the beginning of every meal for its potential help with managing blood sugar.

Herbs, Spices, and Condiments Runner-Up

Black Pepper

Black pepper stimulates the taste buds, which increases production of hydrochloric acid in the stomach, improving digestion. Why would you want more acid, especially if you have heartburn? Many leaders in the field of complementary medicine, such as Jonathan Wright, M.D., argue that heartburn comes from too little stomach acid, not from too much. Pepper's also long been recognized for its ability to stimulate the appetite and produce relief from nausea. It is considered a carminative—an herbal medicine or digestive tonic that can help dispel gas from the intestine.

THE EXPERTS' TOP TEN LISTS

J.J. Virgin, C.N.S., C.H.F.I.

J.J. Virgin is a celebrity nutritionist and the author of the best-selling *The Virgin Diet*, *The Sugar Impact Diet*, and *The Miracle Mindset*.

1. **Apples**: An apple a day keeps the constipation away. The pectin fiber in apples is great for your gut and detoxifying, too.

2. **Freshly ground flaxseed meal**: The fiber will keep the hunger hormone ghrelin suppressed. Flaxseed is a rich source of alpha-linolenic acid, an omega-3 fatty acid.

3. **Green tea**: Drink daily to boost your metabolism and load up on antioxidants. The theanine in green tea is a natural de-stressor.

4. **Extra-virgin olive oil**: Add a few tablespoons to salads and vegetables daily to help lower blood pressure and prevent LDL oxidation.

5. **Berries (all kinds)**: Eat a serving of organic blue, black, or red berries daily for antioxidant protection. They also contain ellagic acid, which is protective against cancer.

6. **Sardines**: A great source of EPA and DHA omega-3 fatty acids, without the heavy metals and toxins found in many large fish.

7. **Lentils**: A great slow-release carbohydrate source that is rich in fiber and moderate in protein. A cup of lentil soup as an appetizer is a great natural appetite suppressant.

8. **Sea vegetables**: Rich in minerals and great at detoxifying heavy metals and pesticides, these are also very alkalizing and can help offset the acid load from the Standard American Diet of grains, meats, and dairy.

9. **Organic eggs**: A great source of complete protein, and yes, eat the yolk—it's rich in vitamins E and A and choline, a nutrient that is important for the brain and nervous system. Eat your eggs soft-boiled or poached to avoid oxidizing the cholesterol in the yolk.

10. **Turkey**: Think of turkey as nature's Prozac. It is rich in tryptophan, which your body uses to make serotonin, the neurotransmitter that helps boost mood and lower sugar cravings.

CHAPTER 13

OILS

As I've mentioned before, one of the great problems with the Western diet is an imbalance in fat intake. We've been oversold on the dangers of saturated fat as well as on the unqualified goodness of polyunsaturated fats. The true picture is more complex and nuanced. All saturated fat is not bad for you (see "Coconut Oil," page 335, for example), and polyunsaturated fat is a large class of fatty acids with many members. Polyunsaturated fats include the proinflammatory omega-6s and the anti-inflammatory omega-3s. The balance between the two is essential to human health. It's as simple as that.

We've heard much about the dangers of omega-6 fats, and how they contribute to inflammation. However, omega-6s aren't, by themselves, bad for you. What is bad for you—very bad, indeed—is overconsuming omega-6s while underconsuming omega-3s, which is exactly what most of us do. Almost all processed foods are made with vegetable oils, restaurants long ago abandoned (healthy) saturated fats for vegetable oils, and health authorities have pounded the message that vegetable oil is good for decades. No wonder research now shows that we typically consume 16 times more of the proinflammatory omega-6s than we do the anti-inflammatory omega-3s.

Omega-6s (linoleic acid) and one of the omega-3s (alpha-linolenic acid) are considered *essential fats* (meaning our body can't make them and we must get them from our diet). The other two omega-3s, which I consider to be the most important of all (docosahexaenoic acid [DHA] and eicosapentaenoic acid [EPA]), can theoretically be made in the body from the first omega-3 (alpha-linolenic acid), but the body does a lousy job of it—only a small percent of alpha-linolenic acid gets converted to DHA and EPA. That's why fish and fish oil are so great—they give you ready-made DHA and EPA so your body doesn't have to make them. But I digress.

What's Wrong with Omega-6s?

The problem of getting far too much omega-6s is compounded by the fact that most of the omega-6s we get are crappy. Omega-6s are like foods at the typical Vegas buffet—the wrong kind of food, and there's so darn much of it! Most of us get our omega-6s from highly refined and processed vegetable oils—safflower, sunflower, soybean, and corn—which are loaded with a refined omega-6 devoid of any of the natural health-promoting antioxidants that are normally found in these oils but are processed out because they shorten shelf life. Commercial, processed, refined vegetable oils are among the worst foods on the planet, and we've been told they're healthy because they are polyunsaturated. Don't believe it for a minute.

It's not that omega-6s don't do any good. They do. A comprehensive review paper on the relationship of fats to coronary heart disease by Frank Hu, JoAnn Manson, and Walter Willett from Harvard—the folks who ran the Nurses' Health Study—points out that omega-6s do lower LDL ("bad") cholesterol and also improve insulin sensitivity. But even that team, gently conservative in its phrasing, point out that "the ratio of omega-3 to omega-6 [fats] is

less than optimal and should be improved." The argument is over whether to improve that ratio by increasing omega-3s, reducing omega-6s, or both. Personally, I think it's both. No one—save theoretically the Eskimos, who eat a ton of omega-3s—is in any danger of getting too much omega-3 and not enough omega-6. In fact, it's the opposite.

BALANCING FATTY ACIDS IS KEY TO HEALTHY BLOOD FLOW

Why is the balance between omega-6 and omega-3 so important? Because these fatty acids are the building blocks of hormones and "minihormones" called *eicosanoids* (also called *prostaglandins*), which control dozens of metabolic processes in the body that need to be in balance for us to stay healthy. For example, some of these prostaglandins control inflammation, some are anti-inflammatory. Some control clotting, some control flow. It's not that they are good or bad—but that they need to be in balance. If you're injured, you want some inflammation and clotting—it's part of the body's healing response to send water and blood to the site of injury and then to allow it to clot. But if you clot too much, you get a stroke. On the other hand, if you don't clot at all, you hemorrhage. Get it? In real estate, it's location, location, location. In fatty acids, it's balance, balance, balance.

Our Paleolithic ancestors—and all known hunter-gatherer societies that have been studied—consumed between a 1:1 and 4:1 ratio of omega-6s to omega-3s. Most nutritionists consider that the ideal intake ratio, and the ones I know lean more toward 1:1. Would you like to know what the average person consuming a Western diet gets? It's between 20:1 and 25:1. (I've heard some estimates as high as 65:1, but even at the lower number, it's completely unhealthy.)

Think I'm being a nervous Nelly about nothing? Consider this: High ratios of omega-6s to omega-3s are associated with increased prostate and breast cancer risk; increased risk of heart disease; and aggravated inflammatory and autoimmune diseases.

In addition, most of our restaurants, in response to the fear of "bad" saturated fat, now cook with "healthy" vegetable oils. And cook. And cook. And recook. New research shows that high amounts of a toxin called HNE (4-hydroxy-trans-2-nonenal), with connections to heart disease and neurological disorders, accumulate in vegetable-based cooking oils that are heated or reheated for hours at a time (fast-food restaurant, anyone?). HNE forms in especially high amounts in polyunsaturated oils—including canola, corn, soybean, and sunflower. (It does not form in saturated fats.) "There's a tremendous literature in biochemistry on HNE, a library of studies going back twenty years. It's a very toxic compound," says lead researcher, A. Saari Csallany, a professor of food chemistry and nutritional biochemistry at the University of Minnesota.

Eating the Right Oils Can Help You Avoid Deadly Diseases

Remember Vioxx and Celebrex? They were COX-2 inhibitors. COX-2 enzymes create inflammation in the body. When our intake of omega-6 fats greatly exceeds our omega-3 fats, guess what happens? COX-2 enzymes increase. High intakes of omega-6 polyunsaturated fats (coupled with low intakes of omega-3s) equal higher levels of inflammation. If you don't think that's anything to worry about, recall the 2004 cover story in *Time* magazine that called inflammation "The Secret Killer." The subtitle: "The surprising link between inflammation and heart attacks, cancer, Alzheimer's and other diseases."

So consider all this when you look at this chapter. Here are the take-home points:

- Some saturated fat is good for us.
- Omega-3s are very, very good for us.
- Monounsaturated fats are good for us.
- Omega-6s are good for us in balanced (usually small) amounts and from sources that haven't been processed and refined to death.
- Reused (reheated) vegetable oils are really, really bad.
- Trans fats are metabolic poison. The acceptable level in the diet is zero.

Keep these points in mind when you read through the fats and oils that have been selected for inclusion in the "world's healthiest foods." Remember as well that in all cases, unrefined, cold-pressed oils beat the pants off the refined kind, even when it's a healthy oil such as olive oil.

Almond Oil

Along with sesame oil, almond oil is probably one of the most popular massage oils, primarily because it smells so darn good. But besides its nonfood uses, almond oil is a really good, healthful oil to use for cooking.

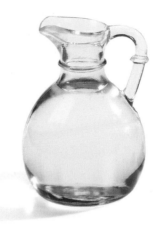

Almond oil is very high in monounsaturated fats—61 to 65 percent of the fat in almond oil is from oleic acid, the same omega-9 monounsaturated fat that makes olive and macadamia nut oils so healthy. Monounsaturated fats (omega-9s) are central to the Mediterranean diet that has been shown in virtually every single research study to be associated with lower rates of heart disease.

Almond Oil Underappreciated for Its Healthy Monounsaturated Fats

Through admirable lobbying on behalf of the olive oil industry, the FDA took a look at the massive evidence for the health benefits of monounsaturated fats and allowed a health claim to be made for olive oil as a result. Understand that the health benefit comes from monounsaturated fat in general, but because it was the Olive Oil Association who petitioned the FDA, the FDA limited its investigation of the research to "monounsaturated fat in olive oil," while recognizing that other oils provide this same fat. It's all political. Monounsaturated fat is monounsaturated fat, and it does good things for you whether you get it from olive oil or almond oil or macadamia oil or avocado oil. True, almond oil doesn't have quite as much as olive or macadamia nut oil, but it's still a good source of this healthy fat.

There are dozens of studies on the potential role of almonds in a healthy diet and on the antioxidant properties of various phytochemicals found in the nut itself. (For more on this, see Almonds, page 165.) How many of these compounds get into the oil is anyone's guess, but it stands to reason that the less high heat, chemicals, and processing used in extracting the oil, the better. (That's why I recommend buying cold-pressed, organic oils whenever possible.)

Though no cooking oils are strong sources of vitamins and minerals, almond oil does have a little bit of vitamin E and vitamin K. It's also got a high smoke point, so it can be used for all kinds of cooking.

And if you use it for the massage I suggested earlier, almond oil can be a terrific stress reliever. Try keeping it at bedside for relaxing times with your loved one.

OILS

Avocado Oil

This oil has become increasingly popular for cooking in the years since the first edition of this book came out—and for very good reasons.

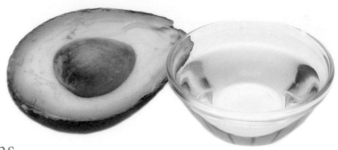

For one thing, avocados have become much more recognized as the superb fruit they are. The fat in them—and in avocado oil—is now universally recognized as a good, heart-healthy fat. The predominant class of fat in avocado oil—monounsaturated fat—is the same kind of fat found in olive oil.) What's more, the smokepoint of avocado oil (approximately 480° to 500°F [250° to 260°C]) is much higher than most other oils, including olive oil.

Important carotenoids such as beta-carotene, lutein, and zeaxanthin need fat to be absorbed well. (That's why they're called fat-soluble nutrients!) And although all fat should theoretically help carotenoids (and fat-soluble vitamins such as vitamin E, K and D) be absorbed more efficiently, researchers actually tested the concept of increased absorption using avocados or avocado oil. They found that it significantly enhanced carotenoid absorption both from salads and salsa by as much as 15 times more than similar foods without avocado oil.

Research published in the April 2005 *Journal of Ethnopharmacology* shows that avocado oil lowers blood pressure. In this animal study, a diet high in avocado oil changed the levels of essential fatty acids in kidneys, causing changes in the way the kidneys respond to hormones that regulate blood pressure. Avocado oil also influenced the fatty acid profile in the heart, causing researchers to conclude that a diet that includes good amounts of avocado oil may improve blood pressure.

Finally, avocado oil possesses anti-inflammatory properties and can be effective as part of a treatment for skin disorders such as psoriasis.

WORTH KNOWING

Most vegetable oils aren't technically from vegetables. They're from seeds—soybean oil, corn oil, safflower oil, etc. Avocado oil is not from seeds, but from the fleshy part of the avocado that you eat. Cold-pressed avocado oil from Hass avocados is a stunning emerald green, believed to be because of high levels of chlorophylls. It's also a naturally low-acidic oil.

Coconut Oil

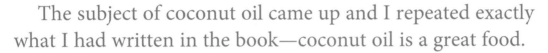

When the first edition of this book was published, the Dr. Oz radio show on SiriusXM was very much in full swing. I was invited to be a guest on the show, and I spent a full hour discussing foods with Mehmet Oz, M.D., his lovely wife Lisa, and his coauthor (and the Cleveland Clinic's chief wellness officer), Michael Roizen, M.D.

The subject of coconut oil came up and I repeated exactly what I had written in the book—coconut oil is a great food.

Roizen did not agree, and we had a disagreement on the air, albeit a polite and respectful one. (Mike Roizen is a great doctor, one of the good guys. He just happened to be wrong about coconut oil.)

Years later, on the Dr. Oz website, I was gratified to see coconut oil listed as number three in a slide-show of Dr. Oz's favorite superfoods. (The article is still online as of this writing, August, 2016.)

Even Dr. Oz had become a convert to coconut oil, which I've been raving about for a decade.

The fat in coconut oil—a form of saturated fat known as MCT (medium-chain triglycerides)—is among the healthiest fats in the world. It contains fatty acids such as lauric acid and caprylic acid, both known to be antiviral and antimicrobial.

And medium-chain triglycerides are more likely to be burned for energy. For many decades this made MCT oil a popular supplement among bodybuilders. Bodybuilders need the calories and energy for their workouts, but can't afford to have an ounce of extra fat on them at contest time. MCTs—the same fat found in coconut oil—provided a source of calories for their workouts that wasn't likely to be stored as fat on their body. (More on MCTs later on.)

Can Coconut Oil Help You Lose Weight?

In a 2009 Brazilian study, 40 women aged 20 to 40 years old with abdominal obesity were given daily dietary supplements of either soybean oil or coconut oil over the course of twelve weeks. All ubjects followed a balanced diet with the same number of calories and were told to walk for fifty minutes a day.

By the end of the study, the coconut oil group had significantly higher HDL ("good") cholesterol and an improved LDL: HDL ratio. Meanwhile, the soybean oil group saw its HDL go down and its cholesterol ratio go up!

Though both the soybean oil group and the coconut oil group had similar reductions in BMI, only the

OILS

coconut oil group saw a reduction in the circumference of their waists.

A very interesting—and unexpected—finding was that those consuming the coconut oil spontaneously reduced their consumption of carbohydrates and increased their consumption of protein and fiber over the course of the study.

"Supplementation with coconut oil does not cause dyslipidemia and seems to promote a reduction in abdominal obesity," write the researchers.

And researchers (St-Onge, 2003) published a study in the *International Journal of Obesity and Metabolic Disorders* stating that "MCT consumption has been shown to increase energy expenditure and lead to greater losses of the adipose (fat) tissue in animals and humans." Translated: It can help with fat loss (under some conditions).

Island Studies Prove the Value of Coconut

The good news on coconut actually started with research back in the 1960s and 1970s. It's long been observed that people from the Pacific Islands and Asia whose diets are very high in coconut oil are surprisingly free from cardiovascular disease, cancer and other degenerative diseases. A long-term, multidisciplinary study was set up to examine the health of the people living in the small, idyllic coconut-eating islands of Tokelau and Pukapuka.

And what it found was astonishing.

Despite eating a high-fat diet (30 to 60 percent of their calories were from fat, mostly saturated fat from coconuts), the Pukapuka and Tokelau islanders were virtually free of atherosclerosis, heart disease, and colon cancer. Digestive problems were rare. The islanders were lean and healthy. There were no signs of kidney disease, and high blood cholesterol was unknown.

Yet when these native people moved to the big cities, changed their diets, and gave up eating coconut oil in favor of the refined polyunsaturated vegetable oils that are believed to be healthier, their incidence of heart disease increased dramatically.

Another Great Benefit of Coconut Oil

If all that weren't enough, coconut oil is great for the immune system.

The predominant medium-chain triglyceride in coconut oil is lauric acid, which has been shown in countless studies to be antimicrobial, antibacterial, and antiviral. The fatty acids in coconut oil are powerful antibiotics. According to well-known naturopath Bruce Fife, N.D., who devoted a book to the subject, bacteria known to be killed by the medium-chain triglycerides in coconut oil include Streptococcus (throat infections, pneumonia, sinusitis), Staphylococcus (food poisoning, urinary tract infections), Neisseria (meningitis, gonorrhea, pelvic inflammatory disease), Chlamydia (genital infections, conjunctivitis, pneumonia, periodontitis), and Helicobacter pylori (stomach ulcers). In addition, there are at least a dozen pathogenic viruses that have been reported to be inactivated by lauric acid. Fife points out that another great thing about lauric acid is that it kills the "bad" bacteria but doesn't harm the friendly intestinal bacteria that we need for healthy digestion. Medium-chain triglycerides also kill Candida and other fungi in the intestinal tract, further supporting healthy gut ecology.

Coconut Oil Is a Natural Remedy with Antioxidant Powers

In his seminal book *Medicinal Plants of the World*, the dean of American herbalists, James Duke, wrote that coconut and coconut oil are used as folk remedies to treat more than thirty-five ailments, from abscesses to wounds. And it's well known that the absorption of calcium, magnesium, and also amino acids has been found to increase when infants are fed a diet using coconut oil. Coconut oil also has substantial antioxidant power. And populations that consume coconuts as a major part of their diets are rarely troubled by osteoporosis.

So do you need to worry about the natural, healthy saturated fat in coconut oil? I don't think so, and neither do many experts. "Coconut oil has a neutral effect on blood cholesterol, even in situations where coconut oil is the sole source of fat," said George Blackburn, M.D., Ph.D., a Harvard Medical School researcher testifying at a congressional hearing about tropical oils back in 1988. "These (tropical) oils have been consumed as a substantial part of the diet of many groups for thousands of years with absolutely no evidence of any harmful effects to the populations consuming them," said the late Mary Enig, Ph.D., who was one of the premier lipid biochemists in the United States and a former research associate at the University of Maryland. Even C. Everett Koop, M.D., former surgeon general of the United States, called the tropical-oil scare "foolishness."

Remember—the saturated fats in fast-food french fries and the saturated fats in healthy, natural foods such as coconut and coconut oil are two completely different animals. Avoid the first like the plague, and enjoy the second to your heart's content.

Coconut Oil, Ketones, and the Brain

Ketones are metabolites of fat, a kind of by-product of fat metabolism. Very low-carb diets force the body to make more of these ketones, which turn out to be an excellent fuel for the brain, the muscles and the heart. Coconut oil is another way to get ketones into your system.

This is not the place to debate the many benefits (and challenges) of a ketogenic diet, or nutritional ketosis. But it's a topic of intense research, particularly when it comes to ketones and the brain. Diets that produce high levels of ketones—(ketogenic diets)—are routinely used as a treatment for childhood epilepsy.

Indeed, the U.S. Navy is researching ketogenic diets with Navy SEALs.

Ketones are a great fuel for the brain. "You can boost the availability of ketones for your brain by simply adding coconut oil or MCT oil to your daily regimen," writes noted integrative neurologist and best-selling author David Perlmutter, M.D. But don't expect to get all the benefits of this added source of rocket fuel if you're still eating a high-sugar diet. Perlmutter hastens to add that to make the addition of ketones from coconut oil effective, "carb restriction is a must."

WORTH KNOWING

Some of the original bad press on coconut oil came from studies in which they used a hydrogenated, inferior product (loaded with trans fats) that behaves very differently in the body than the real thing. When buying coconut oil, go for the best: virgin coconut oil. It's never hydrogenated or partially hydrogenated, and it's processed without high heat and chemicals.

Remember, unrefined coconut oil only has a smoke point of 350°F (180°C), which is fine for many purposes, but it's not as high as, for example, avocado oil. If you want to use coconut oil for much higher heat coconut, you'll have to go for a more refined version. Barlean's, for example, makes both a virgin coconut oil for everything but high-heat cooking, and a slightly refined one for everything else.

OILS

MCT OIL AND COCONUT OIL: WHAT'S THE DIFFERENCE?

Coconut oil is generally billed as a great source of medium-chain triglycerides (MCT), and products called "MCT oil" are everywhere.

This leads to the inevitable question: What's the difference? (Spoiler alert: There's a big one.)

A little background will make it clearer: Every fatty acid—all of them, every one ever invented—is a chain of carbon atoms. When there are fewer than 6 of these carbons chained together, we call them a short-chain fatty acid; when there are more than 14 carbons, it's a long-chain fatty acid. When there are 8–12 carbons, it's a medium-chain fatty acid.

There are three fatty acids that are generally considered medium-chain. Triglycerides—which are three fatty acids joined together with a glycerol backbone—are considered medium-chain triglycerides when they contain these fatty acids:

- Caprylic acid (8 carbons)
- Capric acid (10 carbons)
- Lauric acid (12 carbons)

A fourth fatty acid—Caproic acid (6 carbons)—is sometimes lumped in with the MCTs because it's close in length and also found in coconut oil. Technically it's a short-chain fatty acid and converts (breaks down) into ketones rather quickly. At the other end of the spectrum, the longest of the MCTs—the 12-carbon lauric acid—breaks down more slowly than the others and many think it shouldn't even be counted in the medium category. We'll leave that controversy for another time as it's way too technical and boring to get into now.

The important thing to understand is that the four fatty acids we're talking about have specific uses and advantages. The fatty acids with the shortest chains "burn" the fastest. The lower the number of carbons, the faster the body can turn those fatty acids into ketones, which are a wonderful source of energy for the brain, heart, and muscles. That's the main reason MCT oil manufacturers don't usually include lauric acid in their MCT oil products—at 12 carbons, it's the longest of the medium-chain fatty acids and is processed a little differently (and slower) than the others, making it less of a great source of immediate fuel.

So coconut oil offers a considerably different MCT "profile" than MCT oil.

A product in the store labeled *MCT oil* is most likely to contain either c-8, c-10, or a combination of the two—fast-burning fats right in the middle of the 'middle category. The fat in coconut oil, on the other hand, is mostly lauric acid, with a smattering of the faster burning MCTs.

Lauric acid is wonderful fat with anti-microbal and antibacterial properties, making coconut oil great for the immune system. Athletes using MCTs as a faster burning source of energy, however, may be less interested in the immune-enhancing properties of the lauric acid in coconut oil and more interested in the fast burning energy of the shorter chain MCTs found in MCT oil.

Of course, one could use both—cook with coconut oil, or even take it as a supplement, and still throw some MCT oil in your coffee, the way some coffee companies do.

Both are great, both contain MCTs.

But they're definitely *not* identical.

Extra-Virgin Olive Oil

Tempting though it may be to attribute robust good health to any one factor, the truth is that it's always a combination of things. Unlike lab rats and college sophomores, free-living humans always do a bunch of things together, making cause-and-effect statements much more difficult. In Mediterranean cultures where spend a lot of time outdoors, they eat their big meal in the daytime, and they eat lots of good foods.

And that gorgeous sunny climate can't hurt, either. That said, virtually every nutritional researcher also attributes at least some of the legendary health of those in the Mediterranean to the copious consumption of olive oil.

Olive Oil Joins Omega-3 Fats and Walnuts in an Elite FDA Category

Now don't go running out and start pouring olive oil on your cheeseburgers thinking you're going to get the same results. Obviously, there are a lot of other factors at play here, such as what else besides olive oil is on the menu. The Mediterranean diet is notoriously high in fish, vegetables, and fruits, and it is a lot lower in saturated fats. But all things being equal, a ton of research supports the statement that olive oil has some serious health benefits.

In fact, all that research was compelling enough to cause the FDA to permit olive oil membership in a very select group: foods or food substances whose label may contain a health claim benefit.

So what exactly is in olive oil, and what the heck does it do for you? Well, to start with, olive oil is very high in compounds called phenols, which are potent antioxidants. Olive oil is also mainly made up of monounsaturated fat, the most important of which is

called oleic acid, shown in research to be extremely heart healthy. Compared with carbohydrates, for example, monounsaturated fat lowers LDL cholesterol (the bad stuff) and raises the protective HDL cholesterol. Research in the Archives of Internal Medicine concluded that greater adherence to the traditional Mediterranean diet (including plenty of monounsaturated fat) was associated with significant reduction in mortality among people diagnosed with heart disease. And another study in the same journal compared two groups of people with high blood pressure. One group was given sunflower oil, a typical oil used in Western diets, and one group was given the good stuff: extra-virgin olive oil (more about that in a moment). The olive oil decreased the second group's blood pressure by a significant amount; it also decreased their need for blood pressure meds by a whopping 48 percent. As the English might say, "not too shabby."

Olive Oil Decreases Risk of Colon and Bowel Cancer

Michael Goldacre, B.M., B.Ch.—who researched diet and disease at the Institute of Health Sciences and published his results in the *Journal of Epidemiology and Community Health*—says that olive oil may have a protective effect on the development of colon cancer. And researchers at Oxford found that a diet rich in olive oil was associated with a decreased risk of bowel cancer.

Mark Houston, M.D., director of the Hypertension Institute in Nashville, and my favorite go-to guy for all things related to hypertension, says that monounsaturated fats "make nitric oxide more bioavailable, which makes it better able to keep the arteries dilated," plus they "help combat the ill effects of oxidation and improve endothelial function." Translated from the scientific jargon: The stuff is really good for you. Houston recommends 4 tablespoons (60 ml) a day for his patients.

What Does "Extra-Virgin" Really Mean?

But now the bad news. All olive oil is not created equal. Unfortunately, commercial manufacturers, trying to ride the health hype on olive oil, have rushed to market all kinds of imitation and inferior products that say olive oil on them but have questionable benefits. Here's where being an educated consumer makes a difference. You may have been wondering what this "extra-virgin" designation is all about. Well, here's the deal. Olive oil is almost unique among the oils in that you can consume it in its crude form without any processing. If you had the chance, you could walk around barefoot in barrels of it, and take the resultant oil and use it directly on your salad (something you can't do with most other oils). Not refining the oil has the benefit of conserving the vitamins, essential fatty acids, antioxidants, and other nutrients. On the best family-owned farms, the oil is produced in ways similar to those of the ancient Greeks and Romans: Organic olives are picked by hand so as not to damage the skin or pulp; the oil is separated without the use of heat, hot water, or solvents; and it is left unfiltered. The first pressing produces the best stuff, known as extra-virgin olive oil.

And that's the stuff you want. That's the oil that makes the list of the world's healthiest foods. Once you begin machine harvesting and processing with heat, you start damaging the delicate compounds in olive oil responsible for all those great health benefits. The antioxidant polyphenols are water soluble—they're washed away with factory processing. In fact, that's one reason that factory-produced olive oil has a shorter shelf life—no antioxidants to protect it. Real olive oil—the extra-virgin kind, made with care and love and the absence of heat and harsh chemicals—lasts for years.

So don't fall for the idea that just because an oil in a restaurant says olive, it's necessarily the good stuff. Seek out the extra-virgin stuff. It's worth the extra money and effort to find it.

Your heart will thank you.

WORTH KNOWING

There's been a lot of press about fake olive oil. Much of what we think is extra-virgin olive oil is actually not. It's thinned out with other stuff, or it's deliberately mislabeled. The news show 60 Minutes estimated that 80 to 85 percent of what's sold as extra virgin in the United States is fake—other reports put the number at 70 to 80 percent. Check out *Real Food, Fake Food*, a 2016 book by travel writer and author Larry Olmsted that delves into fake food scandals, including olive oil, Kobe beef, and Parmesan cheese. The deception (and scandal) is real. In 2016, the House Agriculture Committee took steps to address the fraud around olive oil and directed the FDA to take samplings of imported olive oil to determine whether it was adulterated or misbranded. All of which is to say: Buyer be careful. There is genuine extra-virgin olive oil around, and it's worth spending a little time to make sure you're getting the real thing.

★ Flaxseed Oil (flaxseeds)

"Wherever flaxseed becomes a regular food item among the people, there will be better health," said Mahatma Gandhi. He was right. The true nature of flaxseed as a health food has been known for centuries. In the eighth century, Charlemagne considered flaxseed so essential for health that he actually passed laws requiring its use. Flaxseed was one of the original medicines, used by Hippocrates himself.

It's hard to talk about flaxseed and flaxseed oil without discussing essential fatty acids, particularly the omega-3s. You can read about this in more detail beginning on page 330, but briefly, here's what you need to know: Flaxseeds and flaxseed oil are one of the best sources on the planet for the important omega-3 fatty acid called alpha-linolenic acid. Alpha-linolenic acid is considered an essential fatty acid because the body can't make it—it has to be obtained from the diet. The research on the benefits of omega-3 fats is so overwhelming that it would take a book to review them (and many good ones have been written). Flaxseed oil can help protect against cardiovascular disease, cancer, arthritis, and many other degenerative diseases. And though it's primarily a source of omega-3, the oil has the virtue of containing some other fatty acids as well, notably some omega-6s and some heart-healthy omega-9s, providing a nice fatty acid balance.

Lignans in Flaxseed Oil Protect against Hormone-Sensitive Cancers

But the benefits of flax are not limited to the omega-3 content. Far from it. The oil, and especially the seeds, are a great source of something called lignans, which have a whole host of health benefits of their own, for both men and women. Lignans have a protective effect against cancer, especially those that are hormone-sensitive like breast, uterine, and prostate cancers. Lignans increase sex-hormone binding globulin (SHBG), which binds to estrogen and helps get it out of the body. The lignans break down in the gut into two compounds—enterolactone and enterodiol—which interfere with the cancer-promoting effects of estrogen. (Lignans are probably one of the reasons vegetarian women have lower rates of breast cancer.) Researchers have also found that lignans inhibited the growth of human prostate cancer cells in a test tube. Research at Duke University published in the journal

OILS

Urology showed that men with prostate cancer who were given 3 tablespoons (36 g) of flaxseed per day and a low-fat diet had decreased cancer cell growth. And lignans interfere with the production of a nasty testosterone metabolite (DHT, dihydrotestosterone), which is partly responsible for hair loss and benign prostate hyperplasia (the condition that makes men over forty have to go to the bathroom a lot at night).

The flaxseeds—but not, obviously, the oil—also contain soluble fiber. You get all the benefits of the oil, plus the fiber when you eat the seeds. They're ideal for baking, sprinkling on salads, and adding to cereals and smoothies—but you need to break the hard outer coating because the whole seeds can't be digested. Best way: Grind them in a coffee grinder for a few seconds. It's worth the effort. (Or you can buy high-quality pre-ground flax.) That said, 4 tablespoons (28 g) of ground flaxseeds (also known as flaxseed meal) will give you 6 g of protein and 8 g of fiber. And, in addition to all the other good stuff, flaxseeds are also anti-inflammatory and have antioxidant properties as well.

Flax promotes cardiovascular and colon health, can boost immunity, promotes healthy skin, and helps stabilize blood sugar. Because the lignans in flax are actually phytoestrogens (weak estrogenic compounds from plants), they may help relieve menopausal symptoms. In fact, in one study, flaxseed was as effective as hormone replacement therapy in reducing mild menopausal symptoms in menopausal women.

WORTH KNOWING

Certain high-quality flaxseed oils have been specially designed to have a high lignan content. Look for those. And remember, never cook with the oil, just keep it in the fridge and either take it as a supplement or use it on salads or already-cooked vegetables. Cooking damages the delicate omega-3 fats, which don't stand up to heat at all.

One other note: There has been much discussion in the nutritional community about the pros and cons of flaxseed oil vs. fish oil. For those people who are only going to take one or the other, I've generally recommended fish oil. That's because I believe that the two omega-3s found in fish oil (EPA and DHA) are even more important than the one that's found in flax (ALA). That said, the omega-3 fatty acid in flaxseeds and flaxseed oil does have health benefits of its own, and the lignans add enough value to make it worth recommending that you take both.

Hemp Seed Oil

Hemp seed oil (hemp oil) is another of the lesser-known oils that deserves a closer look.

First things first: Don't confuse this nutritious and amazing oil with marijuana. It's not the same. True, they come from the same plant originally, but so do linens, fiber, rope, and tablecloths. In fact, the word canvas is derived from cannabis, which is the Latin name for hemp.

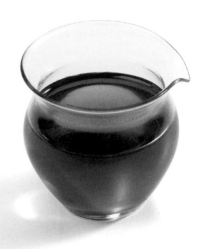

So you won't get high from hemp seed oil. You will, however, get some significant health benefits. And it's perfectly legal.

Hemp seed oil is probably the best balanced of all the oils on the market. What does that mean? Well, remember that every oil is a combination of fatty acids from different families—some are saturated, some monounsaturated, some polyunsaturated. The oils—or fats—tend to get known by their primary fatty acid—for example, olive oil is known as a monounsaturated fat because that's the predominant (but not only) fat it contains. Most oils contain a blend.

Hemp seed oil contains both omega-6 and omega-3 fatty acids. Both omega-6 fatty acids (linoleic acid) and omega-3 fatty acids (alpha-linolenic acid) are considered essential fats because the body can't make them and they have to be obtained from the diet. One of the problems in our diet is too much omega-6 and not enough omega-3, compounded by the fact that most of the omega-6 we get is highly refined and not of good quality. The ratio of omega-6 to omega-3 in hemp seed is the best of all oils. It's balanced in a ratio of 3:1, which is pretty darn good. In addition, this oil hasn't become a commercial favor-

ite, and it's still relatively easy to find the unrefined, cold-pressed, organic oil. Stores and Internet sites that carry it tend to have this nutrient-rich version.

Some of the omega-6 in hemp seed oil is GLA (gamma-linolenic acid), an important omega-6 that we don't get nearly enough of. GLA, the primary ingredient in evening primrose and borage oils, is very helpful for PMS and is a good omega-6; the body can make it, but doesn't always do so efficiently. Hemp seed oil is about 2 percent GLA—as far as I know, hemp is the only edible seed containing GLA.

Hemp Oil Lowers "Bad" Cholesterol and Blood Pressure

So yes, hemp is more dominant in the polyunsaturated omega-6 series of fatty acids, but it is highly beneficial in maintaining cardiovascular health. A comprehensive review paper on the relationship of fats to coronary heart disease by Frank Hu, JoAnn Manson, and Walter Willett from Harvard—the folks who ran the Nurses' Health Study—points out that omega-6s do lower LDL ("bad") cholesterol and also improve insulin sensitivity. As for the omega-3s, hundreds of studies have shown that they lower triglycerides and cholesterol levels. The omega-3 fatty acids in hemp are effective in decreasing blood pressure, platelet stickiness, and fibrinogen levels, a key marker in atherosclerosis. Research has found that for every 1 percent increase in alpha-linolenic acid (omega-3) content there was a decrease of 5 mm Hg in the systolic, diastolic, and mean blood pressure. Omega-3s are also anti-inflammatory and are being studied at Harvard and elsewhere for their effect on mood and depression.

Hemp oil should be stored in the refrigerator, used quickly, and never heated. (There are experts who argue that you can use it at low heat for a short time, but I'd be on the safe side. Omega-3s—such as those in flaxseed, fish oil, and hemp seed oil—are highly unstable and form toxic by-products when they're heated to high temperatures.) Use the nutty-tasting oil on salads and cooked vegetables, or put a tablespoon (15 ml) in your smoothie. You can also mix half-and-half with organic butter for a terrific "essential fatty acid butter."

WORTH KNOWING

Hemp seeds are increasingly becoming available at health food stores, and I can tell you they're delicious. Hemp seeds contain all the essential fats we've been talking about, plus they're about 25 percent protein, 10 to 15 percent fiber, and contain a rich array of minerals, particularly phosphorus, potassium, magnesium, sulfur, and calcium. I love sprinkling them on foods or eating them out of the bag.

Macadamia Nut Oil

Macadamia nut oil probably owes its popularity—at least in this country—to the fact that the noted nutritionist and health author Fred Pescatore, M.D., championed it in his excellent book *The Hamptons Diet*. Pescatore has been a friend of mine for years, and I can tell you this: He's very smart, and he knows his stuff. His program is basically the Mediterranean diet, updated to include macadamia nut oil as the main source of fat instead of the more traditional extra-virgin olive oil. Pescatore, who has become something of an expert on the oils and their manufacturing, worries that there are many highly processed olive oils flooding the market that do not have the health properties of real, extra-virgin, estate-bottled olive oil.

He's a big fan of 100 percent macadamia nut oil, unrefined, of course. Two excellent sources of macadamia nut oil are organic macadamia nut oil from Kenya by Vital Choice, which can be found in the shopping section of my website (www.jonnybowden.com), and MacNut Oil from Australia (www.mac-nut-oil.com).

Macadamia Nut Oil Is Rich in Heart-Healthy Oleic Acid

Macadamia nut oil is even richer in monounsaturated fat than olive oil. The fat in macadamia nut oil is 85 percent monounsaturated, with a predominance of the heart-healthy oleic acid. Oleic acid increases the incorporation of omega-3 fatty acids into the cell membrane, which has all kinds of health benefits. Oleic acid (monounsaturated fats) and omega-3s lower triglyceride levels and raise HDL ("good") cholesterol levels, a very protective combination. (The ratio of triglycerides to HDL cholesterol is even more predictive of coronary heart disease than cholesterol is; anything that lowers triglycerides and raises HDL improves that ratio.) Monounsaturated fats (omega-9s) are central to the Mediterranean diet that has been shown in virtually every single research study to be associated with lower rates of heart disease. The monounsaturated fat in macadamia nut oil, together with a nice intake of omega-3s from fish and fish oil, is a very winning combination guaranteed to provide good health.

Through admirable lobbying on behalf of the olive oil industry, the FDA took a look at the massive evidence for the health benefits of monounsaturated fats. They allow a health claim to be made for olive oil as a result. Understand that the health benefit comes from monounsaturated fat in general, but because it was the Olive Oil Association who petitioned the FDA, the FDA limited its investigation of the research to "monounsaturated fat in olive oil" while recognizing that other oils provide this same fat. It's all political. Monounsaturated fat is monounsaturated fat, and it does good things for you whether you get it from olive oil or macadamia nut oil. Macadamia nut oil is even more monounsaturated-rich than olive oil, so it stands to reason that the cardiac and anticancer benefits would accrue to it as well.

OILS

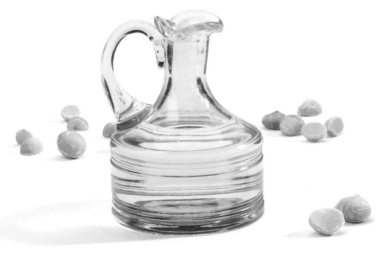

★ Red Palm Oil (Malaysian)

When the first edition of this book came out, palm oil was hardly ever used in the United States. But that was then, and this is now. This wonderful, underappreciated oil is becoming better known every day, and with good reason.

Palm oil is to tropical African cooking what olive oil is to Mediterranean cooking. It's the most heavily consumed dietary oil in the world after soybean oil. The late lipid biochemist Mary Enig, Ph.D., called it "one of the most important edible oils in the world" and with good reason. It's shelf stable, contains absolutely no GMOs, and is trans fat free. Plus, for you cooks, it has a nice smoke point of 450°F (230°C).

What's more, as Enig points out, modern extraction is accomplished with steam, and because 30 to 70 percent of the fruit is oil, solvent (chemical) extraction is not needed and isn't often used. (Contrast that with the darling of the health food set, canola oil, or as Enig called it, "con-ola oil!" Enough said!)

There are other great things about palm oil. First, there's the carotenoid content. The reason palm oil is red is because it's so rich in carotenes (like beta-carotene and its relatives, together known as the carotenoid family). These are powerful antioxidants and have multiple benefits.

Palm oil is also rich in a particular form of vitamin E called tocotrienols, which are the subject of great interest in the nutrition and functional medicine communities because of their rich array of health benefits. Palm oil is actually the richest source of alpha-tocotrienol—which possess unique biological activity even independent of its power as an antioxidant.

What's more, tocotrienols have been found to protect the brain from the damage that can occur after a stroke, possibly because of the neuroprotective properties of alpha-tocotrienol. Chandan K. Sen, Ph.D., associate dean for research at the Ohio State University Medical Center, thinks so much of tocotrienols that he encourages tocotrienol supplementation. In a June 2, 2010, interview with the *Orange County Register,* he said, "Alpha tocotrienol is markedly more potent than the more common available forms of vitamin E in its ability to help protect neurons in the brain from damage or death."

So why has it taken palm oil so long to catch on?

Simple, because of two common beliefs about palm oil, both of which are incorrect.

The first is that palm oil is a saturated fat, which is true. And also meaningless. Here's why.

For the last few decades, conventional wisdom held that saturated fat was one of the bad guys in our diet. This has turned out not to be true, despite the fact that many people (including some doctors) still believe it. We now know, from at least two major peer-reviewed studies in mainstream medical and nutritional journals, that saturated fat does not cause—and never did cause, in my opinion—heart disease. It's not even related to it.

Saturated fat from healthy natural sources such as palm oil, coconut oil, grass-fed beef or butter, are simply no longer fats we have to avoid. I think we'd be much better off substituting some of these healthy saturated fats for the excessive amount of proinflammatory vegetable oil we consume. Many saturated fats are either neutral or have potential benefits— i.e., the tocotrienols in palm oil, the MCTs in coconut oil, and the CLA in grass-fed butter. Although I don't personally believe cholesterol is a big deal (see my book with cardiologist Stephen Sinatra, M.D., *The Great Cholesterol Myth*) for those who might be concerned, plant fats such as palm oil do not actually increase LDL cholesterol (the so-called bad kind), though they often increase HDL (which your doctor would love to see).

The second rap against palm oil has to do with the environment and with animal habitats that are frequently—though not always—destroyed in the making of it. This criticism is valid—but not so in Malaysia and a few other places such as Ecuador.

This is why I always recommend Malaysian red palm oil. Malaysia is environmentally conscious— more than 50 percent of its forests are protected (as opposed to 3 percent of ours). Their palm oil industry is sustainable, and no animal habitats are harmed. That's personally important to me, particularly because I love orangutans, which are the animals most often affected by the deforestation of some palm oil production.

What's more, the Malaysian palm industry even set up a Malaysian Palm Oil Wildlife Conservation Fund, which, among its many functions, safeguards wildlife, deters poaching, and even set up a project specifically to explore orangutan conservation.

Palm oil has a distinct, amazingly rich flavor, and it is popping up at more and more natural food and ethnic food stores.

WORTH KNOWING

Even though virgin palm oil has a relatively high smoke point (about 450°F [230°C]), the longer you use it at high heat the more you will destroy the natural antioxidants. If you're frying with it, definitely don't reuse it.

OILS

Sesame Oil

(unrefined, cold pressed, organic)

The introduction to this section (page 330) was a result of my internal debate over whether to include sesame oil in this book. Sesame oil has a lot to recommend it—but it's high in omega-6s.

Ultimately, I figured by explaining what you need to be aware of regarding omega-6s, I could include sesame oil with a clear conscience; despite being a high-omega-6 oil, it has a lot of potential health benefits. The thing about sesame oil is that it contains a fully developed antioxidant system of its own. Sesame oil and toasted sesame oil contain a powerful antioxidant called sesamol, as well as two related compounds, sesamin and sesamolin. This natural antioxidant system is one reason why unrefined sesame oil doesn't go rancid for a long time. Besides containing antioxidants, these compounds have other benefits. Sesamin inhibits the manufacture of inflammatory compounds in the body. In animal studies, it lowers cholesterol and increases the ability of the liver to burn (oxidize) fat.

Sesame Oil May Lower Blood Pressure

There's also evidence that sesame oil can lower blood pressure. In a report to the American Heart Association's Inter-American Society of Hypertension, Devarajan Sankar, Ph.D., presented evidence that patients with high blood pressure who were taking blood pressure medications (but still had high blood pressure) were able to drop their blood pressure into the normal range by simply switching to sesame oil as their only cooking oil. Sampath Parthasarathy, Ph.D., a biochemist and an expert in antioxidants and metabolism, suspects that the lower blood pressure may be an indirect effect of the

sesamin or sesamol or both.

Though the lion's share of fat in sesame oil (45 percent) is omega-6 fat, sesame oil also is 40 percent monounsaturated fat, the heart-healthy type of fat that makes extra-virgin olive oil so good for us. Annemarie Colbin, Ph.D., author of *Food and Healing*, says that in her experience, "The best-quality fats to use are extra-virgin olive oil (see page 339), unrefined sesame oil, and ghee (see page 198)." I can't emphasize enough how important it is to get cold-processed unrefined oils no matter which oil you're using.

Sesame oil is a popular choice for stir-fries. Fred Pescatore, M.D., author of *The Hamptons Diet*, says sesame oil has a medium smoke point, which makes it good for light sautéing, low-heat baking, and pressure cooking where the temperature stays below 320°F (160°C). Pescatore puts it on his "use rarely" list only because of the high omega-6 content, but we've already covered that issue.

WORTH KNOWING

Sesame oil is called "the most esteemed seed oil in Ayurvedic medicine" and is one of the most popular oils for massage. According to Ann McIntyre, a fellow of the National Institute of Medical Herbalists and the author of twenty books, its chemical structure gives it a unique ability to penetrate the skin easily, nourishing and detoxifying even the deepest tissue layers.

WHAT ABOUT CANOLA OIL?

No, it's not a mistake, nor an omission. Canola oil is not on the list of the world's healthiest foods. It's not even close.

Nutritionists can be divided into two camps on certain controversial issues, soy being one of them, canola oil being another. Conventional wisdom is that canola oil is a wonderfully healthy oil that should be used as much as possible. The minority opinion is that it is an overhyped, unhealthy oil whose success is completely due to brilliant marketing on the part of the industry.

I am firmly in the camp of the second group.

This book is not the place to go into the details of the debate on canola oil. If you're interested, start with the writings of the esteemed lipid biochemist Mary Enig, Ph.D. (For starters, search for "The Great Con-ola," at www.mercola.com and "The Real Story on Canola Oil (Can-ugly Oil)" by Fred Pescatore, M.D., at www.diabetesincontrol.com.

HIGH-TEMPERATURE PROCESSING INCREASES TRANS FATS IN CANOLA OIL

Canola oil was born out of the need for the oil industry to produce an oil high in healthy monounsaturated fats that was more plentiful and less expensive than olive oil. It turned to rapeseed oil, an oil high in monounsaturated fats that has been used extensively in China, India, and Japan and contains a whopping 60 percent monounsaturated fat. Unfortunately, about two-thirds of that fat is from erucic acid, a kind of fatty acid that has been associated with Keshan's disease (fibrotic lesions of the heart). By genetically modifying the rapeseed oil, they were able to produce LEAR (low erucic acid rapeseed). To avoid the ugly connotations of the name rapeseed, the industry settled on canola for "Canadian oil," because most of the new rapeseed came from Canada.

The rapeseed oil used in China, India, and Japan was quite a different oil from the canola oil produced today—Chinese and Indians used oil that was entirely unrefined. Today, the oil is removed from the rapeseed plant by high-temperature mechanical pressing and solvent extraction, and traces of the solvent remain in the oil. As Enig points out, "Like all modern vegetable oils, canola oil goes through the process of caustic refining, bleaching, and degumming—all of which involve high temperatures of questionable safety."

But what about the highly touted omega-3s in canola oil, you ask? Omega-3s are great, but they easily become rancid and foul-smelling when subjected to the high temperatures needed to extract the canola oil. Therefore, they have to be deodorized. The deodorizing process turns a large number of the omega-3 fatty acids into trans fats. (The University of Florida at Gainesville found trans fat levels as high as 4.6 percent in commercial canola oil, even more than in margarine.) Canola oil used in foods (whose manufacturers usually proclaim "made with canola oil!" as loudly as the label will allow) is even worse. Canola oil hydrogenates beautifully, making it ideal for shelf life but not for your life—the hydrogenation increases the trans fat content.

Pescatore knows a lot about oils, and in fact, the section on cooking oils alone is an excellent reason to buy *The Hamptons Diet*. In his list of available oils, here's what he says about canola oil: "This oil is included so that you can compare the profiles more easily. I would never use this oil."

I agree.

THE EXPERTS' TOP TEN LISTS

Dave Asprey

Dave Asprey is the founder of The Bulletproof Executive and the creator of the phenomenally successful Bulletproof Coffee. He's the host of the #1 health podcast, Bulletproof Radio, and is the *New York Times* bestselling author of *The Bulletproof Diet*, *The Bulletproof Cookbook*, and *Head Strong*.

I first met Dave at JJ Virgin's Mindshare Summit, an annual meeting of health professionals and entrepreneurs, and I've since interviewed him several times (and been interviewed by him for his podcast). He's a fascinating guy—a Silicon Valley investor and technology entrepreneur who weighed 300 pounds (136 kg) and spent two decades and more than $300,000 to essentially "hack" his own biology and improve his performance, losing 100 pounds (45 kg) in the process. He overcame severe health problems (not the least of which was being obese) and has become what I call a "high-performance crusader," always looking for cutting edge products (and foods) that can improve stamina, brainpower, and well-being. Here's his list:

1. **Mold-free coffee**. Coffee is the number one source of special antioxidants called polyphenols that are vital to keep the cells in your body at full charge. Mold toxins that are common in coffee inhibit mitochondrial function, so it's critical to get coffee that's completely mold-free.

2. **Grass-fed butter**. It's a rich source of undamaged fat that acts as a building block for your cell membranes and hormones. Grass-fed butter also contains higher amounts of nutrients like CLA, (conjugated linolenic acid) which is associated with weight loss—and butyrate, a special fatty acid that is important for gut health and also reduces inflammation in the brain.

3. **Dark chocolate**. This is another rich source of polyphenols that most people don't get enough of.

4. **Green tea**. Drinking green tea is a terrific way to get antioxidants, such as polyphenols.

5. **Broccoli**. Broccoli contains special enzymes that inhibit cancer. It's best to steam it and have a couple bites raw to get activated enzymes.

6. **Grass-fed beef**. This contains special fat-soluble vitamins that are hard to get anywhere else. Grain-fed beef doesn't do the same thing for you, plus it accumulates toxins that are bad for you.

7. **Sockeye salmon**. This fish contains considerable amounts of the omega-3 fatty acid docosahexaenoic acid (DHA), which is vital for cellular energy production and brain health. Sockeye is lowest in mercury because it lives only a short period of time, making it fully renewable and sustainable.

8. **Avocado**. This terrific fruit is a great source of undamaged monounsaturated fat and polyphenols. And it's delicious!

9. **Seaweed**. This is a rich source of iodine and polyphenols. Just order the salad at a sushi restaurant!

10. **Herbs**. By using a lot of herbs, such as oregano, sage, thyme, and rosemary, you can easily double the amount of antioxidant polyphenols in your diet. So go heavy on the flavor!

CHAPTER 14

FLOUR

Flour. Can't live with it, can't live without it.

Yes, I know that's a paraphrase of an old (and stupid) joke, but in the case of flour, it's true—at least for the majority of people reading this book who are not 100 percent strict Paleo or keto. (And, truth be told, I've had more than a few Paleo-fanatic friends who've been known to sneak a brownie or a chocolate chip cookie now and again. Just sayin'.)

So flour is necessary for just about every baked good on the planet (with the occasional exception like "flour-free brownies"). And here's the problem for nutritionists like me. The very process of making flour renders it pretty useless as a delivery system for nutrients. Flour is basically grain—frequently contaminated with the sprays used to grow it—which is then "purified," and ground into thin, dust-like particles. It is almost the exact opposite of a whole food because it has to be processed a lot to even be usable.

On the other hand, who wants to live in a world without baked goods?

So, for me, flour is a compromise, and in a perfect world—or one where we didn't have taste buds—I'd probably recommend dumping it altogether.

Recently, though, two very interesting types of flour have become available. These were not around when the first edition of the book came out, but they are now, and they're gaining in popularity for good reason.

Cassava Flour

In preparation for the revised edition of this book, I called my dear friend, chef Jeannette Bessinger, a.k.a. the Clean Food Coach. I asked her what foods she'd recommend including in the new edition. One of the first ones she mentioned was cassava flour.

Okay, I admit, I had never heard of cassava flour, but I made a note to look into it. Then, a couple of weeks later, I was speaking at the Paleo f(x) conference in Dallas, and I found myself wandering around the exhibit hall, where dozens of interesting Paleo-friendly food companies were showing their wares. One booth was attracting a lot of people, and when I made my way to the front of the line, it immediately became apparent why everyone was mobbing the booth.

Chocolate chip cookies. But not just any chocolate chip cookies. These were like almost the best chocolate chip cookies I had ever tasted.

But what on earth were chocolate chip cookies doing at a Paleo conference in the first place?

Simple. They were made with cassava flour.

Cassava flour is a resistant starch, which is a special kind of fiber. We generally think of fiber as being either insoluble or soluble, but resistant starch offers the best of both worlds. It's technically an insoluble fiber, but when it reaches the colon, it acts more like a soluble fiber, serving as powerful food for the good bacteria in your gut. The gut bacteria feast on resistant starch, making resistant starch one of the best prebiotic fibers on the planet. (Prebiotics are essential food for probiotics, the live microorganisms that live in your gut.)

Resistant starch like cassava flour and potato starch (see page 354) helps to regulate blood sugar levels and improves insulin sensitivity. And there's good reason to think it may also act as a weight loss tool. Why? Because research has confirmed that the diversity and health of your gut bacteria plays a major role in achieving and maintaining a healthy weight.

Cassava flour can be used in place of wheat flour and many people won't even notice the substitution. (Certainly the people lined up for those amazing chocolate chip cookies weren't missing the wheat!)

Cassava flour has a lot of carbs (like most other grain-based flours), but if you're making something that requires flour, cassava flour seems to be a much better choice than wheat flour.

Why use cassava flour instead of other gluten-free flours? "It has a fine texture, neutral taste, white color, and low fat content compared to almond flour or coconut flour," says my friend Josh Axe. "It's also sustainable for people with allergies who can't consume nuts or coconut." It's also grain-free and nut-free.

A ¼-cup (30 g) serving of cassava flour has 114 calories, 2 g of fiber, and about 28 g of carbs.

Cricket Flour

Cricket flour is made from, well, crickets. But it's not as weird as it might sound. A 2013 report from the Food and Agricultural Organization of the United Nations points out that insects are actually nutritional powerhouses, high in protein, fat, and the essential amino acids lysine and tryptophan. Insects can be farmed with a lot less environmental impact than traditional livestock. And their potential as a food source is very promising.

The story of how cricket flour is pretty interesting. A couple of guys named Gabi Lewis and Greg Sewitz got into the edible insect market while one of them (Lewis) was thinking about taking his homemade protein bars out into the marketplace. Looking for a hook to compete with all the other protein bars, they decided to add crickets, an idea Sewitz got from attending a conference on climate change.

So the two order a few thousand live crickets, get them sent to their house at Brown University, roast them in the oven, and throw them in a food processor.

They played around with it a bit, and the result—now known as cricket flour—got incorporated into the bars to substitute for protein powder from soy.

Cricket flour contains more protein than any other insect source, about 7 g in just two tablespoons (12 g). It's also a great choice for those wanting to avoid gluten. And it's sustainable. Crickets release 80 percent less methane than cattle, and they require much less feed than any other farm animal.

Bitty Foods founder Megan Miller, who has given a TEDx lecture on eating bugs, told National Public Radio (NPR) that her company's blend of powdered crickets and gluten-free starches for baking has quite a following among moms. "There's a need among moms who want to get more protein in their kids' diets, but it can be hard to feed them things like a steak," she said, in an article posted on the NPR website.

In 2012, former president Bill Clinton issued a challenge for those competing for the Hult Prize, the largest student competition in the world for social good. Five MBA students from McGill University in Montreal answered that challenge and came up with the idea that won the Hult Prize for 2013: Farm insects as a sustainable source of protein.

They founded a company—ASPIRE—and bought their first cricket farm in Austin, Texas, and now produce delicious Aketta Crickets and cricket flour in a variety of flavors. Find them at www.aketta.com.

One serving of cricket powder (about 12 g, or 2 tablespoons) contains about 55 calories, 7 g of protein, 2 g of fat, and less than 1 g of carbs.

Potato Starch

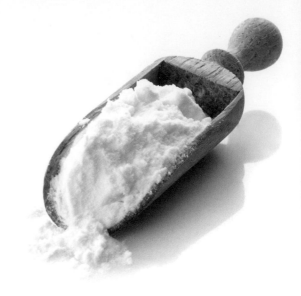

How in the world does potato starch even rate a listing in a book about great foods? Simple. Because it's actually a very fine source of resistant starch (see fiber sidebar page 97). Resistant starch is a form of fiber that is feasted upon by the good bacteria in your colon. That's why it's considered a prebiotic fiber—it's food for the probiotics that live in your gut and that you want to thrive and survive.

Resistant starch improves insulin sensitivity in people with metabolic syndrome. One review paper on the metabolic effects and potential health benefits of resistant starch noted that resistant starch intake seemed to decrease blood sugar and insulin response, lower triglycerides, improve whole body insulin sensitivity, increase satiety, and reduce fat storage. The same paper noted that resistant starch is "an attractive dietary target for the prevention of diseases associated with dyslipidemia and insulin resistance as well as the development of weight loss diets and dietary therapies for the treatment of type 2 diabetes and coronary heart disease."

Like other prebiotic fibers, potato starch is fermented in the large intestine, producing an important short-chain fatty acid called butyric acid, the preferred fuel for colon cells and an important compound for digestive and gut health. Resistant starch in potatoes is formed when you cook the potatoes and then cool them. The cooling transforms some of the digestible starches in potatoes into resistant starches (through a process called retrogradation).

Understandably, many people are loathe to eat a lot of potatoes, because they're high in carbs and are considered high glycemic. (A medium baked potato has a glycemic load of 28—up to 10 is considered low, 10 to 20 is considered medium, and anything over twenty is high.) That's why potato starch is available as a supplement—you get nothing but the resistant starch and none of the high-glycemic carbs. If you're using potato starch as a form of resistant starch, I'd recommend Bob's Red Mill Potato Starch, which is available on Thrive Market for under five bucks, and on Amazon as well. Put a tablespoon or so (12 g) in your smoothie for an extra fiber boost.

CHAPTER 15

SWEETENERS

For centuries, psychologists and philosophers have debated a central question of human existence: How much of who we are is "fixed"("nature")—and how much is the result of learning and socialization ("nurture")? Last time I looked, the debate was still alive and well and raging in the fields of psychology, genetics, behaviorism, and sociology. But one particular taste that seems to be clearly human, one that is hardwired and arrives full-blown and ready to go from the time we're born, is the taste for sweetness.

Watch any infant when you put a sweet-tasting substance on their tongue, and it's hard to debate that their reaction is "learned" behavior. Infants love it.

They come out of the box loving it. Current thinking is that from ability to distinguish sweet and bitter is deeply wired in our DNA as a survival trait, allowing us to avaoid poisonous substances in the wild (usually bitter) from ones that are edible. (Though the relationship between bitter and dangerous isn't perfect, it's pretty reliable.) Another theory is that humans are one of the few creatures on earth unable to make our own vitamin C; we must obtain it from our diet, and it's found most abundantly in sweet things such as fruit. Nature, so the theory goes, gave us a sweet tooth so that we would desire the foods without which we wouldn't survive.

No matter. We humans love sweet things, probably way too much for our own good. In Paleolithic times, a sweet tooth wasn't much of a problem. (There were no twenty-four-hour supermarkets in the caveman era.) The only sweet thing available was the occasional bees nest of honey, which, if you were lucky enough to come upon it, required you to shimmy up a tree to procure its rewards. The fruits and vegetables of the cavemen era were bitter little things, much different from the specially bred, enormous lush fruits of modern time. And the only sugar our ancestors knew was unrefined sugar that came in the original package—fruits, vegetables, plants, and later, sugarcane. Processed sugar came much later. Processed foods loaded with unspeakable amounts of sugar later still. And high-fructose corn syrup, arguably one of the worst inventions of the food science industry, is even more recent.

Are There Healthy Ways to Feed a Sweetness Craving?

So let's recognize that we are sweet-loving folks. The question then becomes how to appease that taste so it doesn't destroy us. Or, put differently, how to feed and mollify the craving while doing damage control.

Now don't misunderstand me. I'm not saying we should never have anything with sugar in it. (Though we'd all probably be a lot more healthy if we did that, even though life wouldn't be as much fun.) I love ice cream as much as anyone on the planet, and life would not be the same without my friend Skye's brownies, or key lime pie, or chocolate chip cookies. But unfortunately, few of the ingredients in those delicious concoctions—at least few of the sweetening ingredients—have any place on the list of the healthiest foods in the world.

Two sweeteners, however, do belong on the list: Blackstrap molasses and raw, unfiltered honey, which we'll get to in a minute

Artificial vs. Alternative Sweeteners (Stevia, Erythritol)

There are other great ways to sweeten and do damage control besides using blackstrap molasses or honey. Stevia, for example. There's absolutely nothing wrong with stevia; in fact, stevoside, one of the sweet compounds in stevia, may help lower high blood pressure. The only problem with stevia—at least, until recently—was the aftertaste, which I personally never liked. Fortunately, since the original publication of this book, there is now an organic, non-GMO stevia product that has zero aftertaste—it's called Pyure, it's available everywhere, and it doesn't cost any more than regular stevia. I make a healthy whipped cream using nothing but real, organic whipping cream and Pyure, blending the two together with an electric hand mixer for about 4 minutes till it turns into the most delicious whipped cream you ever tasted. (I have a video of me making it on my website, www.jonnybowden.com.) I also like xylitol and erythritol (Truvia), but Pyure stevia is my favorite. No calories, and none of the digestive issues that can sometimes arise with sugar alcohols.

In a perfect world, we wouldn't eat sugar, at least not any kind of processed sugar. But this is not a perfect world. The two sweeteners on this list are actual foods, and in my opinion are the best options those who would like additional sweetness in their food.

Blackstrap Molasses

I'm often asked whether there are any sweeteners that are actually good for you. The two that always come to mind are blackstrap molasses and raw, unfiltered honey (see page 358). Blackstrap molasses is very much a food. And a nutritional powerhouse to boot.

Molasses is the by-product of sugar refining that contains all the nutrients from the raw sugarcane plant. Because the roots of sugarcane grow very deep, they are able to receive a pretty broad range of minerals and trace elements usually lacking in the topsoil. During the refining of sugarcane, the plants are boiled to a syrup from which the crystals are extracted. Then they're boiled two more times, both of which produce molasses. Blackstrap molasses, however, comes from the third and final boiling and is essentially the dregs of the barrel. One website innocently described blackstrap molasses as only having commercial value in the manufacture of cattle feed, precisely because it has the least amount of sugar of the three boils.

Blackstrap molasses is very dark and has a robust, somewhat bitter-tart flavor. It's used in a variety of baked goods, particularly meat and vegetable dishes, as a sweetener and coloring agent. It is also widely accepted as a health food. It can be used in any number of recipes and is particularly suitable for gingersnaps, soy-based sauces, licorice, canned baked beans, and fermentation systems.

BLACKSTRAP MOLASSES IS LOW IN SUGAR AND HIGH IN NUTRIENTS

One of the reasons I like it so much is precisely because it has a low amount of sugar and a high amount of nutrients. As the only product from the third and final boil, blackstrap molasses contains the lowest sugar content of the different types, but many more of the vitamins, minerals, and trace elements found naturally in the sugarcane plant, making it more nutritious than most other sweeteners.

Blackstrap molasses is a good source of iron, potassium, calcium, and magnesium, and it is an excellent source of manganese and copper. It also contains a small amount of the cancer-fighting mineral selenium. There are all sorts of claims for the health benefits of taking blackstrap molasses as a nutritional supplement to the tune of a couple of tablespoons (40 g) a day. Some of the claims are probably far-fetched, but where there's that much smoke there's probably a fire somewhere. To my taste buds, blackstrap molasses is completely delicious, and a nutrient-dense sweetener that I wholeheartedly recommend. Best bet: Look for unsulfured blackstrap molasses from organic sugar.

WORTH KNOWING

Blackstrap molasses has a long and storied tradition as a health food and a remedy for all sorts of ailments. One of the most popular legends is that it can reverse gray hair. While I've never seen any scientific proof of this, it's an interesting claim, because a copper deficiency may lead to prematurely gray hair, and blackstrap molasses is very high in copper.

Of the varieties of molasses, blackstrap molasses is richest in nutrients, such as iron, B vitamins, calcium, and potassium.

Raw, Unfiltered Honey

Honey is pure alchemy. And it's precious stuff. One little bee, foraging for nectar over an entire bee-lifetime only produces about one-twelfth of a teaspoon of honey. Bees collect the nectar from flowers; the nectar mixes with enzymes in the bees' saliva; then they carry it back to the hive, and voilà, they make a deposit. Multiply that process by a few hundred bees and before you know it you've got a honeycomb.

Now here's the rub. The stuff you'd find in that hive, if you put your finger in and tasted it, is not the same food you find in a little plastic squeezy bear in the supermarket. Not even close. The honey I'm talking about here is similar—if not identical—to the real, raw, unprocessed, unheated, unfiltered kind you'd get if you took that honeycomb home and ate the contents with a spoon. That's a real food.

PASTEURIZED AND PROCESSED HONEY HAS FEWER NUTRIENTS

This is a very important distinction. Many of the phytonutrients and enzymes that are found in honey are destroyed by pasteurization and high-heat processing. According to some natural foods experts, the best honey has not been heated to temperatures higher than 105°F (41°C), and according to many others, the best honey has not been heated at all. The process of heating and straining the honey makes it look clearer, but also removes a lot of the nutrients and the bee pollen. Some companies—for example, Really Raw Honey—sell unprocessed honey with the bee pollen and part of the comb right in the jar.

THE HARDER THE HONEY, THE BETTER

The type of plants bees forage on determines the color of the honey, the level of nutrients, the fragrance, and the taste. Honey from extremely cold regions is lighter in color than honey from the tropics. According to the website of Tropical Traditions, one reliable company that I particularly like, the strength of crystallization (hardness) determines the level of live-state nutrients and heat-sensitive enzymes. The harder the honey, the better.

Honey contains several members of a class of plant polyphenols called *flavonoids*, which are mentioned throughout this book and are frequently found in fruits and vegetables. (If you're interested, the specific flavonoids found in honey are flavanones, flavones, and flavonols.) Flavonoids are known for their antioxidant activity and are important for human health. At least one study supports the folk wisdom of having some honey in a hot drink when you're sick: A study in the *Journal of Medicinal Food* suggested that honey may stimulate antibody production during primary and secondary immune responses.

HONEY IS A SOURCE OF PROBIOTICS

We've known for a while that honey is helpful for when you're coming down with an illness, probably because of the polyphenols in raw honey that may have immune-stimulating properties, not to mention the ability of honey to soothe and coat the throat. New research is uncovering yet another benefit of this food: a probiotic that's endemic to honeybees.

According to an article in GreenMedInfo, bees produce the probiotic bacterium *Lactobacillus kunkeei*, which has been shown to stimulate the immune system. Remember, that these delicate bacteria are killed when the honey is heated to high temperatures, which is what happens when it is processed. Another reason to consume only raw, cold-processed honey.

In a talk at the 2017 Scripps Conference on Evidence-Based Supplements, Elizabeth Lipski, Ph.D.—an expert on digestive health and the author of *Digestive Wellness*—listed honey as one of the ten best foods for a healthy microbiome.

EVEN RAW HONEY DEMANDS PRECAUTION

Honey is still sugar, if you've got blood sugar issues, proceed with caution. However, because it's a real food and contains nutrients, it's one of the best sweeteners to use, provided you use it judiciously. For the record, one study did show that natural honey lowered blood sugar as well as C-reactive protein (a measure of inflammation) and homocysteine (a risk factor for heart disease) in both healthy and diabetic subjects.

Raw honey doesn't spoil. The nectar that the bees bring to the hive is about 60 percent water, and the bees "cure" it to about 18 to 19 percent water. At this level of water and with a pH of 3 or 4, the honey is very stable and can last for centuries. (It was found in Egyptian tombs.) Of course, if it is left exposed to air, it will eventually ferment and develop an unpalatable taste. The bees prevent the fermentation by sealing the honey in the honeycomb. Pretty cool, huh?

MANUKA HONEY: WHAT'S THE REAL DEAL?

A particular type of honey that's prized among health connoisseurs is manuka honey from New Zealand. Here's why.

All honey—at least the cold, raw, organic kind we're talking about—offers protection against damage caused by bacteria. Some stimulate the production of special cells that can help repair infection-damaged tissue. Honey is also anti-inflammatory when applied to the skin. A component of honey—hydrogen peroxide—gives honey a lot of its antibiotic power.

But not all honey is created equal, and some kinds may be way more potent than others.

Manuka honey has additional components that are antibacterial, such as methylglyoxal (MG). A compound in manuka honey called 5.8-kDa stimulates the immune cells such as TNF-alpha. Honey producers have a scale, the purpose of which is to rate the potency of manuka honey, called UMF for Unique Manuka Factor. The UMF rating corresponds to the level of antibacterial factors in the honey. To be considered potent enough to be therapeutic, the honey needs to have at least a rating of 10 UMF. It can then be marketed as either UMF Manuka Honey or Active Manuka Honey.

Manuka honey is delicious, but it's also very expensive. Remember, the main medical use for it as an antibacterial compound is externally—on top of a wound or burn. Though manuka honey is frequently marketed for all kinds of other conditions (from diabetes to cancer), we don't have a lot of evidence either for or against using it for those conditions. For nutrition purposes only, you're probably just as well off with a high-quality, cold-pressed, organic, locally grown honey. It'll still be more expensive than the processed stuff that comes in a squeezy bear, but not be nearly as expensive as manuka.

WORTH KNOWING

Raw, unfiltered honey is worth seeking out, and many local farms may sell it. You can also find it in natural food supermarkets and on the Internet.

ADDED SWEETENERS:
THE GOOD, THE BAD, THE UGLY

In addition to honey and molasses, there are multiple choices for sweeteners—artificial and not-artificial—that come in packets. Splenda, Equal, Stevia, Sunett, Sweet One, and xylitol all fit the bill, as do a couple of others listed below. Here's what I think of each of them.

SUCRALOSE (SPLENDA) (NO)

The little yellow package is very far from innocuous. Research in the *Journal of Toxicology and Environmental Health*, Part B: Critical Reviews, found that Splenda causes a variety of harmful biological effects in the body. It also alters the amount and the quality of beneficial microbes in your gut, essentially screwing up your microbiome. I would never use this sweetener.

STEVIA (YES)

Stevia is a plant native to South America that has been used for thousands of years as a natural sweetener. It's 200 times sweeter than sugar and it won't raise blood sugar. I like stevia products by Pyure because they have no licorice-y aftertaste and are organic and non-GMO. I have a video on my website of me making delicious and healthy whipped cream with nothing but fresh organic cream and Pyure stevia. Great stuff.

MONK FRUIT a.k.a. LO HAN (YES)

Monk fruit has been used for centuries in China as a remedy for sore throats, colds, and congestion. In southern China, it's considered a longevity aid. It's a low-calorie, low-glycemic food used as a sweetener in beverages and foods. It's also known as Lo Han and, it appears to be perfectly safe.

ERYTHRITOL (YES)

Erythritol, like xylitol, is a sugar alcohol. Sugar alcohols are naturally found in the fibrous parts of different fruits and vegetables. Erythritol itself can be found in pears and melons. Our body can't break it down so it basically provides zero calories and zero glycemic response. I've been using erythritol for years and I've never heard even a word of buzz about any negatives. Definitely okay to use!

XYLITOL (YES)

Xylitol is a sugar alcohol that has a specific benefit—it helps to prevent bacteria from taking a hold on your teeth. That's one reason it's used in tooth-friendly products and recommended by dentists. It also has an ability to strengthen and re-mineralize gums and teeth.

I've always liked xylitol and have used it for over a decade. The only thing to be aware of is that, like many other sugar alcohols, it can have a tendency to cause diarrhea and bloating in some people. It's definitely safe for people with diabetes. okay to use!

ASPARTAME (EQUAL) (NO)

Aspartame is an artificial sweetener, and the debate on whether it's safe has been going on for decades. In 1980, an FDA public board of inquiry confirmed that it "might induce brain tumors." It had been banned, but some behind-the-scenes political maneuvering, it was able to get approval, albeit under a cloud of suspicion. Neurosurgeon Russell Blaylock considers it a neurotoxin. And some people are "aspartame responders," meaning they get intense headaches from consuming it (Lipton, 1989). I would never use aspartame (Equal) and recommend that you don't either.

AGAVE NECTAR SYRUP (NO)

Agave nectar syrup has up to 92 percent fructose, making it dwarf high-fructose corn syrup in terms of its negative impact on your body. (HFCS is about 55 percent fructose). The fact that this has somehow been branded as a healthy sweetener is a testament to the craft of marketing. In very tiny amounts it's probably innocuous, but it's been sold to us as the healthy alternative to sugar. It's not. Stay away.

SACCHARIN (MAYBE)

I grew up thinking that saccharin caused bladder cancer, because that's what we believed throughout the 1970s based on some pretty compelling rat studies. Research has found no such link between cancer and saccharin, however, and the National Cancer Institute points out that the mechanism that caused bladder cancer in rats doesn't exist in humans. That led to a 2000 repeal of the warning label previously required for saccharin. Though it has not been proven to cause cancer, the Center for Science in the Public Interest (a consumer advocacy group) still believes that saccharin may pose a risk. I'd avoid it.

ACESULFAME POTASSIUM (Sunett, Sweet One) (NO)

One of the chemicals found in Acesulfame Potassium (Ace-K) is methylene chloride, a known carcinogen linked to visual disturbances, headache, depression, liver problems, mental confusion, and cancer in humans. The FDA concluded that the methylene chloride in Ace-K is sufficiently low as to be a nonissue. I'm not so sure. I wouldn't use this artificial sweetener.

THE EXPERTS' TOP TEN LISTS

Jeff Volek, R.D., Ph.D., F.A.C.N.

Jeff Volek is one of the world's most respected researchers in the field of low-carb diets. He is a professor in the department of human sciences at Ohio State University, and the author of five books—including the *New York Times* bestseller, *The Art and Science of Low-Carb Living*—and more than 280 peer-reviewed scientific manuscripts.

1. **Whole eggs:** One of the most nutrient-dense foods, meaning it provides a relatively high proportion of essential nutrients per calorie. Egg yolks also contain choline, an important substance necessary for fat breakdown, the membranes of nearly every cell in the body, and production of neurotransmitters.

2. **Salmon:** Salmon is a high-quality source of protein and omega-3 fatty acids.

3. **Yogurt:** An excellent source of high-quality, easily absorbed protein. It has all the nutritional value of milk but with several advantages for individuals with lactose intolerance. Yogurt also boosts the immune system, maintains a healthy gut, and has anticancer effects. Try to find those with the least amount of sugar.

4. **Nuts:** Increasing nut consumption has been associated with reduced risk for heart disease. Nuts also contain about 2 to 3 g of dietary fiber per ounce and several vitamins and minerals, including vitamin E.

5. **Beef:** Beef is an excellent source of biologically available protein and also contains significant amounts of essential vitamins and minerals, including niacin, thiamin, riboflavin, pyridoxine, biotin, folic acid, and vitamin B_{12}. It's also an excellent source of heme iron and zinc.

6. **Olive oil:** Olive oil contains primarily monounsaturated fat, and it is a staple in the diet of individuals living in the Mediterranean region who demonstrate very low rates of chronic disease. When olive oil is the predominant source of lipids, fat intakes greater than 40 percent of total energy are compatible with good health and are associated with no adverse effects.

7. **Water:** Water is second to oxygen in maintaining life. Even minimal changes in body water can impair performance.

8. **Sweet potatoes:** One baked sweet potato provides more than 8,800 IUs of vitamin A, yet it contains only 141 calories. This nutritious vegetable also provides about half your requirement for vitamin C, in addition to smaller amounts of calcium, iron, and thiamine. It is low in sodium and is a good source of fiber and other important vitamins and minerals.

9. **Grapes:** Perhaps the greatest value of grapes is their abundant content of various antioxidants that can help fight free radicals. Grapes are a good source of several natural antioxidants, including vitamin C, as well as phytochemicals and flavonoids, which also offer protection against heart disease and various cancers.

10. **Coffee:** Coffee is full of healthy phytonutrients. Despite popular opinion, overwhelming research suggests that moderate coffee and caffeine consumption causes no adverse health effects.

GLOSSARY

17 beta-estradiol—most potent mammalian estrogenic hormone; can be carcinogenic in cancers that are hormone-related

ACE inhibitors—found in whey protein; reduce blood pressure and improve cardiovascular health

acetylcholine—major neurotransmitter in the body; needed for memory and healthy brain function

acetylenics—component of celery that stops the growth of cancer cells

aldosterone—adrenal hormone that can raise blood pressure

allicin—active ingredient in garlic; produced from interaction between alliin and allinase

alliin—amino acid found in garlic

allinase—enzyme found in garlic; its action on the amino acid alliin produces allicin

allyl isothiocyanate—breakdown product of sinigrin believed to play a role in the prevention of tumors and suppression of tumor growth

alpha-carotene—carotenoid that converts in the body to vitamin A

alpha-lactalbumin—protein fraction with important disease-fighting effects; found in whey protein

alpha-linolenic acid—omega-3 fatty acid that helps reduce inflammation

amino acids—molecules that link together to form proteins

anethole—compound that gives fennel its licorice flavor

anthocyanins—pigment molecules that make blueberries blue, red cabbage and cherries red; improve vision and brain function; guard against macular degeneration; help the body relieve inflammation

anthraquinone—compound in noni fruit that stimulates the synthesis of collagen and may be an antiwrinkle agent

antiemetic—having the property of preventing nausea and vomiting

antimutagen—substance that interferes with cell-changing agents from starting cancer

antioxidants—compounds in food that help fight the process of oxidation, or oxidative stress, a factor in virtually every degenerative disease

antiplatelet activity—helps prevent platelets in the blood from sticking together, thus warding off heart attack or stroke

apoptosis—natural death of cancer cells

arginine—amino acid touted for its role in protecting the inner lining of the arterial walls, making them more pliable and less susceptible to atherogenesis

astaxanthin—natural carotenoid that prevents lipid peroxidation and assists in mending DNA breakdown products; found in salmon

atherosclerosis—disease in which plaque builds up in the arteries, causing them to harden and narrow

avenanthramides—polyphenol antioxidants unique to oats; believed to have anti-inflammatory and heart-healthy properties

beta-carotene—carotenoid that converts in the body to vitamin A

beta-cryptoxanthin—orange-yellow carotenoid that may lower the risk of lung cancer

betacyanin—compound that gives red color to beets

beta-glucans—polysaccharides that stimulate the immune system; e.g., beta-1,6 glucan and beta-1,3 glucan

betaine—metabolite that works synergistically with folate to reduce potentially toxic levels of homocysteine; also known as trimethylglycine (TMG)

beta-lactoglobulin—protein fraction with important disease-fighting effects; found in whey protein

beta-sitosterol—plant compound shown to significantly lower blood cholesterol and protect the prostate

boron—mineral that may be important for bone and joint health, particularly in women

bran—the main source of fiber in whole grains; can also contain nutrients

bromelain—proteolytic enzyme that breaks down amino acids; relieves indigestion; is often extracted from pineapple

butyric acid—fatty acid with antiviral and anticancer properties; raises the level of interferon in the body

caffeic acid—strong antioxidant found in coffee and rosemary; has anti-inflammatory properties

caffeic acid phenethyl ester (CAPE)—active compound in bee propolis known to have anticarcinogenic, anti-inflammatory, and immunomodulatory properties

capric acid—medium-chain triglyceride formed into monocaprin in the human body; found in coconut

capsaicin—active ingredient in hot peppers; common ingredient in pain-relieving creams; vasodilator

carminative—agent that induces the expulsion of gas from the stomach and intestines

carotenoid—antioxidant compound found in plants; associated with a wide range of health benefits

carvacrol—compound with antifungal, antibacterial, and antiparasitic properties; found in oregano and thyme

catechins—very powerful group of polyphenols; found in green tea and cinnamon

chalcone polymers—phytochemicals in cinnamon that increase glucose metabolism in the cells

charantin—compound found in bitter melon that may have antidiabetic properties

chlorogenic acid—antioxidant particularly effective against a destructive free radical called the superoxide anion radical; found in sweet potatoes, apples, and coffee

chlorophyll—substance that makes plants appear green; a natural blood purifier

choline—nutrient found in eggs, needed for healthy brain and liver function and fat breakdown; forms betaine in the body

chromium—trace mineral that helps insulin function

citrate—compound that may help fight kidney stones

conjugated linoleic acid (CLA)—trans fat found naturally in grass-fed dairy and meat

cortisol—adrenal hormone with anti-inflammatory properties

COX-2 inhibitors—drugs that block pain and inflammation messages in the body

C-reactive protein—found in the blood; used as a measure of inflammation

crustacean—only group of arthropods that is primarily marine

cucurbitacins—chemicals in pumpkin seeds that may interfere with production of DHT (dihydrotestosterone), a metabolic by-product of testosterone

curcumin—antioxidant and curcuminoid; has anti-inflammatory and anti-tumor effects; has positive effect on cholesterol

curcuminoids—family of compounds thought to be most responsible for turmeric's medicinal effects and bright yellow color

cyclooxygenase—a compound produced in the body in two or more forms, called COX-1 and COX-2

diallyl disulfide—compound in garlic found to inhibit leukemia cells in a test tube

diallyl sulfide—compound found in onions that increases the body's production of an important cancer-fighting enzyme

dihydrotestosterone—testosterone metabolite partly responsible for hair loss and benign prostate hyperplasia

diosgenin—phytochemical in beans that appears to inhibit cancer cells from multiplying

diterpene—health-promoting plant compound found in rosemary

dithiolethiones—anticancer phytochemicals found in cabbage

dopamine—feel-good neurotransmitter in the brain

eicosanoids—minihormones that control metabolic processes in the body; also called *prostaglandins*

ellagic acid—a naturally occurring phenolic known to be anticarcinogenic and antimutagenic; found in cherries and red raspberries; shown to inhibit tumor growth

enterodiol—breakdown product of lignan in the gut that interferes with the cancer-promoting effects of estrogen

enterolactone—breakdown product of lignan in the gut that interferes with the cancer-promoting effects of estrogen

epigallocatechin gallate (EGCG)—catechin believed to be responsible for the anticancer effects of green tea

eritadenine—active compound in shiitake mushrooms that lowers blood cholesterol

erucic acid—a fatty acid that has been associated with Keshan's disease

essential fatty acids—healthy fats that must be obtained through diet; support many healthy body functions

eugenol—phytochemical with antimicrobial activity that can help stop the growth of bacteria and fungi

fiber—component of food; associated with lower risks of heart disease, diabetes, obesity, and cancer; soluble and insoluble forms

fibrin—sticky, weblike fibers that the body produces to form a structure that stops excess bleeding

fibrinogen—substance in the body that can cause blood clots and strokes

flavonoids—plant compounds with antioxidant, anticancer, and antiallergy properties; more than 4,000 have been identified

flavanols—flavonoids found in cocoa; prevent fatlike substances in the bloodstream from clogging the arteries and modulate nitric acid

folate—B vitamin that helps prevent neural tube defects and helps bring down homocysteine levels

free radicals—destructive molecules in the body; can damage cells and DNA

French paradox—fact that the French have less heart disease than Americans, despite eating far more high-fat foods

fructooligosaccharides—food for good gut bacteria; help maintain healthy gut ecology; also called prebiotics

fucoidan—polysaccharide believed to have anticancer activity; found in kombu and wakame

furocoumarins—compounds found in grapefruit; inhibit a key enzyme that metabolizes and regulates certain drugs; reason to avoid taking drugs with grapefruit juice

gamma-linolenic acid (GLA)—important "good" omega-6 found in hemp seed, primrose, and borage oils; also called GLA

gamma-tocopherol—component of vitamin E that neutralizes the perioxynitrite radical, which destroys cellular endothelial membranes

ganodermic acid—component of reishi mushrooms; benefits blood pressure and liver and adrenal function

geraniol—phytochemical with antimicrobial activity that can help stop the growth of bacteria and fungi

germ—the smallest portion of a grain, rich in vitamins, minerals, and fiber

gingerdiones—antioxidant and active ingredient in ginger

gingerol—phytochemical responsible for the pungent taste of ginger

glucose tolerance factor (GTF)—helps regulate blood sugar levels; found in brewer's yeast

glucosinolates—phytonutrients that are parent molecules of substances that increase human resistance to cancer

glutathione—one of the body's premier antioxidants; required for replication of the lymphocyte immune cells

glutathione-S-transferase—important cancer-fighting enzyme

glycemic index—measure of how much a given food (such as fruit) raises blood sugar

glycemic load—measure of a food's effect on blood sugar that accounts for portion size

glycolipids—substances in butter with anti-infective properties

glycyrrhizin—member of the saponin family and the active ingredient in licorice

goitrogens—naturally occurring substances that suppress thyroid function

haemagglutinin—clot-promoting substance that causes red blood cells to clump together; found in soybeans

hesperidin—predominant flavonoid in oranges; strengthens capillaries; has anti-inflammatory, antiallergic, vasoprotective, and anticarcinogenic actions

homocysteine—naturally occurring amino acid that can harm blood vessels, thereby contributing to the development of heart disease, stroke, dementia, and peripheral vascular disease

host defenses potentiators (HDP)—compounds used as adjunctive cancer treatments throughout Asia; also found in cell structures of mushrooms

husk—inedible outer layer of a grain kernel; also called chaff

hydroxyl radicals—dangerous free radicals

immunoglobulin—protein fraction with important disease-fighting effects; found in whey

indoles—phytochemicals DIM and indole-3-carbinole; protective against prostate, gastric, skin, and breast cancers

inflammation—critical component of virtually all degenerative diseases

insoluble fiber—indigestible part of foods that moves bulk through the intestines

insulin—fat-storing hormone that, if raised high enough, long enough, and often enough, contributes to diabetes, heart disease, and aging

inulin—naturally occurring soluble fiber that feeds the good bacteria in the gut and helps support gastrointestinal health

isoflavones—phytochemicals in soy foods that may help ease menopause symptoms

isothiocyanates—phytonutrients that neutralize carcinogens, reduce their poisonous effect, and stimulate the release of other substances that help combat them

lauric acid—fat that is antiviral, antimicrobial, and important for immune function; found in coconut oil

lecithin—nutritional supplement that is 10 to 20 percent phosphatidylcholine

lectins—substances contained in legumes and grains that originally evolved to fight off insect predators; some lectins can bind with body tissues and create problems

L-ergothioneine—powerful antioxidant in mushrooms that neutralizes free radicals and increases enzymes with antioxidant activity

lignans—plant compounds with protective effect against cancers, especially those that are hormone-sensitive, such as those of the breast, uterine, and prostate

limonene—phytochemical that boosts the body's synthesis of an enzyme that has antioxidant properties and helps detoxify chemicals; found in citrus fruit peels

limonin—limonoid in lemon that seems to be able to lower cholesterol

limonoids—phytochemicals abundant in citrus fruit that account for the scent of fresh lemon or orange peel

linoleic acid—essential fatty acid with anticancer properties; also called omega-6 fatty acid

lipid peroxidation—process by which fats turn rancid

lutein—carotenoid that is a natural antioxidant and maintains eye and skin health

luteolin—flavonoid found in artichokes that prevents LDL oxidation

lycopene—carotenoid associated with lower risk of prostate cancer; found in tomatoes

lysine—amino acid found in quinoa; scarce in the vegetable kingdom

macrophages—white blood cells that devour foreign invaders like fungi and bacteria

magnesium—mineral that helps lower high blood pressure

malic acid—substance in vinegar important for fighting body toxins and inhibiting unfriendly bacteria

manganese—trace mineral essential for growth; reproduction; wound healing; brain function; and metabolism of sugars, insulin, and cholesterol

medium-chain triglyceride (MCT)—healthy class of fatty acids; e.g., lauric acid

metabolite—by-product of the body's metabolic processes

methylhydroxychalcone polymer—active ingredient in cinnamon; seems to mimic insulin function, increasing glucose uptake by cells and signaling certain kinds of cells to turn glucose into glycogen

molybdenum—enzyme-enhancing mineral found in red kidney beans

monocaprin—by-product of capric acid shown to have antiviral effects

monoterpine—plant compound found in rosemary

monounsaturated fats—fats central to the Mediterranean diet, associated with lower rates of heart disease; found in nuts and olive oil; also called omega-9s

mucopolysaccharides—complex sugars mixed with amino acids, simple sugars, and sometimes protein; make up the cell walls of spirulina

myricetin—common flavonoid that may have anti-inflammatory, antitumor, and antioxidant properties; found in raisins

myristicin—volatile oil in parsley that may inhibit tumors

nacre—combination of calcium and protein with which oysters coat any irritating sand or grit that gets trapped within their shells

nasunin—anthocyanin that is a powerful antioxidant; found in eggplant

nattokinase—fibrinolytic enzyme that can help reduce and prevent clots; found in natto

neochlorogenic acid—phytonutrient found in plums and prunes that is particularly effective against a destructive free radical called the superoxide anion radical

neopterin—substance found in humans that appears to play an important role in the immune system; isolated from royal jelly

neoxanthin—carotenoid in spinach that causes prostate cancer cells to self-destruct

nitric oxide—compound in the body that helps relax constricted blood vessels and ease blood flow; synthesized from arginine

nobiletin—citrus flavonoid that may prevent atherosclerosis

octacosanol—compound in wheat germ oil that might help with exercise performance

oleic acid—omega-9 fat found in high amounts in olive oil, macadamia nut oil, and many nuts; increases the incorporation of omega-3 fatty acids into the cell membrane

omega-3 fats—ALA (alpha-linolenic acid), found in flaxseed; DHA (docosahexanoic acid) and EPA (eicosapentanoic acid), found in fish such as wild salmon; keep cell membranes fluid

ORAC value—oxygen radical absorbance capacity; rating system for antioxidant power not used anymore

organosulfur compounds—anticancer substances found in kale

oryzanol—component of brown rice found in its oil that aids in its cholesterol-lowering effect

osteocalcin—compound that anchors calcium molecules inside the bone; activated by vitamin K

oxalate—substance that inhibits calcium absorption

oxidize—damage with free radicals

oxymel—combination of apple cider vinegar and honey widely used to dissolve painful calcium deposits in the body

palmitic acid—fat found in chocolate; shouldn't be eaten in large amounts

pantothenic acid—vitamin B5; found in peanuts; stress reliever

papain—one of a class of enzymes called *proteolytic* enzymes that help break down or digest protein; extracted from papaya and used in digestive enzyme supplements as well as in enzyme supplements used for pain

PCB—polychlorinated biphenyl, a toxin that is sometimes found in farm-raised salmon

p-coumaric acid—polyphenol studied for its antioxidant abilities and its potential as an anticancer agent

pectin—type of fiber that helps relieve constipation, reduce cholesterol, and regulate blood sugar; found in apples and quince

perillyl alcohol—compound that may inhibit tumor growth; found in cherries

phase-2 enzymes—substances that can disarm damaging free radicals and help fight cancer-causing carcinogens

phenethyl isothiocyanate—compound found in cruciferous vegetables that may have anticancer effects

phenolic compounds—natural antioxidants that help neutralize harmful free radicals in the body that are thought to be linked to most chronic diseases, including cancer, heart disease, and diabetes; most belong to the flavonoid group

phenols—plant chemicals that are potent antioxidants and anti-inflammatory agents; also known as phenolic acids

phenylbutazone—anti-inflammatory medicine with effects similar to those of curcumin

phloridzin—phytochemical found in apples that contributes to antioxidant power

phosphatidylcholine—phospholipid with choline as a component; found in eggs; helps keep fat and cholesterol from accumulating in the liver

phthalides—phytochemicals found in celery that increase blood flow and reduce level of stress hormones

phycocyanin—pigment found in spirulina with antioxidant and anti-inflammatory properties; may inhibit cancer-colony formation

phytates—substances that block the absorption of minerals; found in grains and soy foods

phytic acid—phytochemical in beans that can protect cells from genetic damage that leads to cancer

phytoalexins—chemical substances produced by plants as a defense against pathogenic microorganisms

phytoene—antioxidant found in many fruits and vegetables, including tomatoes; along with zera-carotene and phytofluene believed to have strong disease-fighting potential

phytoestrogens—weak estrogenic compounds from plants

phytofluene—antioxidant found in many fruits and vegetables, including tomatoes; along with phytoene and zera-carotene, believed to have strong disease-fighting potential

phytonutrients—nutrients from plants

phytosterols—plant chemicals with numerous health benefits, including lowering cholesterol; also called plant sterols

plant sterols—plant chemicals with numerous health benefits, including lowering cholesterol; also called phytosterols

plasmin—enzyme in the body that dissolves and breaks down fibrin to help prevent blood clots

polyacetylenes—plant compounds that help protect against carcinogens; found in parsnips

polyglutamic acid—compound that makes natto sticky and increases the natural moisturizing factor in skin

polyphenols—powerful antioxidants, many of which have anticancer activity; include flavonoids, anthocyanins, and isoflavones; help protect cells from oxidative stress

polysaccharide—long string of glucose molecules

polyunsaturated fats—large class of fatty acids with many members, including both omega-3s and omega-6s; found in vegetable oils, nuts, and fish

proanthocyanidins—plant compounds helpful in preventing degenerative disease; powerful antioxidants that are several times more potent than vitamins C and E; help protect against the effects of internal and environmental stresses (e.g., cigarette smoking, pollution)

probiotics—good bacteria with positive effects in the digestive system; found in yogurt and naturally fermented foods

prostaglandins—minihormones that control metabolic processes in the body; also called eicosanoids

protease inhibitor—phytochemical in beans that slows the division of cancer cells

proteolytic enzymes—enzymes that break down the amino acid bonds in protein

pterostilbene—powerful antioxidant that is known to lower cholesterol and fight cancer

purines—substances that break down to uric acid in the body; found in cauliflower

quercetin—flavonoid that is a natural anti-inflammatory and has anticancer effects

resistant starch—a type of fiber that serves as food for the good bacteria in your gut

resveratrol— compound found in red wine and the skin of dark grapes; associated with antiaging effects, reduced incidence of cardiovascular disease, and reduced risk for cancer

rhizome—the part of the turmeric plant that is consumed

rhodopsin—purple pigment in the eye; needed for vision in dim light

rosmarinic acid—phenolic acid that is found in oregano and rosemary; has antimutagenic and anticarcinogenic properties

rutin—bioflavonoid found in asparagus; helps protect blood vessels

saponin—health promoting components of vegetables and legumes with strong biological activity, including acting as natural antibiotics; may have anticancer properties

saturated fats—good form found in coconut oil, bad form in fast-food, such as french fries

selenium—essential trace element with protective effect against cancer; found in Brazil nuts and chickpeas

serotonin—feel-good neurotransmitter; helps boost mood and lower sugar cravings

sesamin—member of the lignan family; found in sesame seeds; inhibits the manufacture of inflammatory compounds in the body

sesaminol—phenolic antioxidant; formed when sesame seeds are refined into oil

sesamol—powerful antioxidant found in sesame oil and toasted sesame oil

sesamolin—member of the lignan family; found in sesame seeds

sex-hormone binding globulin (SHBG)—compound that binds to estrogen and helps remove it from the body

shogaols—antioxidant and active ingredient in ginger; have anti-inflammatory properties

silicon—important nutrient for bone health; found in celery

silymarin—plant compound that helps protect and nourish the liver; found in milk thistle and artichokes

sinigrin—chemical found in Brussels sprouts that suppresses the development of precancerous cells

sodium alginate—compound present in strong brown algae; may reduce the uptake of radioactive particles into bones

solanine—compound found in eggplant and other nightshades; may aggravate osteoarthritis

soluble fiber—breaks down as it passes though the digestive tract, forming a gel that traps some substances related to high cholesterol; helps control blood sugar by delaying the emptying of the stomach and retarding the entry of sugar into the bloodstream

stearic acid—fat found in dark chocolate that has a neutral effect on the body

steroidal glycosides—compound found in asparagus root; affects hormone production and possibly and has influence emotions

sterols—fats that serve as the basic molecule for important hormones such as the sex hormones

substance P—chemical that transmits pain messages to the brain

sulfides—smelly sulfur compounds found in onions; may help lower lipids and blood pressure

sulforaphane—member of the isothiocyanate family that protects against prostate, gastric, skin, and breast cancers; found in broccoli and broccoli sprouts

sulfoxides—sulfur compounds found in onions

superoxide dismutase (SOD)—important antioxidant enzyme found in cereal grasses

tannins—group of chemicals in red wine and tea that can cause astringent taste

taraxasterol—hormone-balancing constituent of dandelion

taraxerol—hormone-balancing constituent of dandelion

tartaric acid—found in vinegar; important in fighting body toxins and inhibiting unfriendly bacteria

telomerase—enzyme that "immortalizes" cancer cells by maintaining the end portions of the tumor cell chromosomes

terpenoids—component of licorice

theaflavin—antioxidant in black tea

theanine—substance in green tea that induces the release of a neurotransmitter with a calming effect; triggers the release of dopamine in the brain

thearubigen—antioxidant in black tea

thiosulfinates—smelly sulfur compound found in onions

thujone—compound found in oil of sage that is effective against both *Salmonella* and *Candida*

thymol—powerful antiseptic with antifungal, antibacterial, and antiparasitic properties; found in oregano and thyme

tocopherols—beneficial plant compounds found in olives; part of the vitamin E family

tocotrienols—potent antioxidants and heart-healthy nutrients; found in palm oil extracted from palm fruits; part of the vitamin E family

trans fat—considered metabolic poison, with the exception of CLA (conjugated linoleic acid); partially hydrogenated oil

triglyceride—blood fat that is a risk factor for heart disease

triterpenoids—beneficial component of reishi mushrooms

turmeric—anti-inflammatory spice

tyrosine—amino acid found in oysters that the brain converts to dopamine

umbelliferous—vegetable group that the National Cancer Institute has identified as possessing cancer-protective properties; includes parsnips and parsley

urushinol—toxic resin that can cause contact dermatitis; found in mangoes

xenohormones—toxins that cause hormone disruption

zeaxanthin—carotenoid that is important for eye health

zera-carotene—antioxidant found in many fruits and vegetables, including tomatoes; along with phytoene and phytofluene believed to have strong disease-fighting potential

zingerone—antioxidant and active ingredient in ginger; has anti-inflammatory properties and may be useful in a nutritional program for arthritis and/or fibromyalgia

ACKNOWLEDGMENTS

I love writing acknowledgments pages. They're the most fun of all to write, and I look forward to it every time I do it.

Why, you ask?

Because acknowledging makes everyone feel good, including—or especially—the acknowledger. Everyone loves to be acknowledged, and it's a gift (for me) to be able to thank the people in my life who continue to contribute to me and make such a difference in the quality of my existence on this planet.

Some of them helped a lot with this book. Some of them just increase my joy every day I'm alive. (Some did both.)

All of them—for better or worse—help make me who I am.

So.

I'd like to acknowledge my dear brother Jeffrey, my sister-in-law Nancy, my beloved niece Cadence and her wonderful husband Jared, and my incredibly talented nephew Pace.

My agent and advocate for more than fifteen years, Coleen O'Shea of Allen O'Shea Literary Agency. My friend Mike Danielson and the whole team at Media Relations Agency—Genesis Johnson, Heather Aarre, Tsering Yangchen, Heather Champaigne, Robin Miller, Krista Wigall, Gail Brandt, Sallie Crowe, and Anne Caron. My friend Dean Draznin, and Terri Slater and Diane Chojinowski of Draznin Communications. The brilliant and generous Karl Krummacher of Wellness Media Group. and the equally brilliant and generous Kelly Bakst and Anna Van Tonder of Volcanic Star, Inc. James Goodwin of Black Triangle Media. Danny and Emily Bradey. And, of course, JJ Virgin, and all the friends and colleagues I've met at her annual Mindshare Summit event.

My editors—Nicole Brecha at Better Nutrition, Ann Nix at Amazing Wellness, and Alicia Tyler at Clean Eating. Thanks also to the team at Fair Winds Press— Jess Haberman, the wonderful Cara Connors (my editor on this book and so many others), and the amazing Jenna Patton, Ph.D., who, in addition to being wildly overqualified for the copyediting and fact-checking work she did, was the ultimate Jonny-whisperer.

I'd like to acknowledge my "chosen" family who sustain and nourish me in countless ways: Anja Christy, Andre Davis, Billy Stritch, Brandon Skinner, Christopher Crabb, Christopher Duncan, Danny Troob, Dean and Stephanie Raffelock, Dexter Fletcher, Doug Monas, Glen Depke, Jeannette Bessinger, Kevin Hogan, Lauree Dash, Lauren Trotter, Liz Neporent, Marianna Ricci, Nikki Arguinzoni-Gill, Oliver Beaucamp, Oz Garcia, Peter Breger, Randy Graff, Scott Ellis, Sky London, Susan Wood, Taryn Sena Dunivant, Zack and Bootsie Grakal, and the late Harlan Kleiman.

Except for the four-legged kind, I've never had children. But through a weird trick of fate mixed with irony, I've somehow managed to be lucky enough to have eight of them in my life. I got the best of both worlds, thanks to the parents of Drew Christy (now grown); Luke and Sage Grakal; Charlie Ann, Miles and Brock Duncan; and especially Jade and Zoe Hochanadel, who I could not love more if they were my own. I hope one day you all read this book, happen to notice the acknowledgments section that nobody reads, and remember how much you mean to me.

And to Mark Stockman and Jeff Radich, for everything you do and for the transparency and integrity with which you do it. And, of course, for the hot tub.

A very special thanks to Dana Carpender. And to Dr. Richard Lewis. And to Dr. Beth Traylor.

To my personal, informal mastermind group—Dr. Jade Teta and Esther Blum. I appreciate and admire you so much it's silly. You, too, Mark David.

To my absolutely indefatigable and incredible assistant, Brooke Baird, without whom I can't imagine how I'd get through a day. Anything you touch automatically gets better. You've given me a new understanding of what "got your back" really means. Thank you.

The great, late nutritionist, teacher, author, and humanitarian, Robert Crayhon.

To all my animal companions that bring/have brought such joy into my life—Max, Tigerlily, Woodstock, Allegra, Emily, Lucy, and Bubba.

Allen Stone. Miles Davis. Laura Nyro. Without your soundtrack, it's not the same movie.

The three writers who have influenced me the most: William Goldman, Ed McBain (Evan Hunter), and Dr. Robert Sapolsky.

To Dr. Ernest van den Haag, long forgotten, but never by me.

To Anja Christy, my literary muse through fifteen books and countless articles, who I treasure more than I can possibly say.

Werner Erhard, for starting the process for so very many people, me included.

Michelle Obama for demonstrating time and again what "the better angels of our nature" looks like.

To the entire country of St. Martin—thank you for existing.

And to the universe for—against all odds—bringing me together (at age 63!) with the great love of my life, Michelle Elaine Mosher, with whom I am privileged to be—in the deepest, most passionate, and bashert-y sense of the word—fully and permanently engaged.

ABOUT THE AUTHOR

Jonny Bowden, Ph.D., C.N.S., also known as The Nutrition Myth Buster, is a nationally known, board-certified nutritionist and expert on diet and weight loss. He has appeared on the Dr. Oz Show, Fox News, CNN, MSNBC, ABC, NBC, and CBS and has contributed to the *New York Times*, *Forbes*, the *Daily Beast*, *Huffington Post*, *Vanity Fair Online*, *Men's Heath*, *Prevention*, and dozens of other print and online publications. He is a popular speaker who presents at academic and consumer events all over the world.

Dr. Jonny is the best-selling author of fifteen books, including *Living Low Carb* (now in its fourth edition), *Smart Fat* (with Steven Masley, M.D.), and the controversial best-seller, *The Great Cholesterol Myth: Why Lowering Your Cholesterol Won't Prevent Heart Disease and the Statin-Free Plan that Will* (with cardiologist Stephen Sinatra, M.D.). He lives in Los Angeles, is an avid tennis player, and shares his life with Michelle Mosher, Zoe Hochanadel and Jade Hochanadel, Bubba, Lucy, Emily, Luna, and nine fish.

INDEX